Contents

Foreword

It is an old chestnut that children are not just little adults, but nonetheless it is true. Harvey and Gilmartin's compact book has been a pleasure to read and I am sure that it will be the standard for the paediatric optometry module in many paediatric optometry courses throughout the world. It is also an essential update for optometrists who might be a little out of date in their thinking about paediatric optometry.

Looking after the child as a whole is a vital part of the modern health professional's role. Although optometrists don't often come across many of the conditions discussed within these pages, they can refer to this text when they do, and it gives them an idea of the sort of things that occur outside the optometry clinic.

I particularly like the combination of the various authors, who are either optometrists or ophthalmologists. The optical side of things is very well dealt with and I wish that many paediatric ophthalmologists would read this text as well!

The more academic can update themselves with the appendixes and those whose intellectual honesty is robust can turn to the multiple choice questions. This is a good read and it surely deserves a place at the front of the pile of paediatric optometry books.

David Taylor

Paediatric Optometry

William Harvey MCOptom
Visiting Clinician and Director of Visual Impairment Clinic,
City University, London, UK
Professional Programme Tutor for Boots Opticians Ltd
Clinical Editor of *Optician* Journal
Reed Business Information,
Sutton, UK

Professor Bernard Gilmartin FCOptom, PhD, FAAO
Director of Research, School of Life and Health Sciences,
Neurosciences Research Institute, Aston University,
Birmingham, UK

BUTTERWORTH HEINEMANN | Optician

EDINBURGH LONDON NEW YORK OXFORD PHILADELPHIA ST LOUIS SYDNEY TORONTO 2004

For Heidi, Tallulah, Kitty and Spike, and all the next generation to discover Gong

William Harvey

Butterworth–Heinemann
An imprint of Elsevier Limited

ISBN 0 7506 8792 4

British Library Cataloguing in Publication Data
A catalogue record for this book is available from the British Library.

Library of Congress Cataloging in Publication Data
A catalog record for this book is available from the Library of Congress.

Note
Medical knowledge is constantly changing. As new information becomes available, changes in treatment, procedures, equipment and the use of drugs become necessary. The author/contributors and the publishers have taken great care to ensure that the information given in this text is accurate and up to date. However, readers are strongly advised to confirm that the information, especially with regard to drug usage, complies with the latest legislation and standards of practice.

For Butterworth–Heinemann:
Publishing Director: Caroline Makepeace
Development Editor: Kim Benson
Production Manager: Yolanta Motylinska
Copy Editing/Project Manager: John Ormiston
Design/Layout: Judith Campbell

The Publisher's policy is to use **paper manufactured from sustainable forests**

Printed in Spain

Preface

Whereas all optometrists who read this book will certainly be children of the 20th century, the main beneficiaries of its contents will, we trust, be children of the 21st century. This new century will inevitably witness unremitting development in information and computer technology, such that its children will be exposed to complex visual environments in both educational and leisure pursuits. The ability to engage effectively with these environments will require optimum ocular performance, which will have to be monitored and co-managed by all the eye care professions.

This book presents an optometric perspective of eye care in children and gives comprehensive accounts of current clinical procedures adopted in all the principal areas of paediatric practice. By evaluating current optometric parameters in children's eye care, the material also complements the extensive literature available on the use and efficacy of treatments for specific learning difficulties in children. It is hoped that, by doing so, the book will be useful to all professionals who practice in an area that necessarily requires a multidisciplinary approach.

The content is divided broadly into five areas, whereby specific chapters address aspects of:

- Visual development, terminology and epidemiology;
- Clinical assessment of visual acuity, refraction and binocular vision;
- Paediatric eye disorders and disease relevant to the child patient;
- Specific features of spectacle dispensing, contact lenses and low vision assessment in children; and
- The important areas of clinical communication and vision screening protocols.

Supporting the clinical chapters are two Appendices on the fundamentals of embryology and genetics, topics that represent the essence of neonatal science.

The editors have welcomed the opportunity, first, to assemble formally the substantial expertise of the contributing authors and, second, to produce a text that will inform the debate on how best to optimise eye care for children of the United Kingdom.

Working with the child patient is a challenging and rewarding activity – the child of today is the adult of tomorrow – and will enhance continuity and interest in clinical practice, an outcome well worth the investment in developing additional clinical skills.

William Harvey
Bernard Gilmartin

Contributors

Richard Armstrong
DPhil (Oxon)

Susmito Biswas
FRCOphth

Lisa Donaldson
MCOptom

Alison Finlay
PhD, DIC, MCOptom, DBO. ILMT

Robert Harper
MPhil, DPhil

William Harvey
MCOptom

Jane Henderson
DBO

Andrew Keirl
MCOptom, FBDO

Christopher Lloyd
MB, BS, DO, FRCS, FRCOphth

Nicola Logan
PhD, MCOptom

Gillian Rudduck
PhD, MCOptom

Kathryn Saunders
PhD, MCOptom

Lynne Speedwell
MSc, FCOptom, DCLP, FAAO

Catherine Viner
MCOptom

Chris Wigham
PhD

1
Development of Vision

Gillian Rudduck

It is important that optometrists have an understanding of the age at which different visual functions first appear, as any delay in appearance of a particular function may indicate an underlying delay in maturation.

Visual development is not complete at birth and the early years of life represent a very dynamic period in this process. Changes occur within the anatomy and physiology of the ocular and cortical systems that are reflected in the maturation of visual function.

Visual acuity and contrast sensitivity

The ability of the infant to resolve information about form can be assessed by measuring visual acuity and contrast sensitivity. The development of visual acuity and contrast sensitivity in infants has been investigated using both behavioural and electrophysiological techniques.

The electrophysiological method of evaluating visual acuity uses the visual evoked potential (VEP). The VEP essentially tests the integrity of the visual pathway from the retina to the cortex by recording brain activity through electrodes placed on the scalp. The stimulus used is a pattern-reversal checkerboard or grating and the recorded transient response is time-synchronised to the stimulation.

In studies of acuity, the amplitudes of the VEP to stimuli of reducing size are recorded. An estimation of visual acuity can then be made by extrapolating the amplitude to zero as a function of the spatial frequency (*Figure 1.1*).

The spatial frequency at which no VEP is recordable is the estimated visual acuity.[1] A variation of this, the sweep VEP technique, has also been developed further to determine visual acuity in infants. In this technique, a rapidly reversing stimulus is presented over a range, or sweep, of spatial frequencies and the steady-state response is recorded continually over the range. The visual acuity is then estimated as the spatial frequency at which the VEP amplitude is zero.

For a behavioural estimation of visual acuity the technique of preferential looking (PL) has been employed widely. This technique is based on the observation that

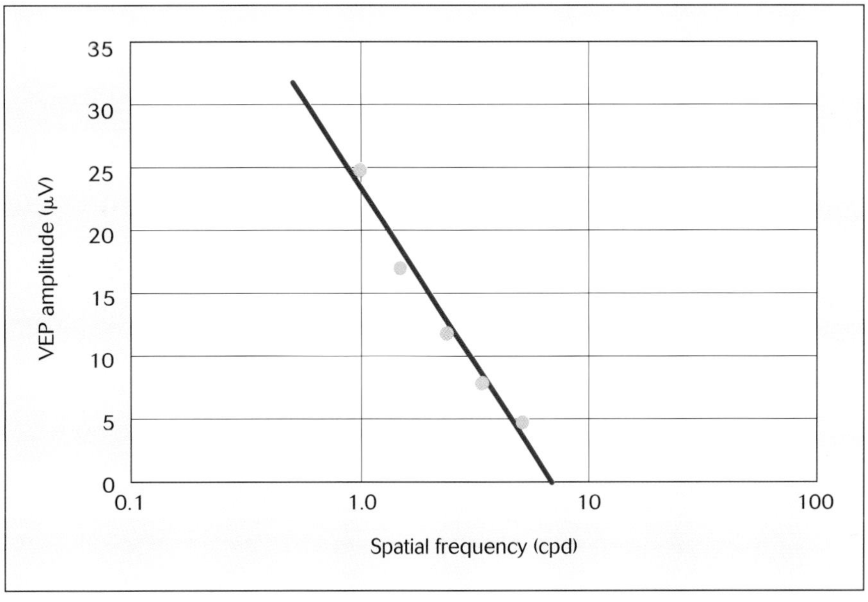

Figure 1.1
Extrapolation of transient visual evoked potential amplitudes (μV) as a function of grating spatial frequency [cycles per degree (cpd)] to determine the visual acuity threshold at 0μV. Acuity estimated from extrapolation in this sample is 7.5cpd

an infant would rather look at a pattern than a blank stimulus.[2] An infant demonstrates no fixation preference when a blank field and the grating pattern appear identical, namely when the grating is too small to be resolved, which gives the estimate of visual acuity. Although these PL techniques are dependent on the examiner's ability and the child's attention, their repeatability and robustness has been demonstrated.[3] It is this technique that has been utilised to develop, for clinical use, the Teller and Keeler Acuity cards and the Cardiff Acuity cards for slightly older children (see Chapter 3 for further discussion of these methods of acuity measurement).

Higher levels of visual acuity can be determined by the VEP technique than by using behavioural studies, and the VWEP method reveals a faster maturation course (*Figure 1.2*). Sokol[4] showed a rapid increase in acuity in the first 6 months of life from 20/150 (or 6/45) at 2 months to 20/20 (6/6) at 6–8 months.[5] PL acuity, in comparison, does not reach adult levels until 36 months, and shows a steady increase with age.[6] Measurement with the PL technique suggests an ability to resolve 20/100 (6/60) by 1 year and 20/20 (6/6) by 3 years.[7] *Table 1.1* gives a summary of PL-measured acuity changes with age. It is generally accepted that estimates of visual acuity for an achromatic stimulus are 1 cpd at birth, 2–5cpd at 2–months, 6cpd at 6 months and 12cpd at 1 year.[8]

The discrepancy in visual acuity data measured with the different techniques may result from the demands of the task. VEP acuity is limited by structural and neural changes in the ocular media and visual pathway, whereas attention and oculomotor development also limit behavioural (PL) acuity.

Whereas visual acuity represents the limit of spatial resolution at maximum contrast, contrast sensitivity gives an overall representation of visual functioning at different spatial frequencies. PL and VEP have been used to assess the development of contrast sensitivity; both techniques show the contrast sensitivity function (CSF) to be extremely immature at birth, but to develop substantially over the first few months of life.

At 2–3 months the shape of the CSF is similar to that of adults, but is shifted to lower spatial frequencies and lower sensitivities. This implies that more contrast is required if a child is to resolve detail. CSF measured using VEP techniques suggests contrast sensitivity reaches adult-like values by 7 months.[9]

Visual acuity is relatively poor at birth and undergoes rapid maturation within the first year of life. There then appears to be a slower fine-tuning to reach adult levels by 3 years of age. Possible limiting factors on infant visual acuity may be optical or neural, so the development of these subsequently improves the transmission of spatial information. The basic optical quality of the infant eye is good, with no evidence of markedly greater aberration than in the adult eye, and hence this cannot be considered a major contributing factor.

When the neural limitations of visual acuity are considered, it is important that the central retina is immature at birth. The cone outer segments are broader, shorter and less densely packed together in a lattice, and this immaturity of the foveal cones limits visual acuity in at least two ways. The low cone density reduces spatial resolution and the shorter length of the cone limits the efficacy of the cone to capture light.[10] The cones become more closely packed as the infant grows, which corresponds to an increase in acuity. Adult levels of cone density are achieved by 4 years of age and occur through cone migration centrally.[11] During the same time period the length of the cone inner segments increases to improve light capture.

The photoreceptor immaturity, however, cannot alone account for the difference between infant and adult levels of acuity and contrast sensitivity. It must, in part, be caused by immaturity at a post-receptoral level.[12] In addition to the growth and differentiation of the retina of the eye post-natally, the central nervous system is also developing. Within the visual cortex the ocular dominance columns, essential for cortical integration of inputs from the two eyes, are segregated at birth until 6 weeks post-natally.[13]

An ongoing change in the number of visual cortex synapses occurs until up to 8 months post-natally.[14]

The myelination of the visual pathways is not complete until 2 years of age,[15] prior to which neural transmission may be impaired somewhat. The time course of anatomical and physiological changes that take place during the first 6–12 months of life appear to be related directly to the improvement of visual function during that period.

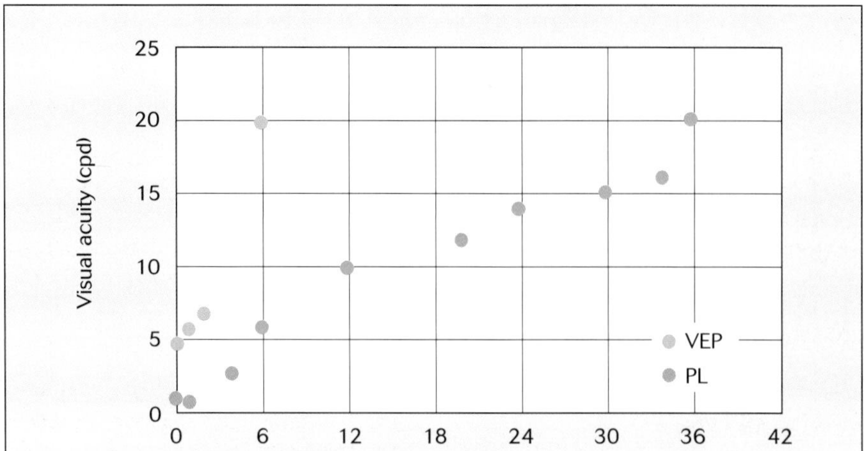

Figure 1.2
Binocular visual acuity as a function of age when assessed by visual-evoked potential and preferential looking

Table 1.1 Change in visual acuity with age using PL

Age	*Approximate Snellen visual acuity*
Birth	6/300
1 month	6/200–6/90
3 months	6/90–6/60
6 months	6/60–6/36
9 months	6/36–6/24
12 months	6/24
18 months	6/18–6/12
24 months	6/12–6/9
36 months	6/9–6/6
5+ years	6/6–6/5

Orientation detection

Newborns can detect changes in the orientation of a stimulus,[16] but show a preference for horizontal rather than vertical gratings.

Sensitivity to oblique orientation is not found until 6 weeks of age,[17] and older infants show slightly better acuity for vertical and horizontal gratings than for oblique gratings. This is also true for adults, so this variation in acuity may be a response to the orientation information within our environment, as we are exposed to more horizontal and vertical information than oblique.

Motion detection

Infants under 2 months of age have poor sensitivity to motion of all velocities.[18] VEP responses to low-velocity stimuli first appear at 10 weeks of age, with responses to speeds four times as fast evident at 13 weeks.

Eye movements

Normal movement of the eyes indicates normal visual development; visually impaired infants demonstrate abnormal movements as a first sign. An infant is able to demonstrate a range of eye movements, although these are less sophisticated than those of an adult. Depending on their level of interest, infants can fixate on stationary objects, follow a moving target or move their eyes towards a stimulus in the peripheral field (*Table 2.2*).

Saccades

While adults use small corrective eye movements of varying size to maintain fixation, the newborn infant can only direct its eyes to a fixation target by a series of small saccades that appear to be of a standard size.

An adult can usually achieve accurate fixation with one saccade, but while the infant's initial saccade towards the target is usually in the correct direction, it only covers a fraction of the distance. The infant takes longer to reach the target and also longer to initiate the first saccade. The ability to control the nerve impulses accurately enough to vary the size of the saccades undergoes marked development during the first 3 months of life, but efficient adult-like saccades are not found until the fifth month of life.[19] Horizontal saccadic eye movements develop before vertical eye movements, which are not seen until 4–6 weeks.

Table 1.2 Development of oculomotor function

Movement	*Age first demonstrated*
Saccades	
horizontal	Birth
vertical up	4–6 weeks
vertical down	3 months
Pursuit	6–8 weeks
Optokinetic nystagmus	Birth
Vestibulo-ocular reflex	Birth

Smooth pursuit

Smooth pursuit movements were not generally thought to be present until 2 months of age, with the infant dependent on using a series of small saccades prior to that. Studies have demonstrated that this is not the case and newborns can produce smooth eye movements under certain conditions.[20] The target velocity must be low enough and with a target of 12° or more, otherwise the infant tracking breaks down into a series of saccades. The maximum speed at which the moving target can be followed by smooth pursuit increases with age. By 10 weeks of age the ability to follow a moving target with reasonable accuracy has developed.

Optokinetic nystagmus

The slow and fast phases of optokinetic nystagmus (OKN) can be induced visually in infants from birth,[21] but an immaturity can be demonstrated in monocular OKN. In monocular OKN there is an asymmetry in the direction of the OKN such that in infants under 2 months of age it can be elicited only in a temporal to nasal direction. Symmetry for both directions is not achieved until 5 months of age.[22] Persistence of an asymmetric response beyond this age indicates a problem in visual development.

Vestibulo-ocular reflex

When a target is presented unexpectedly in the visual field, saccadic eye movements align the eye with the target and the head rotates towards the target. As the head rotates, the semicircular canals of the vestibular system sense a movement and initiate a reflex rotation of the eye in the opposite direction to maintain fixation. This is the vestibulo-ocular reflex and is present at birth.

Accommodation

Early studies of accommodation by dynamic retinoscopy suggested that newborns had a fixed focus and no accommodation.[23] More recent studies have shown that, for resolvable images, adult levels of accuracy in accommodation are present by 2–3 months, with newborns achieving accurate focus over distances of less than 75cm.[24]

The accommodative inaccuracies at 1–3 months are actually within the estimated depth of focus of the visual system. This depth of focus is greater in infants because of the smaller eye and pupil, and hence it appears that an infant has less sensory stimulus to control accommodation accurately.

Convergence

There are two types of vergence, that driven by blur (accommodative) and that driven by diplopia (fusional). Accommodative convergence to a near target is present by 1 month of age, but improves in precision by 2 months.[25] Fusional vergence is intermittent at 2 months, and improves in accuracy with age.

Both vergence mechanisms are involved in convergence, accommodative and disparity detection, and involve pathways between the cortex and the oculomotor centres. Immaturity in the pathways within the visual system underlies poor performance in the task.

Binocular function

The development of binocular function has been assessed widely. Binocular function can be classified into three levels, bifoveal fixation, fusion and stereopsis. The presence of these functions can be used to describe binocular function, but they are not present at birth. Establishing their presence can provide useful information as to the development of binocular function.

Bifoveal fixation is a prerequisite for binocular function. Inaccurate alignment of the eyes results in degradation of stereopsis and fusion. Bifoveal fixation can only occur in a state of orthotropia, which most normal infants achieve between 3 and 6 months of age.

Stereopsis

Stereopsis relates to the visual system's ability to process information about depth perception as a consequence of simultaneous, but slightly disparate, images presented to the two eyes.

Studies of stereopsis using a variety of techniques give comparable results. Behavioural responses to random dot-and-line stereogram techniques, VEP techniques and eye movement analysis have all been used to investigate the development of stereopsis.

Consistent findings across all techniques place the development of stereopsis between 2 and 6 months.[26] Infants have binocular visually evoked responses to random dot stereograms at 3–4 months.[27]

Held *et al.*[28] assessed stereopsis development with uncrossed (behind the plane of fixation) and crossed (in front of the plane of fixation) disparities and showed that crossed emerged earlier (at 12 weeks) than uncrossed (at 17 weeks). The development of stereopsis appears to be almost entirely complete by 6 months, but this appears to take slightly longer when assessed by behavioural methods. Once stereopsis emerges, the time course for improvement in stereoacuity is very rapid, and reaches adult levels of about 1 minute of arc within 5 weeks of onset.

Fusion

Fusion relates to the visual system's ability to combine similar and perhaps non-identical information from two eyes into one image. Fusion development has been investigated using both PL[29] and VEP techniques,[30] and is seen to develop over a similar time course as that of stereopsis. No fusion can be demonstrated before 3.5 months, but it is demonstrated consistently by 6 months. This parallel development of stereopsis and fusion is thought to be a function of the development of the visual cortex.

Colour vision

The emergence of colour vision between the ages of 1 and 3 months has been demonstrated using PL[31] and VEP techniques.[32,33] Infants as young as 2 months of age can discriminate some wavelengths in the absence of luminance information and develop trichromacy by 3 months.

Refractive error

Studies of early refractive development have shown the average newborn refractive error to be hypermetropic with a mean error of 2.00D (±2.00).[34] Premature babies have been shown to be less hypermetropic. Hypermetropia increases from birth to reach a peak at about 6 months of age. This mean gradually decreases towards emmetropia (via the process of emmetropisation) at about 6 years of age (*Figure 1.3*); the adult distribution of refractive error is narrower and centred around emmetropia, with a standard deviation of ±1.00D.[35,36]

The most rapid decline in hypermetropia occurs between 6 months and 2 years of age in normally developing eyes. The emmetropisation process is complete in over 80 per cent of children by 12 months of age.[37] However, children who develop strabismus do not generally show emmetropisation, and demonstrate either increasing hypermetropia or no change in refractive error instead.[38]

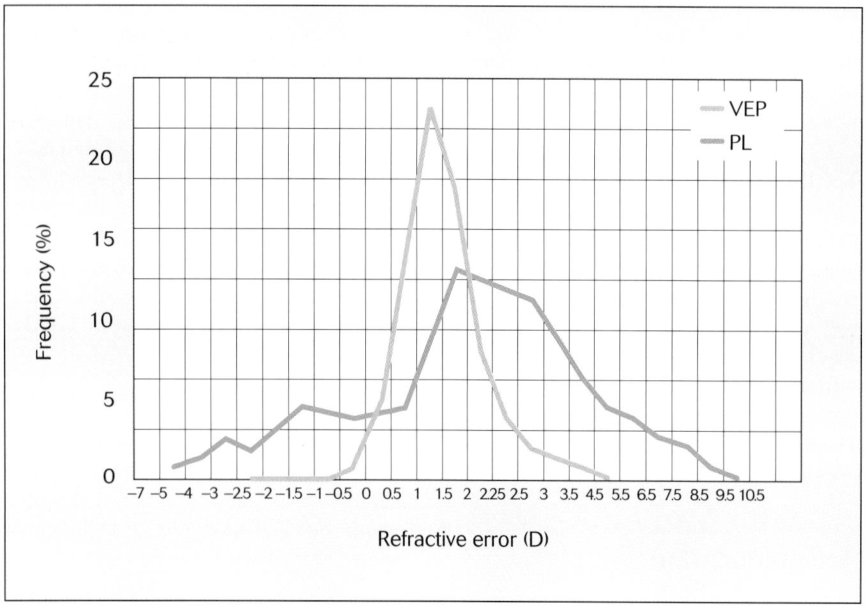

Figure 1.3
Distribution of refractive error in newborns and infants aged 6–8 years of age[35,36]

Emmetropisation refers to the developmental process that co-ordinates growth of the refractive component of the eye in such a manner as to create a non-Gaussian distribution of refractive errors around emmetropia. Emmetropisation is thought to occur as a result of two processes.[39]

One, an active process, suggests that visual experience 'guides' the refractive state towards emmetropia in a visual feedback loop. The eye 'senses' the sign and magnitude of its refractive error and modulates its rate of growth through an active feedback mechanism to reduce the error.[40] For this feedback to work, normal visual stimulation is necessary and any visual deprivation in early life impedes emmetropisation.[41]

A second, more passive, process suggests that post-natal refractive changes are purely a genetically determined continuation of normal eye growth. As the eye grows, its optical power decreases proportionately, which promotes emmetropia.[42]

The majority of emmetropisation is complete within the first year of life,[43] as demonstrated by the reduction in high levels of hypermetropia. The highest rates of emmetropisation seen in the first 12–17 months of life occur in those infants with the highest initial ametropia.[44]

The influences upon myopic progression are considered in Chapter 5. Some researchers have shown that correction of hypermetropia in the first year of life[45] may impede emmetropisation, but correction of 3.50D or more hypermetropia reduces the risk of strabismus and amblyopia.[46]

There is a high prevalence of against-the-rule astigmatism in newborn infants. Astigmatism is more common in infants than in adults and significant amounts are common in children under 3.5 years of age. The mean value of 1.00D reduces from birth to reach adult values by 2–5 years.[47] The age of 3.5 years is an important milestone in the development of astigmatism. The prevalence of astigmatism drops significantly by this age and a shift in the prevalence of against-the-rule versus with-the-rule astigmatism appears . After 5 years of age, with-the-rule gains prevalence. One proposed reason for this change from against- to with-the-rule astigmatism is the pressure exerted by the eyelids.

Summary

Delay in the appearance of a particular function or variation from the reported normal values indicates underlying problems in visual development. For the optometrist, knowledge of the developmental time course of those visual func-

Table 1.3 Summary of vision development with age

	Birth	*1 month*	*2 months*	*3 months*	*4 months*	*6 months+*
Visual acuity (visual evoked potential)	Poor 1cpd		2cpd	3cpd		6–20cpd, 6/6
Visual acuity (preferential looking)						6/24 at 1 year
Orientation	Horizontal and vertical		Present for oblique			
Accommodation		Near accurate <75		Near accurate <150cm	Fine adjustment	Matures at 5–7 months
Motion		Poor		Low velocity at 10 weeks		
Saccades		Fixed amplitude responses	Fixed amplitude responses		Improvement at 3–4 months	Adult-like at 5–6 months
Pursuit		Series of saccades	Smooth pursuit at low speeds			Adult-like at 6 months
Optokinetic nystagmus	Present binocularly and nasalward monocularly			Present monocularly temporalward		
Fusional vergence		Intermittent				Mature
Accommodation vergence			Immature			Mature at 7 months
Stereopsis				Crossed		Uncrossed
Fusion				Nil before 3.5 months		Present at 6 months
Colour			Dichromat	Trichromat		

tions that can be assessed relatively easily in a clinic is important (*Table 1.3*).

Some functions can be affected by environmental factors (e.g., orientation selective cells), while others are unaffected by them, such as colour vision. Some functions are relatively immature at birth and develop rapidly and others have a much slower developmental time course. Accommodation, for example, is almost completely developed by 3 months of age, but requires the improvement in visual acuity to finally refine it by 6 months. Visual acuity and contrast sensitivity have a much longer time course; they improve rapidly in the early stages up to 3 years, but do not actually reach adult values until 5 years of age or later.

References

1 Campbell F and Maffei L (1970). Electrophysiological evidence for the presence of orientation and size detection in the human visual system. *J Physiol.* **207**, 635–652.
2 Fantz RL, Ordy JM and Udelf MS (1962). Maturation of pattern vision in infants during the first six months. *Child Dev.* **46**, 3–18.
3 Heersema DJ and Van Hof van Duin J (1990). Age norms for visual acuity in toddlers using acuity card procedure. *Clin Vis Sci.* **5**, 167–174.
4 Sokol S (1978). Measurement of infant visual acuity from pattern reversal visual evoked potential. *Vis Res.* **18**, 33–39.
5 Norcia AM and Tyler CW (1985). Spatial frequency sweep VEP: visual acuity during the first year of life. *Vis Res.* **25**, 1399–1408.
6 Allen JL (1979). *Visual Acuity Development in Human Infants up to 6 Months of Age.* PhD Thesis. (Seattle: University of Washington).
7 Teller DY, McDonald MA, Preston K, *et al.* (1986). Assessment of visual acuity in infants and children; the acuity card procedure. *Dev Med Child Neurol.* **28**, 779–789.
8 Banks MS and Salapatek P (1978). Acuity and contrast sensitivity in 1-, 2- and 3-month-old human infants. *Invest Ophthalmol Vis Sci.* **17**, 361–365.
9 Norcia AM, Tyler CW and Hamer RD (1990). Development of contrast sensitivity in the human infant. *Vis Res.* **30**, 1475–1486.
10 Yuodelis C and Hendrickson A (1986). A qualitative and quantitative analysis of the human fovea during development. *Vis Res.* **26**, 847–855.
11 Hendrickson A and Yuodelis C (1984). The morphological development of the human fovea. *Ophthalmology* **91**, 603–612.
12 Banks MS and Bennett PJ (1988). Optical and photoreceptor immaturities limit the spatial and chromatic vision of human neonates. *J Opt Soc Am A* **5**, 2059–2079.
13 Le Vay S, Stryker MP and Schatz CJ (1979). Ocular dominance columns and their development in layer IV of the cat's visual cortex: A quantitative study. *J Comp Neurol.* **179**, 223–224.
14 Huttenlocher PR, de Courten C, Garey LJ and Van der Loos H (1982). Synaptogenesis in the human visual cortex. Evidence for synapses elimination during normal development. *Neurosci Lett.* **33**, 247–252.
15 Magoon EH and Robb RM (1981). Development of myelin in human optic nerve and tract. A light and electron microscope study. *Arch Ophthalmol.* **99**, 655–659.
16 Slater A and Sykes M (1977). Newborn infants' visual responses to square wave gratings. *Child Dev.* **48**, 545–554.
17 Braddick OJ, Wattam-Bell J and Atkinson J (1986). Orientation-specific cortical responses develop in early infancy. *Nature* **320**, 617–619.
18 Wattam-Bell J (1991). Development of motion specific cortical responses in infants. *Vis Res.* **31**, 287–297.
19 Atkinson J (1984). Human visual development over the first six months of life: A review and hypothesis. *Human Neurobiol.* **3**, 61–74.
20 Roucoux A, Culee C and Rendlemann P (1983). Development of fixation and pursuit eye movements in human infants. *Behav Brain Res.* **10**, 133–139.
21 McGinnis JM (1930). Eye movements and optic nystagmus in early infancy. *Genetic Psychol Monogr.* **8**: 321–326.
22 Atkinson J and Braddick OJ (1981). Development of optokinetic nystagmus in infants: An indicator of cortical binocularity? In: *Eye Movements: Cognition and Visual Perception*, p. 53–64, Eds Fisher DF, Monty RA and Senders JW. (Hillsdale, NJ: Lawrence Erlbaum).
23 Haynes H, White BL and Held R (1965). Visual accommodation in human infants. *Science* **148**, 528–530.
24 Braddick OJ, Atkinson J, French J and Howland HC (1979). A photorefraction study of infant accommodation. *Vis Res.* **19**, 1319–1330.
25 Aslin RN and Jackson RW (1979). Accommodative convergence in young infants' development. *Can J Psychol.* **33**, 222–231.
26 Fox R, Aslin RN, Shea SL and Dumais ST (1980). Stereopsis in human infants. *Science* **207**, 323–324.
27 Braddick OJ and Atkinson J (1983). Some recent findings on the development of human binocularity: a review. *Behav Brain Res.* **10**, 141–150.
28 Held R, Birch E and Gwiazda J (1980). Stereoacuity of human infants. *Proc Nat Acad Sci USA* **77**, 5572–5574.
29 Birch EE, Shimojo S and Held R (1985). Preferential looking assessment of fusion and stereopsis in infants 1–6 months. *Invest Ophthalmol Vis Sci.* **26**, 366–370.
30 Petrig B, Julesz B, Kropfl W, *et al.* (1981). Development of stereopsis and cortical binocularity in human infants. *Science* **213**, 1402–1405.
31 Teller DY, Peeples DR and Sekel M (1978). Discrimination of chromatic from white light by 2 month old human infants. *Vis Res.* **18**, 41–48.
32 Allen D, Banks MS, Norcia AM and Shannon L (1990). Human infants' VEP responses to isoluminant stimuli. *Invest Ophthalmol Vis Sci.* **31**, S47.
33 Rudduck GA and Harding GFA (1993). Visual electrophysiology to achromatic and chromatic stimuli in premature and full term infants. *J Psychol.* **16**, 209–218.
34 Banks MS (1980). Infant refraction and accommodation. *Int Ophthalmol Clin.* **20**, 205–232.
35 Cook RC and Glasscock RE (1951). Refractive and ocular findings in the newborn. *Am J Ophthalmol.* **34**, 1407–1413.
36 Kempf GA, Collins SD and Jarman EL (1928). *Refractive Errors in the Eyes of Children as Determined by Retinoscopic Examination with a Cycloplegic.* Public Health Bulletin No 182 1928. (Washington DC: Government Printing Office).
37 Ingram RA, Arnold PE, Dally S and Lucas J (1991). Emmetropisation, squint and reduced visual acuity. *Br J Ophthalmol.* **75**, 414–416.
38 Aurell E and Norsell K (1990). A longitudinal study of children with family history of strabismus: factors determining the incidence of strabismus. *Br J Ophthalmol.* **74**, 589–594.
39 Troilo D (1992). Neonatal eye growth and emmetropisation – a literature review. *Eye* **5**, 154–160.
40 Norton TT and Siegwart JT (1995). Animal models of emmetropisation: Matching axial length to the focal plane. *J Am Optom Assoc.* **66**, 405–414.
41 Hoyt CS, Stone RD, Fromer C and Billson FA (1981). Monocular axial myopia associated with neonatal eyelid closure in human infants *Am J Ophthalmol.* **91**, 197–200.
42 Sorsby A (1979). Biology of the eye as an optical system. In: *Refraction and Clinical Optics*, p. ??–??, Ed. Safir S. (Philadelphia, PA: Harper and Row.)
43 Ingram RA, Walker C, Wilson JM, *et al.* (1986). Prediction of amblyopia and squint by means of refraction at age one year. *Br J Ophthalmol.* **70**, 12–15.
44 Saunders KJ, Woodhouse M and Westall CA (1995). Emmetropisation in human infancy: Rate of change is related to initial refractive error. *Vis Res.* **35**, 1325–1328.
45 Ehrlich DL, Anker S, Atkinson J, *et al.* (1996). Changes of refraction with age. *Invest Ophthalmol Vis Sci.* **37**, S730.
46 Atkinson J and Braddick OJ (1988). Infant precursors of later visual disorders: correlation or casualty? *20th Minnesota Symposium on Child Psychology*, p. 35–65, Ed. Yonas A (Hillsdale: Lawrence Eelbaum).
47 Ingram RA and Barr A (1979). Changes in refraction between the ages of 1 and 3.5 years. *Br J Ophthalmol.* **63**, 339–342.

2

Ocular Dysfunction and Disease in Childhood: Terminology and Epidemiology

Lisa Donaldson

Vision plays a huge role in a child's sensory and motor development, and undetected visual or ocular anomalies are liable to impede normal development. It is, therefore, vital that optometrists be aware of the major causes of childhood visual difficulties so that they can correctly detect, prevent or manage them as appropriate.

Incidence and epidemiology of ocular conditions

Refractive error

An emmetropic eye is defined as one in which the fovea lies at the posterior principal focus of the system. All departures from emmetropia can be defined as refractive errors. However, a range of variations from emmetropia can be considered as within normal limits. More than 80 per cent of all children 1–7 years of age have a cycloplegic spherical equivalent refractive error of between +0.50DS and +3.00DS.[1–3] Less than 5 per cent of all 5–7 year olds are more than +5D hyperopic and less than 3 per cent are myopic. These high refractive errors are almost exclusively congenital.[4,5] Only 8 per cent of 5–7 year olds have more than 0.75D of astigmatism, more commonly 'with the rule' (the vertical meridian has maximum refractive power and the cylinder axis is horizontal).[6,7] Juvenile myopia is the most common form of myopia. It can be defined as myopia with onset at any age between 6 and 15 years. Of children in this age group, 15–30 per cent are myopic. Those 5–7 year olds with refraction close to emmetropia (especially those with 'against the rule' astigmatism) are at the greatest risk of developing juvenile myopia. This is because from the age of 8 years there is a myopic shift and mean refractive error drops by an average of +0.25D per year.[8,9] The earlier the onset of juvenile myopia, the higher the ultimate refractive error.[10] There is a slight increase in incidence of 'against the rule' astigmatism with onset and progression of juvenile myopia.

Risk factors for the development of refractive errors

Prematurity

Premature infants are defined as those born before 37 weeks of gestation. In premature infants there are increased incidences of myopia and significant astigmatism (more than 2D) at birth, and frequently both occur together.[11] Prevalence and degree of myopia and astigmatism have been shown to increase with decreasing gestational age (increasing prematurity).[12] Premature neonates with retinopathy of prematurity (a complication of administration of oxygen at birth; see later in this chapter) have a higher incidence still of associated high myopia. In premature infants without retinopathy of prematurity these refractive errors tend to regress in the first year of life, such that they show little variation in ametropia from their normal age peers by 1 year of age. However, in infants with retinopathy of prematurity the associated high myopia is unlikely to regress.[13]

Intra-uterine growth retardation

Intra-uterine growth retardation (IUGR) is diagnosed if a child weighs less than the 10th percentile for his or her gestational age and results in low birth weight. As with premature infants, children of low birth weight are at increased risk of retinopathy of prematurity and high myopia. IUGR is most commonly caused by maternal malnutrition, viral diseases (such as cytomegalovirus, rubella) or fetal alcohol syndrome. Fetal alcohol syndrome occurs through alcohol abuse during pregnancy. It also results in central nervous system dysfunction, such as growth retardation, microcephaly and intellectual impairment.

Maternal disease

High myopia has been shown to be four times more likely in children born to mothers with diabetes.[14–16] Increased incidence of moderate and high myopia is also associated with fetal alcohol syndrome, rubella and toxoplasmosis.

Childhood diseases
Contracting tuberculosis, measles or other febrile diseases before the age of 6 years has been shown to be a risk factor in the development of juvenile myopia.[17,18]

Esophoria
Esophoria has been shown to be a risk factor in the development of juvenile myopia.[18] This may result from increased stress on the accommodation–convergence relationship.

Gender differences
Congenital high myopia is twice as likely to occur in females as in males.[19] As the overall incidence of myopia in the general population has been shown to be distributed evenly between the sexes, this suggests that juvenile myopia is slightly more common in males. High hyperopia is equally prevalent in both sexes. High astigmatism appears to be more prevalent in females than in males.

Ethnic differences
Congenital myopia is of increased incidence in children of Afro-Caribbean origin, whereas juvenile myopia is less common.[20,21] Studies have shown increased prevalence and severity of myopia in Jewish children compared with other children who live in the same geographical area.[22,23] In Jewish children, unlike in other populations, the incidence of congenital high myopia appears to be the same for males and females, whereas the incidence of juvenile myopia has been shown to be significantly greater in Jewish boys than girls. This may result from the high near-vision demands of Jewish boys. Myopia, especially high myopia, has a higher prevalence in Chinese and Japanese children than in Caucasians.[24–27] There do not appear to be large differences between Caucasian ethnic groups, although myopia does appear to be more prevalent in German children.[28] The only study to highlight ethnic differences in astigmatism shows 'against the rule' astigmatism to be the more prevalent type in Chinese infants, the opposite to that of Caucasians.[29]

Socio-economic status
The effect of socio-economic status on refractive error is difficult to isolate. This is partly because children of low socio-economic status are more likely to be born premature, or to have low birth weight or maternal or childhood disease, each of which, as discussed above, increases the risk of congenital refractive error. An increased incidence of myopia has been demonstrated in children who have suffered abuse.[30] In developing countries juvenile myopia is less prevalent than in highly industrialised nations, but high myopia is more common. Juvenile myopia has been shown to be less common in rural communities compared with cities within the same countries.[24,31] An increased prevalence of astigmatism in children of low socio-economic status has been suggested, possibly caused by corneal malleability through poor nutrition.

Genetic predisposition
Juvenile myopia shows a multifactorial inheritance pattern.[32] This means that a number of genes determine the condition, along with environmental factors. It has been shown that if one parent is myopic there is a 22.5 per cent chance of a child developing myopia, the risk increasing to 42 per cent with two myopic parents.[8] Some cases of high myopia may also have a genetic basis.

Childhood ocular trauma
Childhood ocular trauma can, in rare cases, lead to refractive error.[4,17] A comprehensive review of influences on myopic progression is given in Chapter 8.

Genetic conditions
Retinitis pigmentosa is an inherited condition (as discussed in Chapter 8) and usually appears between the ages of 2 and 18 years. Progressive pigmentary degeneration of the retina is associated with poor night vision and progressive field loss. It is associated with increased myopia.

Down's syndrome occurs in one in every 400–600 births, and is caused by an additional or additional part of chromosome 21. Increased incidence of high myopia, hyperopia and astigmatism are among the ocular abnormalities associated with Down's syndrome.[33] Other ocular complications include congenital nystagmus, strabismus, cataract, blepharitis, slightly reduced acuity and colour vision anomalies. Increased incidence of refractive error is also associated with fragile X-syndrome, which occurs in 1/1000 male births and 1/2000 female births. This genetic syndrome is associated with a large range of physical, speech and language difficulties, as well as with other ocular anomalies, notably optic atrophy (28 per cent) and strabismus. Significant refractive error is present in 40–76 per cent of children with cerebral palsy,[34] alongside other visual and ocular complications. Cerebral palsy may be genetic in origin, or result from anoxia, toxaemia, maternal thyroid abnormalities, infections during pregnancy, prematurity, infections (such as mumps and meningitis) or trauma after birth.

Congenital ocular malformations
Congenital ocular malformations are rare, but when they do occur they are very often associated with high refractive error. Buphthalmos (congenital glaucoma) and coloboma are often associated with high myopia. Microphthalmos may be associated with high myopia or hyperopia. Anterior polar and cortical cataracts are commonly associated with high hyperopia. Idiopathic nystagmus is very commonly associated with high astigmatism.

Anisometropia
Anisometropia can be defined as a significant difference in refractive error between the eyes (more than 1.00D in any meridian). It is more common in premature infants, with the incidence increasing further in cases with retinopathy of prematurity. Myopic children are more frequently anisometropic than are hyperopes. Constant unilateral esotropia is very often associated with anisometropia.[35]

Strabismus
Strabismus (heterotropia, squint) is a binocular vision anomaly in which both visual axes of the eyes fail to pass through the point of fixation. It can be constant or intermittent, convergent (esotropia), divergent (exotropia) or vertical (hypertropia and/or hypotropia), affect one eye only or alternate between the eyes. It may be classified as comitant or incomitant. In incomitant strabismus the degree of misalignment varies according to the position of gaze or which eye fixes the target, and results from under or overaction of one of the extraocular muscles. A detailed discussion of strabismus is given in Chapters 9 and 10. Strabismus affects between 3 and 4.8 per cent of children.[36,37] Comparative incidences of esotropia and exotropia vary between studies. About 25 per cent of esotropias are intermittent, compared with around 80 per cent of exotropias.

Risk factors for the development of strabismus
Genetic predisposition
A significantly increased incidence of exotropia and accommodative and partially accommodative esotropia has been shown in children with a family history of squint.[32,38,39] This does not appear to be such a significant factor in the development of infantile esotropia.

Refractive error
Accommodative esotropia is associated with significant hyperopia. The child accommodates to overcome the hyperopia and the resultant convergence leads to esotropia.

Prematurity and birth trauma
Prematurity and birth trauma are linked to an increased incidence of infantile esotropia[38] and hypotropia. These are very common in children who have suffered haemorrhaging caused by hypoxic or hypertensive insults; the more premature the baby, the greater the risk that these complications occur.

Genetic conditions
Strabismus occurs in around 33 per cent of children with Down's syndrome,[33] which means the incidence is up to 10 times that in the general population. Fragile X-syndrome and albinism (see later) are associated with an increased incidence of strabismus.

Maternal drug use
A 24 per cent prevalence of strabismus has been demonstrated in children born to drug-dependent mothers.[40,41] Fetal alcohol syndrome is associated with an increased prevalence of all types of strabismus.[42] Maternal cigarette smoking results in an increased prevalence of esotropia.[43]

Secondary to systemic conditions
Comitant or incomitant strabismus may occur secondary to other systemic conditions, such as infections or inflammations (e.g., meningitis), tumours, as part of a rubella syndrome, in cerebral palsy (34–60 per cent of cases)[44] or after trauma (accidental or non-accidental).[45]

Secondary to ocular conditions
Strabismus secondary to ocular conditions may, in some cases, result from poor acuity, which provides a poor incentive for the development or maintenance of binocular vision. Examples are albinism, toxoplasma chorioretinitis, morning glory anomaly, toxocara retinopathy and retinopathy of prematurity. A recent study found a significant number of all strabismic children examined to have an underlying retinal anomaly, which highlights the importance of a careful fundus examination in children who present with strabismus.[46]

Prevalence and aetiology of incomitant strabismus
Around 15 per cent of all childhood squints have been shown to be incomitant,[47] the most common being overaction of one or both inferior oblique muscles, which is twice as likely to occur in esotropia as in exotropia. Less common causes of muscle underaction are muscle paralysis (most often sixth or fourth nerve palsies), muscle malinsertions, muscle fibrosis (as in Duane's retraction syndrome) and space-occupying orbital lesions.

Amblyopia
Amblyopia can be defined as a non-optical and non-pathological reduction in visual acuity. Incidence is thought to be around 1–2 per cent in schoolchildren.[48] The usual classifications of childhood amblyopia are:

- Strabismic, in the squinting eye in a unilateral strabismus;
- Refractive, in uncorrected refractive error, usually hyperopia or astigmatism;
- Meridional, along the more blurred axis in uncorrected astigmatism;
- Anisometropic, in the more hyperopic eye;
- Deprivational, through the lack of visual stimulus, such as cataract or ptosis.

Amblyopia is discussed further in Chapter 9.

Convergence insufficiency
Convergence insufficiency is diagnosed when the near point of convergence is significantly greater than the normal range (typically less than 10cm). It is a very common cause of asthenopia in the teenage years, but less common in younger children.

Nystagmus
Nystagmus is an involuntary oscillation of the eyes. It may be pendular, with eye movements of equal velocity in each direction, or jerk. Visual deprivation before the age of 2 years always leads to nystagmus (usually pendular and horizontal), and it may develop if there is deprivation before the age of 6 years. Common causes are congenital cataract and albinism. It may also be congenital and of X-linked or autosomal dominant transmission (usually jerk and horizontal). Nystagmus is often associated with strabismus.

Paediatric ocular pathology

Congenital cataract
Congenital cataract may be primary or secondary. Congenital cortical and sutural cataracts arc very common and do not normally interfere with vision. Lamellar cataract is the most common congenital cataract to interfere with vision to markedly. It is often associated with radial spoke-like opacities (a more detailed discussion is found in Chapter 9). About one-third of all congenital cataracts are primary,[49] usually hereditary with a dominant mode of inheritance. Common aetiologies of secondary congenital cataract are Down's syndrome (in around 15 per cent of cases), maternal drug ingestion (notably corticosteroids) and rubella (in around 50 per cent of cases).

Albinism
Oculocutaneous albinism is a hereditary inability to synthesise melanin, which may be partial or total (usually an autosomal recessive trait). Ocular albinism affects the eyes only (usually X-linked). Albinism is commonly associated with strabismus, as there is no foveal differentiation.

Congenital ptosis
Congenital ptosis is drooping of the upper lid, usually caused by dystrophy of the levator muscle. If the pupil is obscured even partly it may lead to amblyopia.

Epicanthus
Epicanthus is a fold of skin, very common in infants, that stretches from the upper to the lower lid and covers the medial canthus, which may give rise to the appearance of an esotropia (pseudo-esotropia).

Congenital optic disc anomalies
Drusen are calcific deposits within the optic nerve head. They are present in about 0.3 per cent[50] of the population and in children they can be difficult to differentiate from papilloedema.

Tilted discs appear oval with an oblique vertical axis, and occur because the optic nerve enters the globe at an oblique angle. They are usually bilateral, are fairly common and are often associated with an inferior crescent, myopia and oblique astigmatism, and a temporal field defect.

Myelinated nerve fibres are common. They are seen as white patches with feathered edges, which usually radiate from the disc and are of varying degree.

An optic disc pit is a dark oval or round pit on the disc, which may lead to retinal oedema. An optic disc coloboma occurs through incomplete closure of the fetal fissure. There is a large, usually inferior, excavation on the disc, often associated with reduced vision and a superior field defect.

Congenital primary optic nerve atrophy may be inherited and of varying severity. Optic nerve hypoplasia is often associated with systemic conditions, such as fetal alcohol syndrome.[42] The optic disc is small and usually pale.

Congenital optic disc abnormalities are often associated with midfacial malformations, such as cleft palate, 'hare-lip' and nasal malformations.

Papilloedema
Papilloedema that results from a space-occupying lesion may be seen in children. Other conditions, such as high hyperopia or buried disc drusen, may mimic papilloedema.

Fundus anomalies

Retinoblastoma is rare, occurring in one in 20,000 live births, but is the most common primary malignant intraocular tumour. Only about 6 per cent of cases have a positive family history. There is an incomplete autosomal dominant transmission. Leukocoria (white 'cat's eye' pupil) is the presenting feature for about two-thirds of cases, whereas strabismus is the presenting feature in 20 per cent of cases.

Retinopathy of prematurity occurs in neonates to whom oxygen is administered. There is retinal neovascularisation. The severity increases with decreasing gestational age, and it is often associated with congenital myopia. Resolution is spontaneous in 80 per cent of cases, but it may lead to retinal detachment.

Congenital toxoplasmosis results from maternal infection with the parasite from the ingestion of carrier raw meat or cat faeces (such as contact with a litter tray). It gives rise to chorioretinitis, which may go unnoticed until a routine fundus examination, or it may be associated with severe brain damage or convulsions.

Ocular toxocariasis occurs as a result of ocular infestation with the intestinal roundworm of cats and dogs. In children between 6 and 14 years of age it usually gives rise to a retinal granuloma, a round, slightly elevated yellowish lesion. Its effect on vision depends on its location. In younger children (2–9 years of age) a more serious chronic endophthalmitis may occur.

Anterior eye infections

Blepharitis is common in childhood and is most often caused by *Staphylococcus aureas* infection (it may also be seborrhoeic). The eyelids appear red, scaly and swollen and give rise to itching, burning and photophobia. It may lead on to an internal or external (stye) hordeolum, a chalazion or bacterial conjunctivitis. Bacterial conjunctivitis is common and associated with hyperaemia and a purulent or mucopurulent discharge.

Viral conjunctivitis is common, most often caused by adenovirus. It is very contagious, initially unilateral with hyperaemia and a watery discharge. It usually resolves spontaneously within 2 or 3 weeks and may be associated with a sore throat (pharyngitis).

Allergic conjunctivitis is usually caused by pollen or animals, and often occurs in association with other atopic conditions (hay fever, asthma, eczema). Acute allergic conjunctivitis is quite common in children and is self-limiting once the allergen is removed.

Corneal anomalies

Dermoid cysts are typically painless, round lesions, usually in the nasal or temporal corner of the orbit. Forceps trauma, metabolic disease and buphthalmos may cause corneal opacities.

Haemangioma

Haemangioma is usually congenital, and may be superficial 'strawberry naevus' or deeper with more reddish blue swelling. It disappears by the age of 5 years.

Malingering

Malingering needs to be borne in mind as a possible explanation for reduced acuity or unexplained symptoms, but only after all other avenues have been explored.

Colour vision anomalies

Normal colour vision
Most people have three types of cone, each of which contain different types of light-absorbing photopigment that have various sensitivities to different wavelengths. Around 10 per cent of cones respond maximally to the short blue wavelengths (around 440nm), with around 45 per cent responding maximally at 545nm (medium, green) and the remaining 45 per cent responding maximally at 565nm (long, yellow). Each single cone can only signal the number of units of light (photons) absorbed by its photopigment. Thus, to determine colour, a comparison of the strength of signal from different types of cone is necessary.

Inherited colour vision deficiencies
Inherited colour vision deficiencies are congenital, lifelong and untreatable. In Europe and the USA around 8 per cent of males and 0.5 per cent of females are affected. Some populations have a lower incidence (about 5 per cent in Japanese and Scottish males).[51,52] Inherited colour vision deficiencies result from the absence or modification of one or more of the cone pigments, usually red or green.

Genetic basis
The inheritance is X-linked as the green and red pigments are encoded on the X chromosome. A male with colour-defective genetic information encoded on his X chromosome is colour defective. If a female has this gene on one X chromosome, she has normal colour vision, but is a carrier. To be affected a female needs colour-defective genes on her two X-chromosomes, which can occur only if a carrier female and affected male reproduce (namely, both her father and maternal grandfather must be affected). This mode of inheritance means that colour-defective men cannot pass the defect onto their sons.

The blue pigment is encoded on chromosome 7.[53] An inherited blue (tritan) defect is very rare (incidence around 0.005 per cent) and not sex linked. Blue defects are much more likely to be acquired.

Classification
The classification of colour vision anomalies is given in *Table 2.1*.

Colour vision tests
Colour vision tests are described in *Table 2.2*.

Practical advice
As colour vision defects are untreatable it is important to identify them early so that children can be counselled as appropriate. This avoids disappointment as a result of limits to career possibilities and allows necessary adaptations to be made at home and at school. The earlier a child and family are aware of a defect, the easier this becomes. Teachers should be informed so that a child is not accused of silly mistakes. In general, saturated and dark colours are easier to differentiate than are pale or light shades. Use of primary colours can be advised. Certain aviation, railway and maritime professions bar those with colour vision anomalies. It may also prove a problem in occupations such as electronics, graphic or interior design and textile and chemical industries in which good colour discrimination is important.

Summary

An initial history and symptoms
Once the incidence of the various influences on normal visual development to which a growing child may be exposed is known, it should be possible to suggest an initial template for questioning the paediatric patient based upon this information. This is further expanded in Chapter 15.

Table 2.1 Classification of colour vision anomalies

Class	*Description*
Achromatopsia	Very rare total absence of colour vision (0.003 per cent incidence).
Anomalous trichromacy	Incomplete loss of sensitivity to certain wavelengths.
Deuteranomalous trichromacy	Most common colour vision defect (accounts for around 60 per cent of all hereditary colour vision defects), and affects 4–5 per cent of all boys. Peak responses of the cones sensitive to long wavelengths are thought to occur at a slightly reduced wavelength, and thus reduce the colour-discrimination ability. Problems are experienced with similar colours to those confused by deuteranopes, with varying degrees of severity.
Dichromacy	Second most common colour vision defect (accounts for about 25 per cent of colour vision defects; affects about 2 per cent of the population). Colour vision is dependent on only two types of cone (the label 'colour blindness', sometimes used, is misleading). Protanopia and deuteranopia are of approximately equal incidence, and affect around 1 per cent of the population each. It is presumed that, as visual acuity is normal, a normal number of cones and amount of photopigment must be present and responding to stimulation, but that sensitivity to certain wavelengths is reduced.
protanopia	Red-sensitive photopigment is absent. Reds are confused with dark browns, dark greys and blacks; purples are confused with blues and light greens with light browns.
deuteranopia	Green-sensitive photopigment is absent. Greens are confused with magenta, reds, oranges and light browns, blues and purples.
Protanomalous trichromacy	Accounts for about 15 per cent of defects (it affects 1–2 per cent of boys). It is believed the peak response of the cones sensitive to medium wavelengths is at a slightly higher wavelength than in normals, which reduces sensitivity to red colours.
Tritanopia	The most common acquired defects, although in children they are very rare. They most often occur as a result of retinal disease (e.g., early retinitis pigmentosa or diabetes).

Table 2.2 Colour vision tests

Test	*Description*
Anomaloscope	Spectral colour-matching instrument based on the property that red and green light, when mixed, appear the same as monochromatic yellow light. The viewer adjusts the controls to achieve a match between two halves of a split field (Nagel anomaloscope). Protanopes and deuteranopes match any red–green mix with yellow. A deuteranomalous trichromat will choose more green and a protanomalous trichromat more red than a normal. Anomaloscopes are expensive and therefore not widely used in clinical practice.
Pseudoisochromatic plates	Best known is the Ishihara. A series of plates are printed as a mosaic pattern of dots arranged to form a number on a coloured background. The first is an orange plate designed so that it can be seen regardless of any colour vision defect. Subsequent plates are designed so that the number may only be seen if colour vision is normal or to identify and classify protan and deutan defects. There are also paths of dots to trace if the patient is not familiar with numbers, but these have been shown to be of very limited use in young children.[54–57] The test has been shown to be effective in identifying defects, but less so in classifying them.
The City University colour vision test	Has 11 plates, each with a central test colour surrounded by four companion colours. The observer must indicate which of these four most closely matches the central plate. Dichromats are identified and classified correctly, but anomalous trichromats frequently pass or are classified incorrectly.[58,59]

Taking symptoms and history

As many visual anomalies are present from birth, a child usually grows up with the assumption that the way he or she sees the world is 'normal', and thus behavioural, and to an extent neurological, development adapts accordingly. For this reason, it is uncommon for a young child to present complaining of blurred vision or, indeed, of any kind of visual difficulty. We must therefore very often rely on parental observations (or those of a teacher) and/or screening (by health visitors, community orthoptists, community medical officers, general practitioners or school nurses) to identify children with a visual anomaly.

As a child has no 'reference' for the standard of vision to expect, the taking of a history necessarily requires careful questioning of the parent(s). The parents' primary cause for concern should be noted. As soon as the child is old enough, which may be as young as 2 years of age, it is also important to address some questions to him or her so that the child does not feel excluded and is put at ease for the subsequent examination.

Obviously, a child's responses may not always be as reliable as those of an adult and there is often a tendency to 'agree' with every question in an attempt to be helpful! In particular, a child's perception of time is often wildly unreliable so that he or she may have no concept of how long a symptom has been present, how often it occurs or how long it lasts. Thus, initially enquiring directly of a child if he or she is experiencing any difficulties and then requesting more detail on any complaints from the parent may be a good way to proceed.

The age of the child determines the level at which the questioning is pitched and the degree to which it is addressed to the parent. Chapter 15 addresses in more detail the expected abilities relative to the age of a child.

With children of school age and above more specific queries should be possible, such as:

- Can you read small writing and/or see the television and or /computer clearly?
- Do you have a board in school?
- Can you read that clearly?
- Do you sit at the front or back of the class?

As with the questioning of adult patients with regard to symptoms, the onset, duration and frequency of any parental observations or patient symptoms as well as any associations should be established where possible. Parents often refer to a child screwing up the eyes as 'squinting' and thus, if this is reported, careful further questioning is necessary. A possible line of questioning would be:

- Does one eye appear to wander?
- Do the eyes appear to move together?
- Does the child follow you with both eyes?

In the case of parental observation of squint

- Is it seen some or all of the time?
- Is it worse when the child is tired?
- Which eye is seen to wander or can either eye?
- Does the eye turn in or out?
- Does it appear more obvious when the child is concentrating and/or reading and/or tired?

Parents may sometimes seem quite vague in their initial concerns, for example, reporting that 'the eyes just don't always look right', but often further questioning along these lines can give better insight into the nature of their observations. If the child is rubbing or screwing up the eyes, when does this happen? Is it associated with reading or other concentrated vision, do the eyes ever look crusty or sticky (blepharitis, allergic conjunctivitis)? Sometimes children develop a nervous habit of frequent blinking (tic) with no underlying cause, but all other possible causes should be explored (refractive error, binocular vision anomaly, external eye problem) before tic is considered as an explanation. The taking of a careful general and ocular history also requires significant adaptation from the routine used with an adult and should include enquiries with regard to the following.

Behavioural or developmental abnormalities

- Are expected milestones being achieved at the appropriate age?
- Is the child making progress at school?

Such abnormalities have been shown to have increased associations with visual anomalies or a visual problem may be their underlying cause; for example, disruptive behaviour, poor concentration or introverted behaviour may stem from a visual problem.

Family history of refractive error, amblyopia or strabismus

Has anyone in the family needed glasses as a child, had a lazy eye or turn in the eye, needed surgery or patching or had any serious problems with their eyes? A positive family history increases the chances of visual or ocular anomalies.

Birth history

- Was the birth normal?
- Was the child premature or of low birth weight? This is associated with an increased incidence of refractive error, strabismus and amblyopia.
- If so, was oxygen given? This is associated with a further increase in incidence of the above as well as retinopathy of prematurity and congenital high myopia.
- Were forceps used at delivery? This is associated with an increased risk of superior oblique (fourth nerve) palsy.
- Was the birth difficult or breach? This is associated with an increased risk of developmental and/or visual problems.

General health

Any systemic anomalies and medication should be noted. Is the child healthy, on any medication or allergic to anything? Systemic anomalies may be associated with increased incidence of visual problems, such as rubella, Down's syndrome, cerebral palsy.

Hearing

- Are there any concerns with regard to the child's hearing?
- Has hearing been screened?

As well as often being associated with developmental and visual anomalies, hearing difficulties may produce similar external signs to visual problems. For example, abnormal head posture (turning a better ear towards a sound source), sitting close to the television, leaning close to people in conversation, apparent poor concentration and poor progress at school, may all be the result of a visual or auditory dysfunction. For these reasons, it is often worth suggesting a hearing check (if one has not been carried out) if a child is assessed visually and found to be normal.

References

1 Mohindra I and Held R (1981). Refraction in humans from birth to five years. *Doc Ophthalmol.* **28**, 19.
2 Atkinson J, Braddick O and French J (1980 Infant astigmatism: Its disappearance with age. *Vis Res.* **20**, 891.
3 Abrahamson M, Fabian G, Anderson AK and Sjostrand J (1990). A longitudinal study of a population based sample of children. I Refraction and amblyopia. *Acta Ophthalmol.* **68**, 428–434.
4 Hirsch MJ (1953). The changes in refraction between the ages of 5 and 14, theoretical and practical considerations. *Am J Optom Arch Am Acad Optom.* **29**, 455.
5 Bercovich L and Donaldson DD (1982). The natural history of congenital sutural cataracts: Case report with long term follow-up. *J Pediatr Ophthalmol Strabismus* **19**, 108.
6 Anstice J (1971). Astigmatism – its components and their changes with age. *Am J Optom Arch Am Acad Optom.* **48**, 1001.
7 Hirsch MJ (1963). Changes in astigmatism during the first eight years of school – an interim report from the Ojai longitudinal study. *Am J Optom Arch Am Acad Optom.* **40**, 127.
8 Gwiazda J, Thorn F, Bauer J and Held R (1993). Emmetropization and the progression of manifest refraction in children followed from infancy to puberty. *Clin Vis Sci.* **8**, 227–344.
9 Tokoro T and Suzuki K (1968). Significance of changes of refractive components to development of myopia during seven years. *Nippon Geka Gakkai Zasshi* **72**, 1472.
10 Baldwin WR (1990). Refractive status of infants and children. In: *Principles and Practice of Pediatric Ophthalmology*. Eds Rosenbloom AA and Morgan M (Philadelphia: J.B. Lippincott Co).
11 Scharf J (1977). Refraction in premature babies: A prospective study. *J Pediatr Ophthalmol.* **15**, 48.
12 Dobson V, Fulton A and Sebris SL (1984). Cycloplegic refraction of infants and young children: The axis of astigmatism. *Invest Ophthalmol Vis Sci.* **25**, 83.
13 Mukherji R, Roy A and Chatterjee SK (1983). Myopia in newborn. *Indian J Ophthalmol.* **31**, 705.
14 Breidahl HD (1966). The growth and development of children born to mothers with diabetes. *Med J Aust.* **12**, 268.
15 Cummins M and Norrish M (1980). Follow-up of children of diabetic mothers. *Arch Dis Child.* **55**, 259.
16 Tuncer M (1974). A long term study of children born to diabetic mothers. *Turk J Pediatr.* **16**, 59.

17 Hirsch MJ (1957). The relationship between measles and myopia. *Am J Optom Arch Am Acad Optom.* **34**, 28.
18 Jain IS, Jain S and Mohan K (1983). The epidemiology of high myopia – changing trends. *Indian J Ophthalmol.* **31**, 723.
19 Krause U, Krause K and Rantakillio P (1982). Sex difference in refractive error. *Acta Ophthalmol (Copenh.)* **60**, 917.
20 Sperduto RD, Seigal D and Roberts J (1983). Prevalence of myopia in the United States. *Arch Ophthalmol.* **101**, 405.
21 Kantor DW (1932). Racial aspects of myopia in compositors (racial factors in degree of myopia). *Br J Ophthalmol.* **16**, 45.
22 Sorsby A (1933). Race, sex and environment in the development of myopia. LCC Report, vol IV, II London 55.
23 Sourasky A (1928). Race, sex and environment in the development of myopia (preliminary investigation). *Br J Ophthalmol.* **12**, 197.
24 Zhan MZ Saw, SM Hong RZ, *et al.* (2000). Refractive errors in Singapore and Xiamen, China – a comparative study in school children aged 6 to 7 years. *Optom Vis Sci.* **77**, 302–308.
25 Edwards MH (1999). The development of myopia in Hong Kong children between the ages of 7 and 12 years: A five-year longitudinal study. *Ophthalmic Physiol Opt.* **19**, 286–294.
26 Otsuka J (1956). Genesis of myopia. *Bull Tokyo Med Den Univ.* **3**, 1.
27 Rasmussen OD (1936). Incidence of myopia in China. *Br J Ophthalmol.* **20**, 350.
28 Tenner AS (1915). Refraction in school children: 4800 refractions tabulated according to age, sex and nationality. *NY Med J.* **102**, 611.
29 Sato T (1957). *The Causes of Acquired Myopia.* (Tokyo: Kanahara Shuppan).
30 Yoo R, Logani S, Mahat M, Wheeler NC and Lee DA (1999). Vision screening of abused and neglected children by the UCLA Mobile Eye Clinic. *J Am Optom Assoc.* **70**, 461–469.
31 Saw SM, Hong RZ, Zhang MZ, *et al.* (2001). Near-work activity and myopia in rural and urban schoolchildren in China. *J Pediatr Ophthalmol Strabismus* **38**, 149–155.
32 Fatt HV, Griffin JR and Lyle VM (1992). *Genetics for Primary Eye Care Practitioners*, Second Edition. (Oxford: Butterworth–Heinemann).
33 Woodhouse JM, Pakeman VH, Cregg M, *et al.* (1997). Refractive errors in young children with Down syndrome. *Optom Vis Sci.* **74**, 844–851.
34 Maino JH (1979). Ocular defects associated with cerebral palsy: A review. *Rev Optom.* 69–72.
35 Friedman Z, Neumann E, Hyams SW, *et al.* (1976). Ophthalmic screening of 38,000 children age 1 to 2 years in child welfare clinics. *J Pediatr Ophthalmol Strabismus* **17**, 261.
36 American Academy of Ophthalmology (1994). *Basic and Clinical Science Course in Pediatric Ophthalmology and Strabismus.* Section 6 (San Francisco: American Academy of Ophthalmology).
37 Abrahamsson M, Magnusson G and Sjostrand J (1999). Inheritance of strabismus and the gain of using heredity to determine populations at risk of developing strabismus. *Acta Ophthalmol Scand.* **77**, 653–657.
38 Matsuo T, Yamane T and Ohtsuki H (2001). Heredity versus abnormalities in pregnancy and delivery as risk factors for different types of comitant strabismus. *J Pediatr Ophthalmol Strabismus* **38**, 78–82.
39 Schworm HD and Rudolph G (2000). Comitant strabismus. *Curr Opin Ophthalmol.* **11**, 310–317.
40 Block SS, Moore BD and Scharre JE (1997). Visual anomalies in young children exposed to cocaine. *Optom Vis Sci.* **74**, 28–36.
41 Nelson LB, Ehrlich S, Calhoun JH, Matteucci T and Finnegan LP (1987). *Am J Dis Child.* **141**, 175–178.
42 Stromland K (1987). Ocular involvement in the fetal alcohol syndrome. *Surv Ophthalmol.* **31**, 277–284.
43 Hakim RB and Tielsch JM (1992). Maternal cigarette smoking during pregnancy. A risk factor for childhood strabismus. *Arch Ophthalmol.* **110**, 1459–1462.
44 Duckman RH (1979). The incidence of visual anomalies in a population of cerebral palsied children. *J Am Optom Assoc.* **50**, 1013–1016.
45 Aurell E and Norrsell K (1990). A longitudinal study of children with a family history of strabismus: Factors determining the incidence of strabismus. *Br J Ophthalmol.* **74**, 589–594.
46 Berk TA, Oner HF and Saatci OA (2000). Underlying pathologies in secondary strabismus. *Strabismus* **8**, 69–75.
47 Flom MC (1963). Treatment of binocular anomalies of vision. In: *Vision in Children*, p. 214. Eds Hirsch MJ and Wick RE (Philadelphia: Chilton).
48 Flom MC and Bedell HE (1966). Prevalence of amblyopia (Reprint of US Public Health Reports 81:329,341). *Am J Optom Arch Am Acad Optom.* **43**, 732.
49 Maumenee IH (1979). Classification of hereditary cataracts in children by linkage analysis. *Ophthalmology* **86**, 1554–1559.
50 Rosenberg MA, Savino PJ and Glaser JS (1979). A clinical analysis of pseudopapilloedema. *Arch Ophthalmol.* **97**, 71–75.
51 Thuline HC (1964). Color-vision defects in American school children. *J Am Med Assoc.* **188**, 514–518.
52 Walters JM (1984). Portsea modified clinical technique: Results from an expanded optometric screening protocol for children. *Aust J Optom.* **67**, 176–186.
53 Tovee MJ (1992). Colour blindness. *Psychol: Bull Br Psychol Soc.* **5**, 501–503.
54 Verriest G (1981). Colour vision tests in children, Part I (1981). *Attiv Fond G Ronchi.* **XXXVI**, 83.
55 Verriest G (1981). Colour vision tests in children, Part V (1981). *Attiv Fond G Ronchi.* **XXXVI**, 111.
56 Verriest G, De Coninck MR and Uvijls A (1981). Colour vision tests in children, Part IV. *Attiv Fond G Ronchi.* **XXXVI**, 106.
57 Cox BJ (1971). Validity of a preschool colour vision test. *Can J Optom.* **33**, 22.
58 Hill AR, Heron G and Lloyd M (1982). An evaluation of some colour vision tests for children. In: *Colour Vision Deficiencies, VI.* Ed. Verriest G, *Doc Ophthalmol Proc Series* **33**, 183.
59 Verriest G and Caluwaerts MR (1978). An evaluation of three new colour vision tests. *Med Probl Ophthalmol.* **19**, 131.

3
Assessment of Visual Acuity

Kathryn Saunders

Types of visual acuity
Visual acuity tests
Expected norms for age
Repeatability of acuity tests
Significant interocular acuity differences

Visual acuity is poor at birth. In addition to poor control of eye movements, the immature optics, retinal anatomy and cortical architecture restrict visual performance, increase visual noise and reduce spatial sensitivity. During the first 6 months post-natally, the anatomical and physiological changes that occur in the normally developing visual system result in a dramatic improvement in visual performance, including visual acuity. The size, shape and distribution of the photoreceptors on the retina mature to maximise visual efficiency[1] and the cortical connections and processes required for adult-like visual processing develop.[2] The infant becomes better able at the fine control of eye movements, and both accommodation and stereopsis mature.

It is not clear when visual acuity is fully mature. The use of various methods to establish this is discussed in Chapter 1. The age at which adult-like acuity estimates are achieved is largely dependent on the test used to access this information. The visual evoked potential (VEP) records electrical responses from visual stimuli at the level of the primary visual cortex. All it requires is for the subject to look at a computer monitor that presents visual stimuli. VEP provides an objective measure of visual acuity, is minimally affected by attentional and motivational factors, and is therefore highly suitable for infant subjects. It is also suitable for subjects with profound neurological impairment who are unable to respond to other forms of acuity testing.

While this technique may be useful in hospital and research environments, it is rarely applicable in general optometric practice. VEP studies have demonstrated adult-like acuity responses at 12 months, which suggests that the majority of the anatomical and physiological changes responsible for refining visual acuity are complete by this age.[3] VEPs assess function only to the level of the primary visual cortex, so it is unclear from such studies what further refinements to processing (if any) are required beyond this level.

For other types of acuity test more applicable to optometric practice, attentional and motivational factors are likely to influence the acuity estimates achieved. These techniques, which include preferential looking (described below), are sometimes referred to as 'behavioural' acuity measures. While the influence of attentional and motivational factors may be viewed as a disadvantage, it may be argued that behavioural techniques provide a more complete picture of a child's visual function, including processing beyond the level of the primary visual cortex. Using preferential looking (PL) techniques, adult levels of visual acuity may be recorded during the third year of life.[4,5] More complex tests, such as those that involve letter recognition and matching and/or naming, may not produce adult acuities until about 6 years of age.[6]

Types of visual acuity

Methods used to measure acuity are diverse and the principles that underlie them need to be understood so that they can be used appropriately and to maximal effect. The four basic types of acuity measure are:

- Detection (minimum visible);
- Resolution (minimum resolvable);
- Recognition/identification (minimum recognisable);
- Hyperacuity (minimum discriminable).

Detection (minimum visible)

Detection refers to the smallest test object that can just be detected. Under ideal conditions a dark line of width 0.5 seconds of arc can just be detected.[7]

Tests such as the Stycar Balls and the 'Hundreds and Thousands' tests, traditionally used by health visitors in routine infant visual screening, are examples of detection acuity tests. Detection tasks such as these are often less affected by visual impairment than are more complex acuity tasks, such as those discussed below. Use of these tests may grossly overestimate visual acuity in visually impaired children. Children may also fail tests such as the 'Hundreds and Thousands' one because of a motor problem that reduces their control of fine hand movements, rather than an inability to detect the individual sweets.

Although detection acuity tasks may be cheap and quick to use, their use is limited, even as a screening tool.

Resolution (minimum resolvable)

Resolution measures the smallest angular separation between adjacent targets that can be resolved. Resolution acuity is probably limited by the optical limitations of the eye and the retinal photoreceptor spacing; it is usually in the region of 30 seconds of arc.

PL tests and VEPs are examples of resolution acuity tests. Resolution acuities are a more useful and sensitive measure of visual acuity than are detection tests. They can be successful in estimating acuity in infants from birth.

Recognition and/or identification (minimum recognisable)

Recognition is the type of acuity measured with the Snellen chart and with other acuity tests that use letters or other optotypes. It refers to the ability to identify a form or its orientation.

Children from about 2.5 years of age can be tested successfully with some forms of recognition tests (e.g., Kay picture test, uncrowded logMAR test). Recognition acuity differs from resolution acuity in several ways:

- Resolution acuity stimuli tend to subtend a larger area than recognition targets. While the resolution stimuli may contain detail as fine as the smaller recognition targets, their overall size is larger.
- Resolution acuities are less degraded in the normal and pathological peripheral retina than are resolution acuities.[8,9] Strabismic amblyopes demonstrate falsely high acuities with resolution targets because the larger size of the resolution targets stimulates parafoveal areas in which resolution acuity is less degraded than is recognition acuity.
- Recognition acuity tasks are affected by contour interaction, whereas resolution stimuli are not. The ability of recognition acuity tasks to reveal the crowding phenomenon in which acuity thresholds increase (i.e., visual acuity decreases) when contour interaction is present means they are more effective than resolution acuity at detecting and monitoring amblyopic deficits.

Overall, recognition acuities are more sensitive to pathological and physiological degradation than are resolution acuities.

Hyperacuity (minimum discriminable)

Hyperacuity describes the ability to determine differences between two stimuli (e.g., vernier acuity). Relative size, orientation and position can be judged with an accuracy of 3–6 seconds of arc.[10]

Hyperacuity is limited less by optical and retinal factors than is resolution acuity, and it is believed to reflect cortical processing. Stereoacuity may also be considered a type of hyperacuity.

Visual acuity tests

In all cases, the value we record with an acuity test is referred to more accurately as an acuity estimate. The estimate obtained depends not only on the acuity present, but also on the type of test used, the motivation and attention of the child, the presence of pathology and the skill of the examiner.

As optometrists we aim to measure visual acuity in such a way that we can detect those children with reduced binocular acuity and those with interocular acuity differences. We aim to monitor effectively the change in acuity that result from spectacle correction or other intervention. The visual acuity tests below are discussed in terms of their ability to fulfil these aims. The age group for which they are appropriate and other advantages and disadvantages are also examined. Some of the most commonly used and most well-designed commercially available tests are discussed. Detection tests such as the Stycar Balls and the 'Hundreds and Thousands' tests are not covered, as their use is considered to be limited. VEP measures of acuity are also not included, as these are rarely used in optometric practice.

Preferential looking tests

PL tests measure resolution acuity. They are designed around the principle that an infant looks towards a pattern rather than a blank stimulus.[11]

The patterns utilised in PL tests are generally square-wave gratings (alternating black-and-white lines of equal thickness and length). These gratings are described in terms of their spatial frequency (i.e., the number of black-and-white pairs in each degree of visual angle). The higher the spatial frequency the finer the grating.

Gratings of increasing spatial frequency are presented to an infant and their looking responses recorded. The highest spatial frequency (finest grating) that elicits an appropriate looking response may be used to estimate visual acuity. Commercially available grating PL tests include the Teller acuity cards and the Keeler acuity system. The Keeler acuity system is the most commonly available grating PL test in the UK (*Figure 3.1*). It is available in two formats, the 'Screening' set and the 'Additional' set. Both sets are required for an estimate of acuity to be obtained.

Another type of stimulus used in PL tests is the vanishing optotype. Vanishing optotypes are based on similar principles to the grating stimuli, but use pictures constructed of black-and-white lines (*Figure 3.1*). The black and white lines used to form the picture are made finer and finer to allow the assessment of acuity. The Cardiff acuity test uses vanishing optotypes.[5]

Three important aspects of the design and administration of PL tests are:

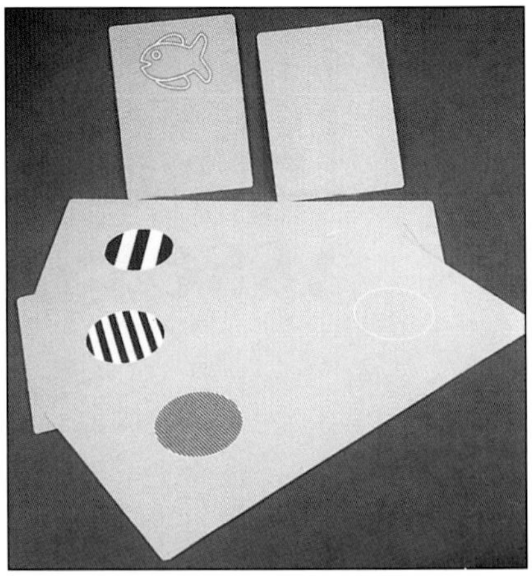

Figure 3.1
Preferential looking acuity tests: The Cardiff acuity test (top) and Keeler acuity system (bottom)

- Firstly, the stimulus must be isoluminant (equal average luminance) to the grey background (Cardiff acuity test) or to the blank stimulus (Keeler acuity system). This means that when the stimulus is beyond the resolution limit of the viewer the Cardiff acuity card looks uniformly grey and the Keeler acuity card appears to have two grey patches of equal luminance within the white circles. Under these circumstances the infant shows no looking preference. This design feature ensures that the acuity estimated is based on the ability to detect and resolve the grating rather than on a preference for one shade of grey over another.
- Secondly, when a PL test is administered, it is important for the examiner to be unaware of the position of the stimulus when presenting it to the infant. This allows the examiner's judgement of the infant's eye movements to be unbiased by any knowledge of the stimulus position (*Figure 3.2*).
- Thirdly, judgements regarding the position of the stimulus must be made using eye movements rather than pointing or verbal responses. Whereas pointing and naming can be encouraged to maintain the attention of a toddler, these are not as reliable as eye-movement responses.

The Keeler acuity system and the Cardiff acuity test are administered in much the same way. A gross target, expected to be above threshold, is presented first. This not only ensures that a gross level of resolution acuity is present, it helps to familiarise the examiner with an individual infant's mode of response to a seen target and to demonstrate to the infant what the test is about.

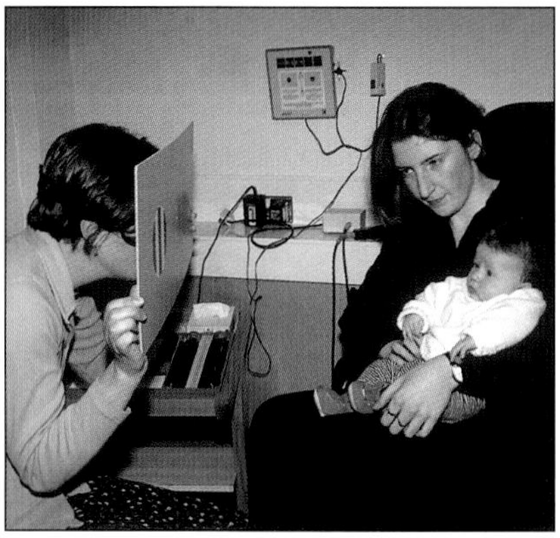

Figure 3.2
Estimating preferential looking acuity of a 3-month-old infant

The examiner must correctly identify the position of the grating and/or optotype on three or more of four presentations for that particular stimulus to be regarded as seen. Increasingly fine targets are presented until the point at which the examiner is no longer able to judge correctly the position of the target from the infant's eye movements.

PL tests can be used from birth and are the most appropriate acuity test in optometric practice for children under 2.5 years. Beyond this age, letter- (or optotype-) matching tests should be introduced if the child is intellectually and physically capable of these more challenging tests. The Keeler acuity system is very successful for estimating acuity in the youngest infants because the wide separation of the stimuli makes the judgement of eye movements easier. The short attention span of toddlers tends to be held for longer by the picture targets presented in the Cardiff acuity test, and may be more appropriate for those over 1 year of age.

The Cardiff acuity test was designed such that the target is positioned at either the top or bottom of the card. This design feature optimises the Cardiff acuity test's potential for acuity estimation in patients with nystagmus. Discriminating vertical PL eye movements from horizontal nystagmus eye movements is relatively straightforward. The Keeler acuity system's cards can also be presented vertically for the same reason.

As discussed above, resolution acuity measures, such as those obtained from PL tests, are limited in their sensitivity when compared with recognition tests. However, given the limits of attention, motivation and cognitive ability of infants and very young children, these are the only available measures. As soon as a child is developmentally able to co-operate with a recognition test, this should become the test of choice.

Optotype-matching and naming tests

Prior to a child knowing and being able to relate accurately the letters of the Snellen acuity chart, recognition acuity can be assessed using letter-matching tests or picture-naming or matching tests. For matching tests, the child has a key card that displays the same elements as presented in the acuity test.

The examiner presents the letter or picture targets at a specified distance from the child (usually 3m or 6m), and the child chooses a match from the key card (*Figure 3.3*). Older children can name the picture or letter. Optotype tests can present either an isolated letter or picture in an 'uncrowded' format, or a line of letters or pictures close enough together to introduce contour interaction and reveal the 'crowding' phenomenon. Crowded or linear presentation of targets should improve the test's ability to detect amblyopic eyes, for which acuities are overestimated with single target presentation.

Young children from 2.5–3 years of age may be able to co-operate with single optotype matching, but find the more complex crowded tests difficult. Success with the latter is usually better with children from 3.5–4 years of age.

Many letter-matching and picture-matching or naming charts to assess visual acuity are available. Some of the more commonly used are discussed below.

Kay picture test

The Kay picture test is designed for children 2–3 years of age. It presents a series of isolated pictures at either 3m or 6m in a flip-card format. The pictures can be either matched or named. A useful near version of the test to assess near visual acuity is also available. The test was designed around Snellen principles and the use of pictures rather than letters improves the test's ability to obtain recognition acuity estimates from younger children because of the increased familiarity of the targets. However, pictures are difficult to standardise in terms of the amount of detail and different spatial frequencies they contain. Many targets that supposedly test a single level of acuity consist of lines of different spatial frequency and are of varying overall size. This lack of uniformity in targets at the same acuity level reduces the sensitivity of the test and is a problem common to many other picture-naming and matching tests (*Figure 3.4*). However, an improved crowded version of the Kay pictre test was marketed recently, and its results have been shown to compare well with the crowded LogMar acuity test when acuity is scored per picture identified correctly.[12]

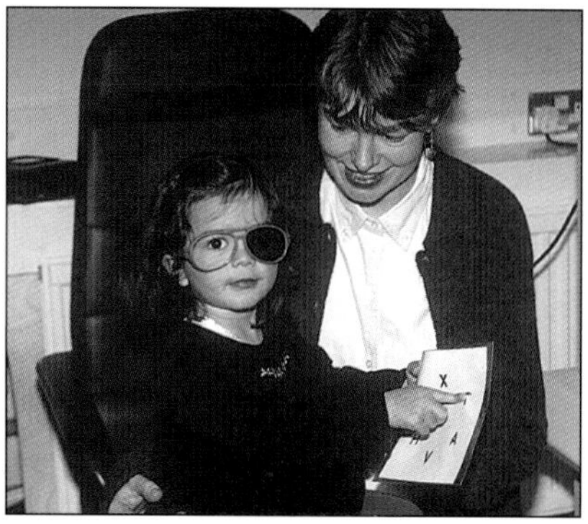

Figure 3.3
A 3-year-old performs a letter-matching acuity test

LH symbols

LH symbols – a house, heart (or apple), circle and square – can be either matched or named. They are suitable for children 2–3 years of age and come in both single and crowded format. Unlike those in the Kay picture test, the symbols are uniform in terms of detail, line width and overall size, which provides a more standardised acuity task.

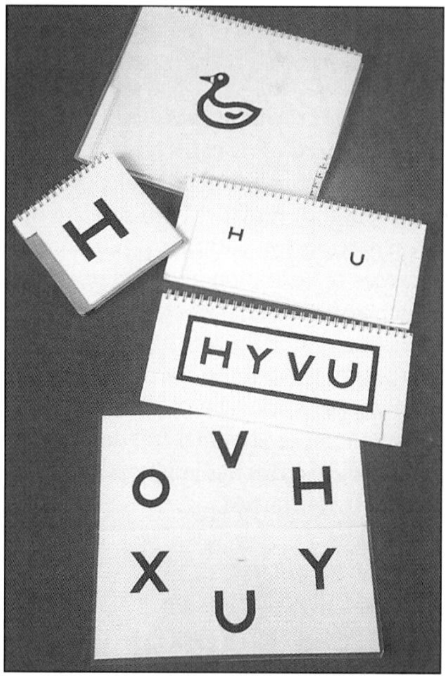

Figure 3.4
Letter and picture-matching acuity tests: the Kay picture test (top), Sheridan–Gardiner single-letter test (left) and the logMAR uncrowded and crowded charts (right). At the bottom is an example of a letter-matching key card held by the child

Illiterate, tumbling E and Llandolt C
Illiterate, tumbling E and Llandolt C are familiar tests that use Snellen letters E or C in different orientations. The child has to identify which direction the prongs of the E are pointing or where the break in the C is. Both are rather repetitive tests and the interpretation of acuity scores should be based largely on the child's discrimination of vertical positions, as frequently left–right orientations are confused by young children. These tests are suitable for children 3 years of age and older, by which age a letter-matching test is often possible and probably more appropriate.

Sheridan–Gardiner
Most optometric practices have a Sheridan–Gardiner test lurking in the drawer (*Figure 3.4*). This test can be used at either 3m or 6m and is suitable from about 2.5–3 years of age. The Sheridan–Gardiner test is based on the Snellen chart and suffers from many of its design faults (see below). In addition, it does not provide crowded letter presentation and may over-estimate acuity in amblyopia.

Sonksen–Silver
The faults of the Sheridan–Gardiner test are addressed in this test, which is suitable from about 3.5 years of age and presents letters in linear format. Its improved design includes letters that are spaced at intervals equal to the width of one letter, in an attempt to introduce contour interaction in the horizontal direction.

Cambridge crowding cards
Cambridge crowding cards are another letter-matching test that contains contour interaction. It provides both single-letter presentation for younger children and crowded presentation in a neat briefcase, which also contains occluding spectacles to assess monocular acuities. One disadvantage of the Cambridge test is that the acuity scale is based on the Snellen chart, such that letter size does not decrease in uniform steps. This has implications for the sensitivity of the test.

LogMAR acuity test
The logMAR acuity test, previously known as the Glasgow Acuity Cards,[13] was designed to address the problems present in the majority of children's acuity tests by utilising the principles of the 'gold standard' Bailey–Lovie Acuity test.[14] The Bailey–Lovie chart presents letters such that the subject's task at each acuity level only varies with regard to the level of acuity required to identify the target. All other variables are the same, regardless of acuity. This is not true for Snellen acuity charts, in which the spacing between letters and lines, the number of letters presented on each line and the change in letter size between lines all vary with acuity level.

The logMAR test applies the Bailey–Lovie principles. Letter size decreases in logarithmic fashion, which allows each letter to be scored individually with a score of 0.025. The scoring system gives a value of 1.0 logMAR to 6/60 and 0.0 logMAR to 6/6, with letters below 6/6 given a negative score. It comes with three charts: an 'uncrowded' acuity flip chart, on which isolated letters are presented, and two crowded acuity flip charts, each of which present four letters in crowded format, surrounded by a box to maintain vertical and horizontal contour interaction for all letters (*Figure 3.4*). Two crowded acuity charts are included in the test to avoid memorising of letters on repeat testing. Children from 2.5–3 years of age can be tested using the uncrowded version of this test, and for those from 3.5–4 years of age the crowded version is suitable. The careful design of the logMAR test means it may be preferable to continue with its use through childhood, using it as a letter-naming test once the child is able.

Near vision testing
Children generally have ample accommodation and few near vision problems when distance refractive errors are corrected. However, those with neurological impairment or low vision may have reduced accommodation, so it is important to assess near visual acuity. Several tests, such as the Kay picture and the Sheridan–Gardiner tests, have near vision charts that consist of single letters or pictures rather than words. These are appropriate for children as young as 2.5–3 years of age.

Expected norms for age

With increasing maturation of the visual system, we can expect to measure increasing levels of visual acuity with age. It is useful for optometrists to know what level of acuity can be expected from a child of a particular age when using a specific test. These data are difficult to obtain, but some are produced in *Table 3.1* for the Cardiff acuity and Sonksen–Silver tests. Those for the Sonksen–Silver tests may be applied cautiously to other crowded letter-matching acuity tests; likewise, those for the Cardiff acuity test may be applied to the Keeler acuity system. Where age norms are not available they can be calculated by individual practitioners collecting their own normative data from visually normal subjects with a range of ages. It might be useful to compare these values with those of *Table 1.1* in Chapter 1 to see the difference when PL is used.

Repeatability of acuity tests

In addition to a knowledge of age norms, it is important that optometrists understand the repeatability of the acuity test used and the relevance of this when acuity is assessed.

The repeatability of a test reflects the amount of inherent variability within a technique and hence its precision. Poorly designed tests with a low level of repeatability do not detect small differences and/or

Table 3.1 Age norms for PL acuity using the Cardiff acuity test and for letter-matching acuity with the Sonksen–Silver acuity test

Age	*Binocular acuity*	*Monocular acuity*	*Test type*
12 months	0.21–0.73		LogMAR Cardiff[a]
18 months	0.01–0.45		LogMAR Cardiff[a]
25 months	0.00–0.21		LogMAR Cardiff[a]
12–<18 months		0.40–0.80	LogMAR Cardiff[b]
18–<24 months		0.10–0.70	LogMAR Cardiff[b]
24–<30 months		0.10–0.50	LogMAR Cardiff[b]
30–36 months		0.00–0.30	LogMAR Cardiff[b]
2.5–<3.5 years	3/6	3/6	Sonksen–Silver[c]
3.5–<5.0 years	3/4.5	3/6	Sonksen–Silver[c]
5.0–<6.0 years	3/4.5	3/4.5	Sonksen–Silver[c]
6 years and over	3/3	3/4.5	Sonksen–Silver[c]

[a]Based on data from Deves *et al.*[4]
[b]Based on data from Adoh and Woodhouse[5]
[c]Based on data from Salt *et al.*[6]

changes in acuity reliably. Once the repeatability of a test is established, the practitioner can assess whether differences in acuity between two eyes or between visits are real or rather a product of test and/or retest variability. For a change or difference to be real or significant it must be greater than the limits of repeatability of the test. The most precise and accurate measures of acuity are likely to be achieved by tests designed to limit variability and with high levels of repeatability.

In a study of adult subjects, Lovie-Kitchin[15] demonstrated that the Snellen chart has a relatively low level of repeatability, such that the acuity measured on two occasions must differ by two lines (e.g., 6/18 compared with 6/9) before the measure can be said to differ significantly. By contrast, the improved design of the Bailey–Lovie chart results in a higher level of repeatability. A difference in acuity of five letters or more between two measures can be regarded as significant. Unfortunately, these data are scarce for most commercially available picture- or letter-matching tests. McGraw *et al.*[16] demonstrated a repeatability value for the crowded logMAR test of five letters (0.125 logMAR). Differences of five letters or more on repeat testing of an eye can be regarded as real or significant. When examining interocular acuity differences, they found that a difference of 0.1 logMAR (four letters) indicated a real interocular acuity difference.

Significant interocular acuity differences

One of the most important aspects of acuity testing for the optometrist is to detect significant interocular acuity differences. Binocular acuity values allow the optometrist to rule out a gross visual impairment, but monocular visual acuities provide much greater insight into the state of the developing visual system. During early infancy, transient interocular acuity differences are not uncommon, but persistent interocular acuity differences beyond the first year of life are cause for concern and require further investigation. They may signal amblyopia, other pathology or anisometropia.

Optometrists must also be able to judge whether acuity between visits or after treatment or spectacle correction has changed significantly. As discussed above, when attempting to detect significant acuity differences, knowledge about the repeatability of an acuity test is vital. The level of repeatability and the availability of these data should be of concern to optometrists when choosing an acuity test. A poorly designed test is less repeatable and less sensitive to real interocular and test–retest acuity differences, so such differences need to be large before they can be detected reliably. Unfortunately, this type of information is not readily available for all tests, but figures for some are given in *Table 3.2*. These figures were obtained by testing large populations of visually normal children.

Assessment of monocular acuities can be particularly difficult during the second year of life, as occlusion reduces the toddler's attention and co-operation. Patching is a useful method of occlusion in infancy, but toddlers and older children often co-operate better when occluded with brightly coloured, occluding spectacles, which can be made from cheap, plastic, children's sunglasses (*Figure 3.5*).

Armed with this information, the individual optometrist must choose which tests he or she prefers to use in practice, bearing in mind their advantages and limitations. To test a wide range of infants, pre-school and older children, the author's choice would be to purchase the Cardiff acuity test, the logMAR acuity test and the near Sheridan–Gardiner test. This choice is based on the design features of the tests as well as their cost, ease of use and storage and availability. The type of acuity test utilised should always be noted alongside the recorded acuity, so that results can be reviewed and interpreted with this knowledge. In addition to their utility in assessing the acuity of young patients, these types of acuity test also provide a valuable alternative to Snellen acuity for patients with communication difficulties, either as a result of congenital or acquired neurological impairment or because of a language barrier.

Table 3.2 Significant acuity differences for various acuity tests

Test name	*Test type*	*Significant difference*
Keeler acuity system	Preferential looking grating	Two cards
Cardiff acuity test	Preferential looking optotype	Two cards
Kay picture test	Isolated picture naming/matching	Two lines
Sheridan–Gardiner singles	Single letter matching	Three lines
Sonksen–Silver acuity system	Crowded/linear letter matching	Two lines
Cambridge Crowding cards	Crowded letter matching	Two lines
LogMAR acuity test	Crowded letter matching	Four letters

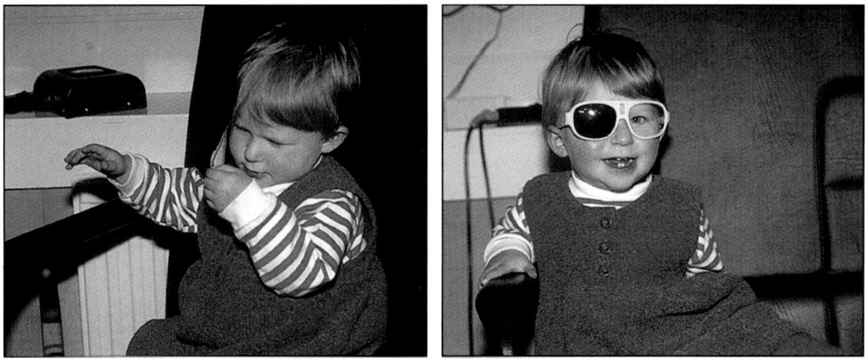

Figure 3.5
Toddlers may be more co-operative for monocular acuity testing when bright spectacles rather than a patch is the occlusion

References

1 Banks MS and Bennett FJ (1988). Optical and photoreceptor immaturities limit the spatial and chromatic vision of human neonates. *J Opt Soc Am.* **5**, 2059–2079.
2 Wilson HR (1988). Development of spatiotemporal mechanisms in infant vision. *Vis Res.* **286**, 611–628.
3 Norcia AM and Tyler CW (1985). Spatial frequency sweep VEP: Visual acuity during the first year of life. *Vis Res.* **25**, 1399–1408.
4 Deves S, Williams C, Parker J, *et al.* (1996). Visual acuity in children up to age 3: normal ranges and comparisons between tests from the 'ALSPAC' study. *Invest Ophthalmol Vis Sci.* **37**, S730.
5 Adoh T and Woodhouse JM (1994). The Cardiff Acuity Test used for measuring visual acuity development in toddlers. *Vis Res.* **34**, 555–560.
6 Salt AT, Sonksen PM, Wade A, *et al.* (1995). The maturation of linear acuity and compliance with Sonksen–Silver Acuity System in young children. *Dev Med Child Neurol.* **37**, 505–514.
7 Hecht S and Mintz EU (1939). The visibility of single lines of various illuminations and the retinal basis of visual resolution. *J Gen Physiol.* **22**, 593–612.
8 Loshin DS and White J (1984). Contrast sensitivity: The visual rehabilitation of the patient with macular degeneration. *Arch Ophthalmol.* **102**, 1303–1306.
9 Mayer DL, Fulton AB and Rodier D (1984). Grating and recognition acuities of paediatric patients. *Ophthalmology* **91**, 947–953.
10 Klein SA and Levi DM (1985). Hyperacuity thresholds of 1 second: Quantitative predictions and empirical validation. *J Opt Soc Am A* **2**, 1170–1190.
11 Fantz R, Ordy J and Udelf M (1962). Maturation of pattern vision in infants during the first six months of life. *J Comp Physiol Psychol.* **55**, 907–917.
12 Jones D, Westall C, Averbeek K and Abdolell M (2003). Visual acuity assessment: A comparison of two tests for measuring children's vision. *Ophthalmic Physiol Opt.* **23**, 541–546.
13 McGraw PV and Winn B (1993). Glasgow Acuity cards: A new test for the measurement of letter acuity in children. *Ophthalmic Physiol Opt.* **13**, 400–404.
14 Bailey IL and Lovie JE (1976). New design principles for visual acuity test charts. *Am J Optom Physiol.* **53**, 745–753.
15 Lovie-Kitchin JE (1988). Validity and reliability of visual acuity measurements. *Ophthalmic Physiol Opt.* **8**, 363–370.
16 McGraw PV, Winn B, Gray LS and Elliott DB (2000). Improving the reliability of visual acuity measures in young children. *Ophthalmic Physiol Opt.* **20**, 173–184.

4
Refractive Examination

Catherine Viner

Refraction of a child can result in immense frustration, but it can also provide an inordinate amount of satisfaction to the practitioner, potentially improve the well-being of the child and offer an opportunity for clarification and understanding to the parent or guardian.

An accurate refraction can help establish whether the child's visual system is developing normally. It offers an opportunity to correct any ametropia, and so allow the child to achieve the maximum possible visual acuity. It can also help highlight the cause of a number of irregularities in the development of good binocular vision.

In the refractive examination of a child, it is important to gather information about the child by taking a thorough history and symptoms. Not only does this allow a preliminary assessment of how likely it is that the child is at risk from an abnormally developing visual system, but also it gives an initial opportunity to interact with the child and to start designing a strategy for the rest of the examination. An initial model for history and symptoms with a child patient is developed in Chapter 2.

During the consultation the visual acuity and level of binocularity should be established. The health of the eyes must be examined and the refractive state should also be investigated and compared with the expected age-related norm. This chapter considers refraction techniques suitable for use with infants and children.

Investigation of refractive state

With adult patients, the practitioner can normally place reasonable confidence in the answers given to questions asked in the subjective part of the refraction. These answers can help substantiate the objective findings. With a child, the objective findings are critical in determining the true refractive state. With very young children, subjective questioning is, of course, impossible. Even with older children, who may respond to limited questioning, the practitioner is wise not to rely too heavily on the replies.

Although autorefraction can be used reasonably successfully on older children (they may even find the instrument intriguing and fun), unsatisfactory accommodation control and the daunting size of the instrument rules out its use on younger patients. Having said this, more recent instruments, such as the Welch Allyn Suresight Vision Screener, have been developed as hand-held autorefractors specifically to screen large numbers of children in a short period of time by non-specialist staff. Another instrument worthy of mention is the Powerrefractor from PlusOptix, which is able to carry out a rapid full dynamic binocular or monocular refraction within a spherical range of +5.00 to −7.00D and has proved valuable in screening children. Autorefraction may, therefore, still play an important role in the initial screening before more accurate intervention by an eye care professional.

The most useful objective technique, therefore, in determining the refractive state of a child is retinoscopy. In infants, individual trial lenses held in the hand (or in a lens rack) in front of the eyes is the most satisfactory technique to use when attempting to neutralise any movement seen (*Figure 4.1*). As most infants are hypermetropic, it is necessary to relax the accommodation in the fixating eye by holding up a fogging lens while performing retinoscopy on the other eye. As the pupillary distance is small, it is

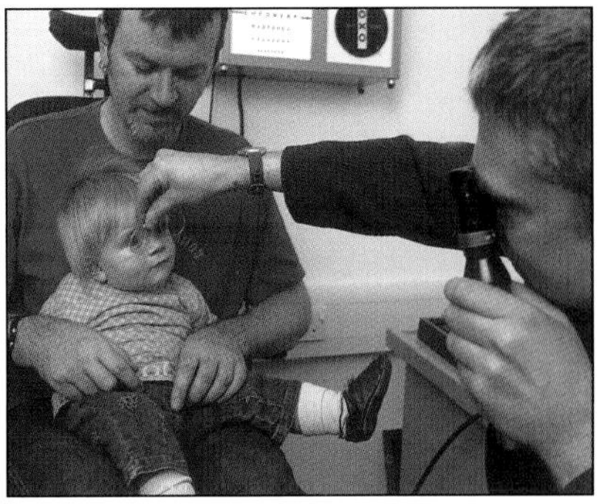

Figure 4.1
Holding the lenses before the child's eye removes the need for an impositional trial frame

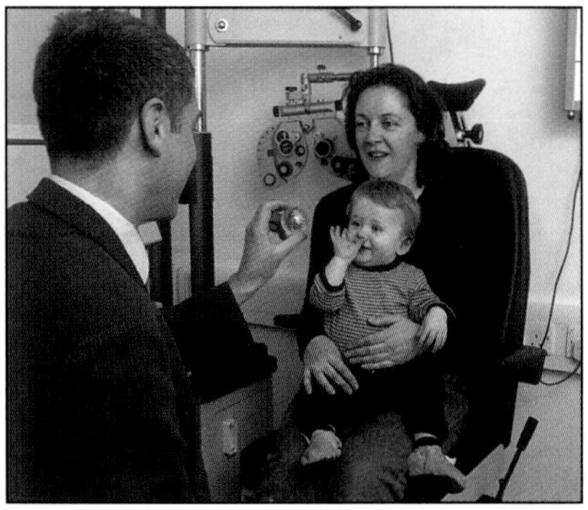

Figure 4.2
Interaction with the child is important throughout

possible to hold two trial lenses in one hand, one in front of each eye. In an astigmatic eye, each meridian should be neutralised separately. With slightly older children who tolerate wearing a trial frame, the use of a paediatric trial frame and full aperture trial lenses, to enable eye movements to be seen more easily, makes the procedure more comfortable for the child and therefore easier for the practitioner.

Static retinoscopy

The word 'static' refers to the patient's accommodation. In static retinoscopy the accommodation should be 'static' in its relaxed state. This state is achieved by encouraging the child to fixate on a target at a distance of at least 6m. An exciting target, such as a video, picture, interesting toy or useful assistant, helps keep the child's attention. The parent or guardian can sometimes help out here.

It is necessary for the practitioner to keep talking to the child, asking questions about the target: 'What can you see on the picture?' or 'Is mummy waving to you?' (*Figure 4.2*). This will ensure that the child's attention is held at the correct distance. Infants do not fixate a distance target readily, and the retinoscope light is likely to be of more interest to them. This can be used as an advantage with the Mohindra technique, which is described later. However, if the infant is asleep, providing Bell's phenomenon has not occurred, it is possible to refract the eyes by lifting the eyelids and approaching the visual axes to as close as possible. The exact accommodative state is not known, but if it is assumed to be the same in each eye, a useful comparison between the two eyes can be made.

Dynamic retinoscopy

Dynamic retinoscopy, in contrast, is a method whereby the patient's accommodation is kept in an active state by encouraging him or her to fixate an accommodative target at his or her working distance. The aim is to measure the effectiveness of the accommodation rather than the refractive error itself. Theoretically, if nothing hinders the child's accommodation and it is working accurately, neutral should be found at the same position at which the target is being held. Realistically, even with emmetropia and normal accommodation, a small 'with' movement is seen on retinoscopy when the retinoscope is used in this position. This is known as the dynamic or objective lag and, in normal individuals, usually falls between +0.25D and +1.00D. The lag can be explained simply as an inexactness of focusing. It can be measured by keeping the target still at a known distance, while the practitioner moves the retinoscope further away from the patient until neutral is seen. This distance is then measured and the two distances converted into dioptric values to work out the amount of lag present.

For example, if the child has a working distance of 25cm (equivalent to 4.00D), and if neutral is seen at 33cm (equivalent to 3.00D), the lag of accommodation is 4.00D – 3.00D, that is 1.00D.

Alternatively, lenses can be placed binocularly in front of the patient's eyes to neutralise the movement seen. This point is called the low neutral point and is equivalent to the dynamic lag. No allowance for the working distance needs to be made with either technique.

Of course, a number of factors can influence the effectiveness of the accommodation. A greater lag than normal can indicate a level of uncorrected hypermetropia with which the child cannot cope. A lag that appears different between the two eyes indicates that the effectiveness of the accommodation is different in each eye, possibly because of uncorrected anisometropia. A lag that appears different between the two meridians of the same eye could indicate a different effectiveness of the accommodation in each of the meridians, because of a different level of uncorrected hypermetropia in each of these meridians (i.e., astigmatism).

So, although an exact measure of any refractive error is not found, this technique is useful to use, in conjunction with other types of retinoscopy, to alert a practitioner to the possibility of the presence of uncorrected hypermetropia, anisometropia and astigmatism.

Mohindra technique

The Mohindra technique is a modification of near-fixation retinoscopy and benefits from the fact that an infant may well be attracted to the retinoscope light in a darkened room. Calling to the infant can also help keep his or her attention, as can feeding the infant at this moment. It is also thought that feeding helps relax the accommodation. Mohindra suggests that one eye should be occluded. It would seem sensible to ask the parent to do this if the practitioner does not feel comfortable occluding one eye while holding individual trial lenses in front of the other eye.

Retinoscopy is carried out on one eye at a time from a distance of 50cm. It is assumed that the retinoscope light provides no stimulus to accommodation and the eye is at its resting accommodative level. A correction of –1.25DS is added to the findings. Mohindra initially established this figure from experimental results. However, Owens *et al.*[1] suggest that this correction is derived by subtracting 2.00DS, because of the 50cm working distance, and then adding 0.75DS to account for a small amount of myopia induced by the lack of visual stimulus in the darkened consulting room.

Opinions vary as to the accuracy of this technique. If, during retinoscopy, the retinoscope light does not provide a stimulus to accommodation and the eye assumes its normal resting state of accommodation (known as tonus), it would seem that the results should have reasonable reliability. Two studies, by Mohindra and Molinari[2] (involving children between the ages of 5 and 7 years), and Borghi and Rouse,[3] found that there was a credible correlation between the results from retinoscopy using the Mohindra technique and those using a cycloplegic. However, Wesson *et al.*[4] found that results from these two different types of retinoscopy were not particularly close when they were compared for infants (which, of course, may well be the group on whom this technique would be most used). Maino *et al.*[5] felt that results from children with higher refractive errors had a poor correlation. It is thought that tonic accommodation may be dependent on the type of refractive error present, with hypermetropes having a greater amount. This would result in an underestimate of the amount of hypermetropia seen on retinoscopy using the Mohindra technique.

Cycloplegic refraction

Indications

Some practitioners argue that a cycloplegic examination should be carried out on all new child patients. Indeed, in the Paediatric Clinic at the University of Manchester Institute of Science and Technology (UMIST), all children undergo a cycloplegic refraction at their first visit. However, it is possible to highlight certain groups of children on whom a cycloplegic refraction is essential:

- Those in whom a satisfactory standard of acuity is not demonstrated;
- Those in whom a satisfactory level of stereopsis is not demonstrated;
- Those who present with a manifest squint, particularly an esotropia;
- Those who have an esophoria that appears significant or unstable;
- Those with a family history of squint, amblyopia or high hypermetropia;
- Those in whom pseudomyopia is suspected;
- Those who have a history of an 'eye turn' observed by the parent or guardian;
- Those who have anisometropia greater than 1.00D;
- Those in whom poor accommodation is found.

Of course, a cycloplegic agent can always be used as an aid to refraction for a patient who shows poor co-operation during a standard routine refraction. The child may not be able to co-operate fully because of mental or physical constraints or through an obstreperous disposition.

There are, of course, pros and cons to the use of a cycloplegic, which should always be borne in mind before proceeding. In a healthy, co-operative child, with satisfactory acuities, accommodation and stereopsis for his or her age, no notable family history and no binocular vision problems, it could be argued that there is no significant gain in performing a cycloplegic examination.

Advantages

The advantages of cycloplegic refraction are:

- Reveals latent hypermetropia;
- Aids fundus examination;
- Accurate fixation for static retinoscopy is less crucial.

Disadvantages

The disadvantages of cycloplegic refraction are:

- Photophobia caused by dilated pupils;
- Decreased ability in close work tasks because of cycloplegia;
- Distress to child on instillation of drops;
- Risk of adverse and allergic reactions.

Photophobia may be overcome by the use of sunglasses, which are now more readily available for children. It is prudent to warn the parent or guardian and school-age child that close work tasks may prove more difficult until the effects of the drug have worn off. Appropriate timing for a cycloplegic examination of a school-age child might be immediately after school, so the cycloplegic effect of the drug can wear off that evening and overnight, to allow full scholastic participation the next day.

Distress to the child on instillation of the drops can be minimised by careful explanation of what is going to happen. To tell the child that 'this won't hurt' when it surely will is to lie to the child and risk the loss of respect and co-operation. Avoidance of the words 'hurt' and 'painful', while mentioning that the drops might 'feel a bit funny' or 'feel a bit like fizzy lemonade', can help maintain the child's tolerance of you. Some practitioners advocate the use of a local anaesthetic, typically proxymetacaine 0.5% (as it stings considerably less than other anaesthetics) prior to the instillation of the cycloplegic agent. The purpose of this is twofold. Firstly, if the cornea is anaesthetised, the stinging of the next drug will not be felt. Secondly, the local anaesthetic may increase the absorption of the cycloplegic agent. The disadvantage of this method is that if the child does not like the first set of drops, he or she may make it extremely difficult for the second (more important) set of drops to reach their correct target.

The risk of an adverse reaction may be reduced by occluding the puncta while instilling the drops, thus reducing systemic absorption via the gut. Also, a careful history should be taken to ensure that a previous reaction has not occurred.

Adverse reactions to atropine are typically described as rendering the patient:

- 'As blind as a bat', because of the cycloplegia;
- 'As dry as a bone', through inhibition of sweat and salivary glands;
- 'As red as a beetroot', through increased vasodilation of the blood vessels of the skin as the body tries to reduce its temperature by an alternative means;
- 'As mad as a hatter', as the central nervous system (CNS) effects, including hallucinations, ataxia and psychotic reactions, manifest themselves, which indicates an advanced stage of poisoning.

CNS effects following the use of cyclopentolate have also been reported, usually after the administration of a higher than recommended dose. Confusion, difficulty in speaking, restlessness and hallucinations, fortunately, do not seem to last for more than a few hours and leave no permanent problems.

Local allergic reactions to both atropine and cyclopentolate are known. If these occur, future use of the drug should be avoided and parents or guardians should be warned of potential allergic responses to other anticholinergic agents, such as preparations to combat motion sickness.

Children with Down's syndrome and cerebral palsy show increased sensitivity to cycloplegics, which can lengthen the period over which the drug is effective. Some writers also feel that the use of a cycloplegic in a child with Down's syndrome is contraindicated because of an idiosyncratic cardio-accelerator response. Taking a full history should highlight whether or not the Down's child has experienced heart problems.

Cycloplegic agents

Cycloplegic agents are antimuscarinics. They work by blocking the muscarinic receptors in the ciliary muscle. These are normally stimulated by the release of acetylcholine from the nerve endings of the parasympathetic system. When stimulated, the ciliary muscle contracts, and so pulls the ciliary body forward. This relieves the tension in the suspensory ligaments, which support the lens. Consequently, the lens can become more convex, which results in an increase in refractive power to produce accommodation.

While the receptors of the ciliary muscle are blocked by an antimuscarinic agent, they are no longer receptive to acetylcholine and accommodation is not possible. In the eye, there are also muscarinic receptors in the iris sphincter. These, too, are blocked with the use of antimuscarinics, which results in mydriasis.

An ideal cycloplegic would have no ocular or systemic side-effects. It would be able to produce a rapid onset of cycloplegia, inhibit accommodation completely for an adequate period of time and then swiftly restore effective accommodation. These are demanding requirements, but the three most common cycloplegics (atropine, cyclopentolate and tropicamide) between them cover most of these ideals. Their properties are considered below and in *Table 4.1*.

Atropine

Atropine sulphate 1.0%, whereas useful when cyclopentolate has failed to produce a satisfactory cycloplegia, is not widely used today. Its potentially fatal adverse reactions, coupled with its slow action and long-lasting effects, make it a less favourable choice. Indeed, its length of action rules out its use completely in infants under the age of 3 months, because of the risk of stimulus-deprivation amblyopia. There is also a risk that the use of atropine in a child with a large heterophoria or an intermittent strabismus could lead to a permanent squint being established by the time the cycloplegia wears off.

A practitioner who wishes to use atropine on a child must rely on accurate parental administration of the drug, or be prepared to administer it him- or herself, twice a day for 3 days prior to the examination. The use of atropine also generally requires a tonus allowance of about −1.00DS to be made to the final prescription, because atropine completely abolishes all accommodative tonus, and when this returns, if no allowance is made, the resultant prescription is over plussed.

Cyclopentolate

Cyclopentolate hydrochloride 0.5% and 1.0% is probably today's most popular choice of cycloplegic. It does not produce complete cycloplegia, but leaves a residual amount of accommodation of about 1.50D or less. However, this depth of cycloplegia is adequate for the majority of cases and also means that a tonus allowance does not normally need to be considered when calculating the final prescription.

To avoid administering an overdose, one drop of the 0.5% solution should always be used with infants of 3 months and younger. The 0.5% solution can also be useful when a cycloplegic refraction is carried out on a fair-skinned individual over the age of 12 years. In all other cases, one drop of the 1.0% solution offers the most useful amount of cycloplegia in a reasonable time frame. In particularly dark-skinned patients, a second drop may need to be instilled if little effect is seen after the first 15 minutes.

Cyclopentolate is available in a multi-dose preparation (Mydrilate), but is principally used in single dose form (Minims Chauvin). Ismail *et al.*[6] found that spraying cyclopentolate onto the eyelashes of a gently closed upper lid resulted in an easier application with no compromise of the cycloplegic effects.

Tropicamide

A 1.0% solution of tropicamide can provide useful short-acting cycloplegia in patients in their late teens or older. Two drops may need to be instilled, separated by 5 minutes. If retinoscopy is delayed beyond 35 minutes after instillation, a third drop should be used. Although tropicamide is traditionally thought to be less advantageous for cycloplegic refractions on younger patients, Manny *et al.*[7] in their Correction of Myopia Evaluation Trial (COMET) concluded differently. They found that two drops of a 1.0% solution of tropicamide, instilled 4–6 minutes apart and after an initial drop of topical anaesthetic, provided an effective cycloplegic agent in myopic children between 6 and 11 years of age.

Table 4.1 Comparison of atropine, cyclopentolate and tropicamide

Agent	*Onset of adequate cycloplegia*	*Duration of cycloplegia*	*Duration of mydriasis*	*Tonus allowance needed*
Atropine	36 hours	7–10 days	1 0–14 days	Yes
Cyclopentolate	30–60 minutes	Up to 12 hours	24–48 hours	No
Tropicamide	30 minutes	2–6 hours	8–9 hours	No

Commencing retinoscopy

As can be seen from the above, the onset of adequate cycloplegia varies according to which drug is used. Also, the different time spans involved in continued cycloplegia and continued mydriasis indicate that, although these two actions are linked, the presence of one does not necessarily indicate the presence of the other. Initially, to confirm that there has been some corneal absorption and transfer of the drug to the muscarinic receptor sites, a check of pupil size before and 10 minutes after drug instillation can prove useful.

However, to ensure paralysis of the ciliary muscle is occurring, a regular check on the accommodation should be made. It is usually thought to be satisfactory to start retinoscopy when the residual accommodation is below 2.00D. In an older child, the RAF rule is used at 10 minute intervals to check when this level has been reached. As the accommodation ability falls, the use of a pair of +2.50DS lenses helps keep the end point on the RAF rule. Dynamic retinoscopy, which shows an increasing dynamic lag, can be used in younger children.

When performing retinoscopy, it is still preferable that the child fixates a distance target, because of the residual accommodation. With an increased pupil diameter it can be difficult to determine the direction and size of the moment. It is important to concentrate only on the central 3–4mm of the pupil and to ignore the aberrations of the light movements in the peripheral annulus. Traditionally, cycloplegic retinoscopic results are recorded in red.

When and what to prescribe

In considering whether or not to give a spectacle correction and, if so, what that spectacle correction should be, the practitioner needs to be aware of the expected refractive errors in children. It is well known that the average refractive error at birth is one of hypermetropia, in the region of +2.50DS. We also know that this refractive error decreases to an average of +0.50DS as the child approaches 5 or 6 years of age, because of the process of emmetropisation.

An astigmatic error in infants of approximately 1.00–1.50DC, which reduces in the first couple of years of life, is not uncommon. Clearly, any child with a refractive error that falls within these ranges appears to be developing as normal for his or her peer group and, providing acuity, motor status and sensory status are also within normal limits, no prescribing is necessary.

Prescribing under the age of 6 months

During this early developmental period, relatively large refractive changes can be encountered. Any concerns an optometrist may have about an infant's refractive error, particularly if accompanied by a positive history, should be referred to a paediatric ophthalmologist.

Prescribing from 6 months onward

Hypermetropia

The easiest recommendation to give is in the case of a fully accommodative esotrope, who should be given the full cycloplegic correction to keep him or her straight.

Hypermetropes whose prescription falls just outside the normal range should be monitored to look for any reduction in acuity, stereopsis or a change in motor status. Should any of these present themselves, a prescription should be given and any resultant amblyopia must be treated.

Hypermetropic prescriptions that vary greatly from the age-related norm are usually accompanied by a positive history and decrease in the expected acuity and stereopsis results. A prescription should always be given in these cases and any amblyopia treated.

It is common practice not to give the full value of the prescription to allow some blur to remain, which encourages good compliance and therefore acuity development. The author favours reducing the prescription by 1.00–1.50DS.

Myopia

Myopes are less at risk from developing amblyopia as a child's world is closer to him or her, but clear. Low prescriptions, such as those of −1.00DS or less, simply can be monitored regularly. However, any prescription greater than −3.00DS should be given to a child over the age of 1 year. At approximately 3 years old, the child's visual world becomes larger, and, taking into account any falling unaided vision, a myopic correction over −1.00DS may well be of some benefit to the child. As indicated in Chapter 2, however, preliminary data found that 44 per cent of children have an ocular or systemic condition associated with myopia greater than 5.00D, which indicates that detection and prompt referral of these cases by community health care services may, in some cases, prolong vision and possibly life expectancy.

Astigmatism

As evidence suggests that astigmatism is common in children under the age of 2 years, moderate cyls of up to 2.00–2.50DC can be monitored up until this age, provided there is no reduction in acuity. If the cyl is stable and over 2.50DC, it should be prescribed for infants younger than 12 months old. Any cyl greater than 1.50DC should be given to a child over 1 year old if the cyl is stable and causes a reduction in acuity. The axis of the cylinder is important, as oblique cylinders, if uncorrected, are likely to induce meridional amblyopia, so warrant correction at an earlier stage; 1.00DC is advisable for oblique cylinders.

Anisometropia

A transient level of anisometropia can be demonstrated in neonates, but a difference in refractive error of a dioptre or more between the two eyes can be considered significant after 12 months of age. This is particularly so when it is accompanied by a corresponding difference in visual acuity. Hypermetropes with even small levels of anisometropia are at risk from developing amblyopia.

When comparing non-cycloplegic and cycloplegic results, if a difference in anisometropia is found, the amount found under cycloplegia should be used when prescribing, as this will indicate the true amount present under a stable accommodative state. If a partial correction is to be given, the full difference in prescription between the two eyes should be maintained.

For example:

Cycloplegic Rx:	RE +5.50DS
	LE +4.00DS
Rx given:	RE +4.50DS
	LE +3.00DS

Any amblyopia that persists after spectacle correction should be treated accordingly. Myopes are less likely to be at risk from developing amblyopia from any anisometropia, as both eyes are able to receive a clear retinal image. Therefore, less intervention is needed.

Summary

Refraction of children requires a good working knowledge of expected age-related norms. Flexibility in working practices enables the practitioner to take full advantage of opportunities as they arise. An understanding of different types of retinoscopy arms the practitioner with an opportunity to double-check the findings. A familiarity with cycloplegics and feeling comfortable with their use enables a more relevant and accurate result to be obtained in a great number of cases.

References

1 Owens D, Mohindra I and Held R (1980). The effectiveness of a retinoscope beam as an accommodative stimulus. *Invest Ophthalmol Vis Sci.* **19**, 942–949.

2 Mohindra I and Molinari JF (1979). Near retinoscopy and cycloplegic refraction in early primary grade schoolchildren. *Am J Optom Physiol Opt.* **56**, 34–38.

3 Borghi RA and Rouse MW (1985). Comparison of refraction obtained by 'near retinoscopy' and retinoscopy under cycloplegia. *Am J Optom Physiol Opt.* **62**, 169–172.

4 Wesson MD, Mann KR and Bray NW (1990). A comparison of cycloplegic refraction to the near retinoscopy technique for refractive error determination. *J Am Optom Assoc.* **61**, 681–684.

5 Maino JH, Cibis GW, Cress P, Spellman CR and Shores RE (1984). Non-cycloplegic versus cycloplegic retinoscopy in pre-school children. *Ann Ophthalmol.* **16**, 880–882.

6 Ismail EE, Rouse MW and De Land PNA (1994). Comparison of drop instillation and spray application of 1% cyclopentolate hydrochloride. *Optom Vis Sci.* **71**, 235–241.

7 Manny R, Hussein M, Scheiman M, Kurtz D, Neiman K, Zinzer K and the COMET Study Group (2001). Tropicamide (1%): An effective cycloplegic agent for myopic children. *Invest Ophthalmol Vis Sci.* **42**, 1728–1735.

5

Myopia: Prevalence, Progression and Management

Nicola Logan

Global prevalence of myopia
Myopia; theories on apparent increased prevalence
Summary of research into myopia intervention
Prediction of future myopes
Summary

Management of myopia is generally undertaken by the optometrist and accounts for around 35 per cent of his or her clinical work. Around 18 per cent of patients seen by optometrists are under 16 years old and, of these, approximately 15 per cent present with myopia.[1]

Considerable evidence shows that refractive errors are distributed normally at birth.[2–4] However, by the age of 6 or 7 years the refractive state of the majority of children is close to emmetropia.[5] At this age, when many of the children are emmetropic, why do a significant proportion go on to develop myopia? Optometrists are often asked questions by patients about the onset and development of myopia. However, the myopia research literature often reveals conflicting results or equivocal opinions. Various studies have suggested several interventions that may retard the progression of myopia in children.

These studies include the use of atropine to paralyse accommodation,[6] bifocal and progressive addition spectacle lenses to reduce defective accommodative responses at near,[7–10] contact lenses either to flatten the cornea or retard axial elongation,[11] and β-blocker drugs to reduce raised intraocular pressure (IOP).[7] At present, there are no definitive answers and as such optometrists are unable to recommend any particular measure to prevent or retard the progression of myopia in children.

Global prevalence of myopia

Study of the prevalence of myopia reveals a wide variation in the figures reported in the published literature. These variations arise from differences in population samples and from discrepancies in methodology. The prevalence of myopia has also been found to change significantly with age.

Refractive error has a wide distribution in newborn infants, with myopia present in approximately 19 per cent of Caucasian infants.[2] However, the refractive status of the infant does not appear to differ significantly between races or different geographical locations.[12,13] As refractive error development depends, in part, on visual feedback,[14] it is not surprising that there is little variation in infant refraction across races, as presumably the near world of infants is similar everywhere.

Premature infants demonstrate a higher frequency of myopia compared with full-term infants.[15,16] In pre-school children an emmetropisation process is thought to reduce the prevalence of myopia to 2–3 per cent (for Caucasian children), but by the age of 6 years the prevalence rises to approximately 6 per cent[17–19], and approximately 25 per cent of Caucasian young adults have developed myopia (*Figure 5.1*).[20]

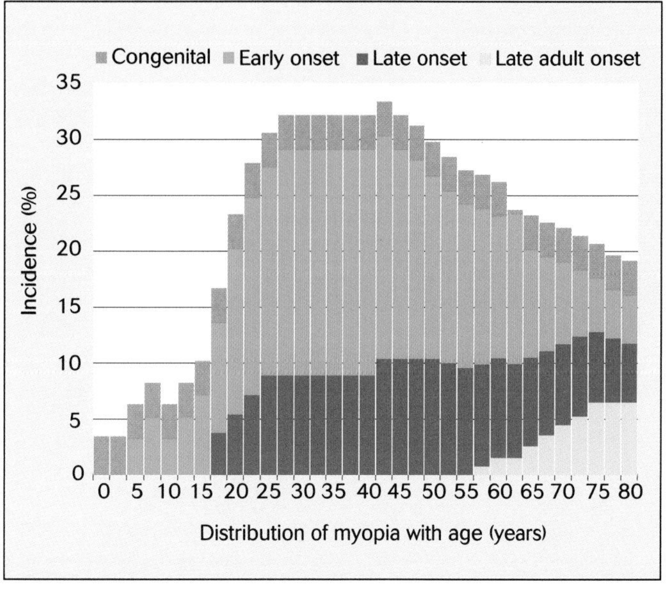

Figure 5.1
The early onset class of myopia constitutes the largest number of myopes and its prevalence now approaches 25 per cent of the young population in modern industrialised Western societies; it reaches 75 per cent in some Far Eastern countries. (Reproduced with permission[21]; © American Academy of Optometry)

The prevalence of myopia varies considerably with race; much higher values are reported for Chinese,[22] Japanese and Singaporean[23] populations. For example, myopia has been found in 30 per cent of Chinese children 6–7 years of age, and in up to 70 per cent of Chinese males 16–17 years of age.[24] Similarly, 15–20 per cent of Japanese 7 year olds are myopic and a prevalence of 66 per cent has been reported in Japanese 17 year olds.[25] Other Chinese population studies also recorded a high prevalence of myopia; values of 11.8 per cent for 6-year-old Taiwanese children have been reported.[26] This prevalence was found to increase to 55.5 per cent by the age of 12 years and to 75.9 per cent at 15 years of age. In Taiwanese medical students 18–21 years of age, 92.8 per cent were myopic (≥0.25D).[3]

Not all Asian populations have a high prevalence of myopia; in Tibet and Melanesia the prevalence of myopia in children has been found to be much lower than that in Hong Kong, Japan and Taiwan. In Tibetan children 6–16 years of age, a prevalence of myopia of 3.9 per cent has been reported,[27] with a similar finding in Melanesian children.[28] Epidemiological studies on remote populations in Arctic regions revealed an inordinately high increase in myopia prevalence in the present generation compared to previous generations.[29]

Even within a single racial or cultural group, the prevalence of myopia has been found to vary greatly with occupation;[30] students have a greater prevalence of myopia than people whose work entails little near vision activity.[31] A longitudinal study on the development of myopia in a specific occupational group (clinical microscopists) recorded that 45 per cent of the people in the study became myopic (≥0.37D) during the 2 year period.[32]

Comprehensive data on myopia prevalence in the UK date back approximately 40 years to the work of Sorsby *et al.*,[33] and the prevalence of myopia in the UK is extrapolated principally from findings in the USA and Scandinavia. However, recently, as part of an ongoing study in the UK, The Avon Longitudinal Study of Parents and Children,[34] the prevalence of myopia was found to be 0.9 per cent in a birth cohort of 7600 children 7 years of age. The prevalence of myopia differs by geographical location (*Table 5.1*), but the data are also confounded by a variety of other factors, which include ethnicity, age, occupation and socio-economic status.

Myopia: theories on apparent increased prevalence

Over the years, considerable evidence has accumulated that indicates both genetic and environmental components in the aetiology of myopia.

Genetic factors

Evidence exists that suggests genetics is a fundamental determinant of the refractive state. The distribution of myopia among races and ethnic groups, its prevalence in families and comparative studies in twins all support the idea that hereditary factors influence the development of ocular refraction.[35]

Molecular genetic studies[36,37] of US families with two or more individuals with –6.00D or more of myopia have found significant links with regions on chromosome 18p and 12q. Interesting candidate genes in these regions include ones for the alpha subunit of laminin and decorin, both components of the sclera. The Family Study of Myopia is a current study at Cardiff University, Wales, that aims to identify genes responsible for high myopia in the UK population. Preliminary results suggest that a gene on chromosome 12q is responsible for high myopia in at least 25 per cent of people in the UK.[37] As the study progresses and data from more families are included, further information hopefully will be identified. Genetic analysis of DNA from children and their families who participated in a longitudinal US study on myopia, the Orinda Study, revealed that the genetic loci for high myopia were not associated with the lower levels of myopia more commonly seen in children.[39]

An important population study by Young *et al.*[40] reported a dramatic increase in the prevalence of myopia in the generation of Alaskan Eskimos first exposed to compulsory education and a 'westernised' environment during their childhood. In the Eskimo families the parents were illiterate, whereas the children attended schools that followed a similar curriculum to the rest of the USA. Only two of the 130 parents were myopic, whereas 60 per cent of the children were myopic. The cause of the increase in myopia cannot be attributed solely to the introduction of formal schooling, as both diet and lifestyle changes occurred.

Similar studies that examined other isolated communities exposed to changes in their environment corroborated the findings of greater myopia among the younger generation.[29,41]

Human clinical data also support a genetic basis for myopia. Myopic parents tend to have myopic children in higher proportions than do non-myopic parents.[42–45] The prevalence of myopia in children with two myopic parents is 30–40 per cent, decreasing to 20–25 per cent in children with only one myopic parent and to less than 10 per cent in children with no myopic parents. A higher number of myopic parents increases the odds of being myopic, with odds ratios of between 5 and 7.3[39,42] reported for having two myopic parents versus no parents with myopia.

The relative effect of heredity and environment on refractive error can best be investigated using co-twin controls. Identical twins are single-ovum (monozygotic) individuals, the product of a single conception; the ovum splits in two at an early stage within the womb, and thus leads to two individuals with identical genetic make-up.

Binovular twins develop from two separately fertilised ova (dizygotic). Their genetic make-up tends to be as similar as that of ordinary siblings. The general consensus is that if a significant amount of similarity, or concordance, exists between a pair of twins, this indicates genetic background as a major factor in determining ametropia.[46]

Monozygotic twins tend to resemble each other, in both ocular component values and refractive error, more than dizygotic twins do. Twin studies have provided high values for refractive error heritability (0.82 or greater), that is the proportion

Table 5.1 Prevalence of myopia in children of different races and ages

Study	*Age (years)*	*Prevalence of myopia (%)*
CLEERE, USA (n = 2583)[19]	6–14	9.3
Australian (n = 2571)[18]	4	1
	12	8.7
Singapore (n = 1453)[23]	7 to	29 to
	9	53
Hong Kong[22]		
Local school (n = 335)	13–15	80 in Chinese
		65 in mixed Chinese
International school (n = 789)		43 in non-Chinese

of phenotypic variance that may be accounted for by genetic factors, and imply that the environmental impact on refraction is not significant.[47,48]

However, the epidemiological association between near work and myopia, the increase in myopia prevalence within a few generations and the theory of gene–environment interaction suggest that some individuals may be genetically susceptible to myopia if exposed to certain environmental factors.

Environmental factors

In the development of myopia, evidence from 'form-deprivation' myopia suggests that environmental factors appear to override genetic factors. Form-deprivation myopia occurs when clear vision is compromised severely during a critical period of post-natal development. This has been shown with both animals[49] and human infants.[50]

Furthermore, experimental findings from animal studies show that the refractive state of the eyes of young chicks or rhesus monkeys adapts to compensate for refractive errors induced by spectacle lenses.[49] Human clinical data also contain evidence for the influence of environment. The prevalence of myopia in Hong Kong Chinese has increased from approximately 30 per cent to 70 per cent in just one generation, which provides strong evidence of an environmental causal factor.[24,51,52]

One assumed link between animal and human studies is that the human accommodative response is inaccurate, and creates a hyperopic defocus during near work that simulates the effect of blur induced by spectacle lenses in animal experiments.[53–55] This hyperopic blur is a hypothetical stimulant to eye growth, which increases the rate of axial elongation and myopia progression. The major correlate of myopia in children is an increase in axial length of the eye.[33]

However, the significance of hyperopic blur as a risk factor may need to be re-examined. Recent clinical trials in children and young adults aimed at reducing the exposure to hyperopic defocus through the use of bifocal spectacles or progressive lenses produced only a modest reduction in the progression of myopia, which was not of clinical significance.[8,9]

Association with near work

Excessive and sustained near work has been cited for many years as a factor that predisposes a child to myopia, especially if combined with high levels of cognitive demand. The association between myopia and near work has been comprehensively reviewed in the book *Myopia and Nearwork*,[31] which concludes that although near work does not appear to cause myopia, an association between the two does exist.

Level of education is often used as a surrogate measure for near work, with a higher prevalence of myopia found among the more educated.[20,56,57] Researchers in Asia have suggested that their rigorous schooling system with the long hours that the children spend studying is responsible for the high rates of myopia in Asia.[58,59]

The complexity of examining and quantifying near work is further confounded by the association between myopia and intellectual ability. Children with myopia have been found to have higher intelligence test scores and higher achievement test scores, with better grades in school, than those of non-myopes.[60–63] Unravelling the relative importance of near work, intelligence and heredity is impossible without examining all three factors in the same subjects.

In the Orinda longitudinal study on myopia the association between children's myopia and parental myopia, children's visual activities and children's performance on a standardised achievement test has been evaluated.[43] Both heredity and near work were found to be significantly associated with myopia, with heredity being the more important factor.

Visual display units

There has been a dramatic increase in use of computers in recent years, and with this there is often an assumption that visual display unit (VDU) use may be associated with the development of myopia. A review of the literature[64] revealed a high prevalence of asthenopia among computer users, but no clear evidence of any association with myopia progression.

Night lighting

One study that has been much publicised relates the use of night lights to the development of myopia.[65] We know from research in animals that post-natal eye growth and refractive development are governed by a vision-dependent retinal mechanism.[66,67] The basis for the night-light study in humans was research on chick eyes that showed eye growth was modified by the duration of the light cycle,[68] with myopia progressing with light exposure and less ocular growth in the dark. The human study found that exposure to ambient lighting at night before 2 years of age indicated a tendency for myopia development.[65] The researchers found that 55 per cent of the children who slept with some light before the age of 2 years were found to be myopic. Other researchers have been unable to confirm this link between myopia development and ambient lighting at night.[45,69,70] However, these researchers found that myopic parents are more likely to use night-time lighting aids for their children, possibly to aid their own poor acuity in the dark. The well-documented association between parental myopia and their child's myopia was not taken into consideration in the initial study.

Under-correction of myopia

Recent work reported that under-correction of myopia increases myopia progression.[71] The researchers assessed the progression of myopia over a 2 year period in 94 Malaysian and Chinese myopic children between 9 and 14 years of age. The children were randomly assigned to a group in which the myopia was corrected fully or to a group in which the myopia was under-corrected. The children's myopia was under-corrected by approximately +0.75D, blurring their visual acuity to 6/12. After 2 years the myopia progression in the fully corrected group was −0.77D, whereas in the under-corrected group the myopia had progressed by −1.00D. Controversially, the authors stated that under-correction of myopia was a common procedure in clinical practice. Discussions with many optometry colleagues and academic optometrists, responsible for teaching the modules of refraction and prescribing to students, have not revealed any evidence of under-correction of myopes in UK optometry practice.

These research findings are contrary to the findings in animal studies, in which under-correction of the myopia slows myopia development.[72] Previous studies on children did not find any effect on myopia progression if spectacles were not worn for close work.[73,74]

High myopia

Currently, there is much interest in risk factors for the development of myopia,[43,75] and recent studies investigated the amelioration of progression of low to moderate myopia by optical[8,76] and pharmaceutical methods,[77,78] with some degree of success (*Tables 5.2* and *5.3*). However, the importance of myopia greater than 6D as a category is evident from Curtin[35] and from the work of Marr *et al.*,[84] who found high myopia to be associated strongly with ocular and systemic diseases in young children who attended a hospital eye department.

Ocular problems associated with high myopia include retinal dystrophies (e.g., achromatopsia, congenital stationary night blindness), lenticular or zonular abnormalities (e.g., microspherophakia, ectopia lentis, lenticonus) and amblyopia.[35,84] In addition, there are important systemic ramifications: Marfan's syndrome is probably the disorder most frequently thought of in association with high myopia, but other disorders include homocystinuria, Stickler's syndrome and Down's syndrome.[35,84,85] High myopia in early childhood is not identified specifically in current ophthalmology, optometry or orthoptic protocols for screening, referral or investigation. An ongoing study[86] in the West Midlands, UK, is investigating high myopia that presents to community health care clinics, with the aim of compiling guidelines for assessment and subsequent referral. Preliminary data show that 44 per cent of the children had an ocular or systemic condition associated with myopia greater than 5D. The study highlights that detection and prompt referral of these cases by community health care services may, in some cases, prolong vision and, possibly, life expectancy.

Summary of research into myopia intervention

As already mentioned, the prevalence of myopia in most Western industrialised societies is now approaching 25 per cent of young adolescents, and Far Eastern societies, such as Hong Kong and Taiwan, have levels that exceed 70 per cent. If, as is likely, the prevalence of myopia in the UK matches those reported for mainland Europe and the USA, appropriate consideration must be given to various modes of myopia treatment.

The suggested mechanisms for the development of myopia outlined above have given rise to a wide variety of studies to investigate several different forms of intervention that may retard the progression of myopia in children and thus decrease the severity of myopia in adulthood.

Spectacle lens studies

The rational for the use of bifocal or progressive addition lenses in myopia control is normally to reduce accommodative demand. The precise mechanism whereby accommodation might lead to the development of myopia is unclear. One suggestion is that myopia occurs from an increased lag of accommodation during near work,[54] and the resultant retinal blur leads to an increase in ocular growth.

Several studies of the effects of bifocal lens wear on myopia progression have not shown any benefit.[7,73,87] The Houston Myopia Control Study[87] examined 207 children 6–15 years of age, who were assigned to one of three groups (bifocals with +1.00 add, bifocals with +2.00 add or single-vision lenses). After a follow-up period of 3 years no evidence was found for a reduction in myopia progression with bifocal lenses. Similarly, a study on 240 Finnish children 9–11 years of age found no difference in progression of myopia between a bifocal group (wearing +1.75 add) and a single-vision lens group who took their spectacles off for near work.[73]

Another study examined children between the ages of 7 and 13 years who were allocated to a bifocal lens (+2.00 add) group, a single-vision group or a single-vision group who also received timolol drops twice a day.[7] There was no statistically significant difference between the groups after 2 years. Furthermore, bifocal lenses may be less acceptable cosmetically, difficult to adapt to and compliance with spectacle wear may be a problem. In addition, it is not known whether children actually use the lower segment of the lens for reading and there is no direct evidence to suggest that children accommodate less through the bifocal segment.

Progressive addition multifocal lenses are more acceptable cosmetically and allow children to have clear vision at all distances without accommodating. In young myopes, however, the progressive addition lens must be fitted high to facilitate the use of the reading addition. A study using progressive addition lenses in two groups of Chinese children between 9 and 12 years of age (+1.50 add in 22 subjects and +2.00 add in 14 subjects) found less progression in myopia compared with 32 children in an age-matched single-vision control group.[79] A dose-related effect was also observed, with least myopia progression in the +2.00 add group.

A more recent Hong Kong study[8] did not find any evidence that myopia progression was retarded in children 7–10.5 years of age who wore progressive addition lenses (+1.50 add in 121 children) compared with single-vision lenses (160 children). However, the results for myopia progression using progressive addition lenses in 21 esophoric children are equivocal. A similar result was found by a US study[9] on esophoric myopic children treated with a +1.50 addition bifocal. The small reduction (0.25D) in myopia progression is not of clinical significance. The Correction of Myopia Evaluation Study (COMET), currently in progress in the USA, may provide further evidence for the efficacy of multifocal lenses in esophoric myopic children.[76] *Table 5.2* summarises this work.

Contact lens studies

Although previous studies to control myopia development with contact lenses indicate that rigid contact lenses slow the progression of myopia in children, they have all suffered from limitations that challenge the significance of their results (reviewed by Saw *et al.*[88]). The US National Institute of Health is currently conducting the Contact Lens and Myopia Progression (CLAMP) study, which will provide more information on the beneficial relationship between gas-permeable lenses and the reduction of the progression of myopia.[89]

Ophthalmic drug studies

Cycloplegic agents, such as the non-selective muscarinic antagonist atropine, have been found to have some success in pre-

Table 5.2 The effect on control of myopia progression using multifocal (PAL) and bifocal (B/F) spectacle lenses

Spectacle lenses	*Subjects*		*Duration (year)*		*Rate (D/year)*	
	T	C	T	C	T	C
B/F, +1.75 (Parssinen *et al.*[73])	80	80	3	3	–0.56	–0.49
B/F, +2.00 (Jensen[7])	48	48	2	2	–0.48	–0.57
PAL, +1.50 (Leung and Brown[79])	22	32	2	2	–0.38	–0.62
PAL, +2.00	14				–0.33	
PAL, +1.50 (Edwards *et al.*[8])	121	133	2	2	–0.56	–0.63
PAL, +2.00 (Gwiazda *et al.*[80])	235	234	3	3	–0.42	–0.49

T, treatment group (bifocal or multifocal spectacles); C, control group, with single-vision spectacles).

venting the progression of axial myopia in both adolescent humans[6,81,82,90] and animal models of myopia development.[91,92] The rationale for using cycloplegic agents was based on the hypothesis that myopia resulted from excessive or chronic accommodation.

The success of these studies in preventing myopia progression has given strong support to a role for accommodation in the development of myopia. However, the side-effects of cycloplegia and mydriasis result in poor compliance and high drop-out rates in human myopia trials. Further research on the long-term side-effects of atropine and on the progression of myopia after atropine therapy has been stopped is required before atropine intervention can be considered a viable form of myopia intervention.

More recent evidence questions a primary role for accommodation in the development of myopia, as research suggests the visual signals that control eye growth and myopia development proceed directly from the retina to the choroid and/or sclera, and not primarily via higher central visual-processing centres.[93–95] Research, in animals, has demonstrated that atropine prevents myopia via a non-accommodative mechanism.[96,97] The use of selective antagonists with affinities for specific muscarinic receptors makes it possible to target a particular class of receptor[98,99] and thus provide further information regarding the site of myopia development.

In the eye, M1, M2, M3 and M4 receptor subtypes have been identified in the chick retina[100] and M2 and M3 muscarinic receptors have been detected in the iris and ciliary complex.[101] Recent evidence[102] disputes the presence of M1 receptor in the chick eye, although it has been identified in mammalian eyes. The relatively selective M1 antagonist pirenzepine has been found to block axial elongation of the eye in animal models of myopia[103–106], whereas M2 and M3 antagonists had no effect,[104] which suggests the retina as a site for myopia development.

Several centres worldwide are investigating the drug pirenzepine for topical ocular use to moderate and/or halt the progression of myopia in children. Administration of a 2 per cent strength gel was found to be comfortable and safely tolerated by myopic children.[107] After 1 year of treatment, the initial results from two separate studies show that the progression of myopia has been reduced by up to 50 per cent in the pirenzepine-treated myopic children compared with a placebo.[77,78] However, the results from both studies are modest, with a reduction in myopia progression of 0.26D[77] and 0.37D,[77] respectively. A third phase of the trial is due to be implemented.

A simple explanation for eye growth could be the interaction between IOP and scleral rigidity. If the scleral walls of myopic eyes were equally or more susceptible than those of emmetropic eyes to stretch under the influence of IOP, and if IOP were greater in myopes than in emmetropes, this could lead to excessive eye enlargement and the development of myopia.

A logical extension of this theory leads to the prediction that IOP-lowering drugs should reduce or prevent eye enlargement and thus myopia progression. Several studies have investigated the relationship between IOP and myopia with equivocal results. A study of children found that IOP was slightly higher in the myopic eye.[108] However, another study measured the IOP in anisometropic Chinese children with a refractive error difference of 2D or more between a pair of eyes,[109] and found no difference in IOP between the more myopic and less myopic eyes, which suggests that the inter-eye difference in refractive error may result from discrepancies in scleral structure. Based on the theory that a higher IOP could lead to myopia development, the effect of the IOP-lowering drug, timolol, on myopia progression has been investigated in children.[7] No reduction in the rate of myopia progression was found. *Table 5.3* summarises this work.

Prediction of future myopes

If, indeed, a mode for intervention of myopia progression is realised, proper consideration must be given to a method to predict future myopes. One study found that a refractive error of less hyperopia than +0.75D measured at 8 years of age predicted the onset of myopia by 13 years with a sensitivity of 86.7 per cent and specificity of 73.3 per cent.[110] However, this model would not identify 13.3 per cent of future myopes, and 26.7 per cent of non-myopes would have been treated unnecessarily if a mode of successful intervention existed. Similarly, parental myopia is not specific enough to identify future myopes.

Summary

Little new advice can be offered to the optometrist on the management of myopia in children. The majority of myopic children will fall into the 7–14 years of age category, and thus full correction should be given to these children. Regular monitoring of the myopia development is also required.

The optometrist is no doubt fully aware of the paucity of information that can be given to the concerned parent regarding progression of myopia. There is a greater risk of myopia developing in a child if both parents are myopic and also in children for whom the refractive error is less than +0.75D hyperopia at 8 years of age. If the first child becomes myopic, the parents should be advised to have the child's siblings checked. A new finding is that high myopia (≥5D) in a child under 10 years of age may indicate the presence of a systemic or ocular disorder and warrants referral to an ophthalmologist.

Although the evidence of myopia development and VDU use is not clear, it is

Table 5.3 The effect on control of myopia progression using topical instillation of antimuscarinic drugs

Treatment	*Subjects*		*Duration (years)*		*Rate (D/year)*	
	T	*C*	*T*	*C*	*T*	*C*
Pirenzepine 2.0% (Tan *et al.*[77])	140	70	1	1	–0.47	–0.84
Pirenzepine 2.0% (Siatkowski *et al.*[78])	117	57	1	1	–0.26	–0.53
Atropine 1.0% (Brodstein *et al.*[81])	253	146	2.75	6.56	–0.16	–0.23
Atropine 0.5% (Shih *et al.*[82])	66	61	1.5	1.5	–0.28	–0.93
Atropine 1.0% (Chua *et al.*[83])	152	179	2	2	–0.13	–0.60

T, treatment group; C, control group.

advisable to avoid prolonged VDU use. The increased use of virtual reality will no doubt place extra demands on the ocular system with unknown effects on the visual and oculomotor systems. The preliminary results from the pharmacological control of myopia with pirenzepine are promising, and more comprehensive results are awaited with interest.

References

1 College of Optometrists (1995). *Clinical Survey*. (London: College of Optometrists).

2 Cook RC and Glassock RE (1951). Refractive and ocular findings in the newborn. *Am J Ophthalmol*. **34**, 1407–1413.

3 Mohindra I and Held R (1981). Refraction in humans from birth to five years. *Doc Ophthalmol Proc*. **28**, 19–27.

4 Saunders KJ, Woodhouse JM and Westall CA (1995). Emmetropisation in human infancy: Rate of change is related to initial refractive error. *Vision Res*. **35**, 1325–1328.

5 Hirsch MJ (1962). Relationship between refraction on entering school and rate of change during the first six years of school – an interim report from the Ojau longitudinal study. *Am J Optom Arch Am Acad Optom*. **39**, 51–59.

6 Gimbel HV (1973). The control of myopia with atropine. *Can J Ophthalmol*. **8**, 527–532.

7 Jensen H (1991). Myopia progression in young schoolchildren. A prospective study of myopia progression and the effect of a trial with bifocal lenses and beta blocker eye drops. *Acta Ophthalmol (Copenh.)* **200**, S1–S79.

8 Edwards M, Wing-hong Li R, Siu-lin Lam C, Kwok-fai Lew J and Sin-ying Yu B (2002). The Hong Kong progressive lens myopia control study: Study design and main findings. *Invest Ophthalmol Vis Sci*. **43**, 2852–2858.

9 Fulk GW, Cyert LA and Parker DE (2000). A randomized trial of the effect of single-vision vs. bifocal lenses on myopia progression in children with esophoria. *Optom Vis Sci*. **77**, 395–401.

10 Goss DA and Grosvenor T (1990). Rates of childhood myopia progression with bifocals as a function of nearpoint phoria: Consistency of three studies. *Optom Vis Sci*. **67**, 637–640.

11 Chew SJ, Saw SM, Rajan U, *et al*. (1997). RGP contact lenses in the control of myopia progression. *Invest Ophthalmol Vis Sci*. **38S**, 1157.

12 Fulton AB, Dobson V, Salem D, *et al*. (1980). Cycloplegic refractions in infants and young children. *Am J Ophthalmol*. **90**, 239–247.

13 Edwards MH (1991). The refractive status of Hong Kong Chinese infants. *Ophthalmic Physiol Opt*. **11**, 297–303.

14 Smith EL and Hung LF (1999). The role of optical defocus in regulating refractive development in infant monkeys. *Vis Res*. **39**, 1415–1435.

15 Dobson V, Fulton AB, Manning K, Salem D and Peterson RA (1981). Cycloplegic refractions of premature infants. *Am J Ophthalmol*. **91**, 490–495.

16 Saunders KJ, McCulloch DL, Shepherd AJ and Wilkinson AG (2002). Emmetropisation following preterm birth. *Br J Ophthalmol*. **86**, 1035–1040.

17 Robinson BE (1999). Factors associated with the prevalence of myopia in 6-year-olds. *Optom Vis Sci*. **76**, 266–271.

18 Junghans B, Crewther SG, Kiely P and Crewther DP (2002). The prevalence of hypermetropia and myopia amongst a large multicultural population of school children in Sydney. Presented at *Ninth International Conference on Myopia, Hong Kong and Guangzhou*.

19 Zadnik K, Jones LA, Mitchell GL and Mutti DO (2002). *Baseline ocular component data from the Collaborative Longitudinal Evaluation of Ethnicity and Refractive Error (CLEERE) study*. Presented at *Ninth International Conference on Myopia, Hong Kong and Guangzhou*.

20 Sperduto RD, Seigel D, Roberts J and Rowland M (1983). Prevalence of myopia in the United States. *Arch Ophthalmol*. **101**, 405–407.

21 Grosvenor T (1987). A review and suggested classification of myopia on the basis of age-related prevalence and age of onset. *Am J Optom Physiol Opt*. **64**, 545–554

22 Lam CSY, Goldschmidt E and Edwards MH (2002). *Prevalence of myopia in local and international schools in Hong Kong*. Presented at *Ninth International Conference on Myopia, Hong Kong and Guangzhou*.

23 Saw S-M, Carkett A, Chia K-S, Stone RA and Tan DTH (2002). Component dependent risk factors for ocular parameters in Singapore Chinese children. *Ophthalmology* **109**, 2065–2071.

24 Lam CSY and Goh WSH (1991). The incidence of refractive errors among school children in Hong Kong and its relationship with the optical components. *Clin Exp Optom*. **74**, 97–103.

25 Matsumura H and Hirai H (1999). Prevalence of myopia and refractive changes in students from 3 to 17 years of age. *Surv Ophthalmol*. **44S**, 109–115.

26 Lin LL-K, Shih Y-F, Tsai C-B, *et al*. (1996). Epidemiological study of ocular refractions among school-children. *Invest Ophthalmol Vis Sci*. **37S**, 1002.

27 Garner LF, Yap MKH, Kinnear RF and Firth MJ (1995). Ocular dimensions and refraction in Tibetan children. *Optom Vis Sci*. **72**, 266–271.

28 Garner LF, Kinnear RF, Klinger JD and McKellar MJ (1985). Prevalence of myopia in school children in Vanuatu. *Acta Ophthalmol*. **63**, 323–326.

29 Johnson GJ (1988). Myopia in arctic regions. *Acta Ophthalmol*. **66**, 13–18.

30 Goldschmidt E (1968). On the etiology of myopia. *Acta Ophthalmol*. **98**, S1–S172.

31 Rosenfield M and Gilmartin B (1998). *Myopia and Nearwork*. (Oxford: Butterworth–Heinemann).

32 McBrien NA and Adams DW (1997). A longitudinal investigation of adult-onset and adult-progression of myopia in an occupational group. *Invest Ophthalmol Vis Sci*. **38**, 321–333.

33. Sorsby A, Benjamin B and Sheridan M (1961). *Refraction and its Components during the Growth of the Eye from the Age of Three*. (London: Medical Research Council).

34 Barnes M, Williams C, Lumb R, *et al*. (2001). The prevalence of refractive errors in a UK birth cohort of children aged 7 years. In *2001 Annual Meeting Abstract and Program Planner*. Abstract 2096. Accessed at www.arvo.org. (Association for Research in Vision and Ophthalmology).

35 Curtin BJ (1985). *The Myopias: Basic Science and Clinical Management*. (Philadelphia: Harper & Row).

36 Young TL, Ronan SM, Drahozal LA, *et al*. (1998). Evidence that a locus for familial high myopia maps to chromosome 18p. *Am J Hum Genet*. **63**, 109–119.

37 Young TL, Ronan SM, Alvear AB, *et al*. (1998). A second locus for familial high myopia maps to chromosome 12q. *Am J Hum Genet*. **63**, 1419–1424.

38 Farbrother JE, Kirov G, Owen MJ and Guggenheim JA (2003). Linkage analysis of 18p, 12q and 17q high myopia loci in 51 UK families. In *2003 Annual Meeting Abstract and Program Planner*. Abstract 4780. Accessed at www.arvo.org. (Association for Research in Vision and Ophthalmology).

39 Mutti DO, Semina E, Marazita M, *et al*. (2002). Genetic loci for pathological myopia are not associated with juvenile myopia. *Am J Med Gen*. **112**, 355–360.

40 Young FA, Baldwin WR, Box RA, Harris E and Johnson C (1969). The transmission of refractive error within Eskimo families. *Am J Optom*. **46**, 676–685.

41 Alsbirk PH (1979). Refraction in adult West Greenland Eskimos. *Acta Ophthalmol*. **57**, 84–95.

42 Pacella R, McLellan J, Grice K, *et al*. (1999). Role of genetic factors in the etiology of juvenile-onset myopia based on a longitudinal study of refractive error. *Optom Vis Sci*. **76**, 381–386.

43 Mutti DO, Mitchell GL, Moeschberger ML, Jones LA and Zadnik K (2002). Parental myopia, nearwork, school achievement and children's refractive error. *Invest Ophthalmol Vis Sci*. **43**, 3633–3640.

44 Mutti DO and Zadnik K (1995). The utility of three predictors of childhood myopia: A Bayesian analysis. *Vis Res*. **35**, 1345–1352.

45 Saw S-M, Zhang ML, Hong RZ, *et al*. (2002). Nearwork activity, night lights and myopia in the Singapore–China study. *Arch Ophthalmol*. **120**, 620–624.

46 Chen C-J, Cohen BH and Diamond EL (1985). Genetic and environmental effects on the development of myopia in Chinese twin children. *Ophthalmic Paediatr Genet*. **6**, 113–119.

47 Hammond CJ, Snieder H, Gilbert CE and Spector TD (2001). Genes and environment in refractive error: The Twin

Eye Study. *Invest Ophthalmol Vis Sci.* **42**, 1232–1236.
48 Lyhne N, Sjolie AK, Kyvik KO and Green A (2001). The importance of genes and environment for ocular refraction and its determiners: A population based study among 20–45 year old twins. *Br J Ophthalmol.* **85**, 1470–1476.
49 Wildsoet CF (1997). Active emmetropization – evidence for its existence and ramifications for clinical practice. *Ophthalmic Physiol Opt.* **17**, 279–290.
50 Mohney BG (2002). Axial myopia associated with dense vitreous haemorrhage of the neonate. *J Am Assoc Paediatr Ophthalmol Strabismus* **6**, 348–353.
51 Lam CSY, Goh WSH, Tang YK, *et al.* (1994). Changes in refractive trends and optical components of Hong Kong Chinese aged over 40 years. *Ophthalmic Physiol Opt.* **14**, 383–388.
52 Goh WSH and Lam CSY (1994). Changes in refractive trends and optical components of Hong Kong Chinese aged 19–39 years. *Ophthalmic Physiol Opt.* **14**, 378–382.
53 Goss DA (1991). Childhood myopia. In: *Refractive Anomalies – Research and Clinical Implications.* Eds Grosvenor T and Flom MC, p. 81–103 (Boston: Butterworth–Heinemann).
54 Gwiazda J, Thorn F, Bauer J and Held R (1993). Myopic children show insufficient accommodative response to blur. *Invest Ophthalmol Vis Sci.* **34**, 690–694.
55 O'Leary DJ and Allen PM (2001). Facility of accommodation in myopia. *Ophthalmic Physiol Opt.* **21**, 352–355.
56 Angle J and Wissmann DA (1978). Age, reading and myopia. *Am J Optom Physiol Opt.* **55**, 302–308.
57 Rosner M and Belkin M (1987). Intelligence, education and myopia in males. *Arch Ophthalmol.* **105**, 1508–1511.
58 Au Eong KG, Tay TH and Lim MK (1993). Education and myopia in 110,236 young Singaporean males. *Singapore Med J.* **34**, 489–492.
59 Zhao J, Pan X, Sui R, *et al.* (2000). Refractive error study in children: Results from Shunyi District, China. *Am J Ophthalmol.* **129**, 427–435.
60 Hirsch MJ (1959). The relationship between refractive state of the eye and intelligence test scores. *Am J Optom Arch Am Acad Optom.* **36**, 12–21.
61 Grosvenor T (1970). Refractive state, intelligence test scores, and academic ability. *Am J Optom Arch Am Acad Optom.* **64**, 482–498.
62 Teasdale TW, Fuchs J and Goldschmidt E (1988). Degree of myopia in relation to intelligence and educational level. *Lancet* **ii**, 1351–1354.
63 Young FA, Leary GA, Baldwin WR, *et al.* (1970). Refractive errors, reading performance and school achievement among Eskimo children. *Am J Optom Arch Am Acad Optom.* **47**, 384–390.
64 Mutti DO and Zadnik K (1996). Is computer use a risk factor for myopia? *J Am Optom Assoc.* **67**, 521–530.
65 Quinn GE, Shin CH, Maguire MG and Stone RA (1999). Myopia and ambient lighting at night. *Nature* **399**, 113–114.
66 Wallman J, Gottlieb MD, Rajaram V and Fugate-Wentzek LA (1987). Local retinal regions control local growth and myopia. *Science* **237**, 73–77.
67 Wildsoet CF and Schmid KL (2001). Emmetropisation in chicks uses optical vergence and relative distance clues to decode defocus. *Vis Res.* **41**, 3197–3204.
68 Stone RA, Lin T, Desai D and Capehart C (1995). Photoperiod, early post-natal eye growth, and visual deprivation. *Vis Res.* **35**, 1195–1202.
69 Zadnik K, Jones LA, Irvin BC, *et al.* (2000). Myopia and ambient night-time lighting. *Nature* **404**, 143–144.
70 Gwiazda J, Ong E, Held R and Thorn F (2000). Myopia and ambient night-time lighting. *Nature* **404**, 144.
71 Chung K, Mohidin N and O'Leary DJ (2002). Undercorrection of myopia enhances rather than inhibits myopia progression. *Vis Res.* **42**, 2555–2559.
72 Hung L-F, Crawford MLJ and Smith EL (1995). Spectacle lenses alter eye growth and the refractive status of young monkeys. *Nature Med.* **1**, 761–765.
73 Parssinen O, Hemminki E and Klemetti A (1989). Effect of spectacle use and accommodation on myopia progression: Final results of a three-year randomised clinical trial among schoolchildren. *Br J Ophthalmol.* **73**, 547–551.
74 Ong E, Grice K, Held R, Thorn F and Gwiazda J (1999). Effect of spectacle intervention on the progression of myopia in children. *Optom Vis Sci.* **76**, 363–369.
75 Saw S-M, Nieto FJ, Katz J and S-J C (1999). Distance, lighting and parental beliefs: Understanding near work in epidemiologic studies of myopia. *Optom Vis Sci.* **76**, 355–362.
76 Gwiazda J, Marsh-Tootle WL, Hyman L, Hussein M and Norton TT (2002). Baseline refractive and ocular component measures of children enrolled in the Correction of Myopia Evaluation Trial (COMET). *Invest Ophthalmol Vis Sci.* **43**, 314–321.
77 Tan DT, Lam D, Chua WH, Crockett RS and Group APS (2003). Pirenzepine ophthalmic gel (PIR): Safety and efficacy for pediatric myopia in a one-year study in Asia. In *2003 Annual Meeting Abstract and Program Planner.* Abstract 801. Accessed at www.arvo.org. (Association for Research in Vision and Ophthalmology).
78 Siatkowski R, Cotter S, Miller J, *et al.* (2003). Pirenzepine 2% ophthalmic gel retards myopic progression in 8–12 year old children. In *2003 Annual Meeting Abstract and Program Planner.* Abstract 4778. Accessed at www.arvo.org. (Association for Research in Vision and Ophthalmology).
79 Leung JTM and Brown B (1999). Progression of myopia in Hong Kong Chinese schoolchildren is slowed by wearing progressive lenses. *Optom Vis Sci.* **76**, 346–354.
80 Gwiazda J, Hyman L, Hussein M, *et al.* (2003). A randomised clinical trial of progressive addition lenses versus single vision lenses on the progression of myopia in children. *Invest Ophthalmol Vis Sci.* **86**, 1306–1311.
81 Brodstein RS, Brodstein DE, Olson RJ, Hunt SC and Williams RR (1984). The treatment of myopia with atropine and bifocals. *Ophthalmology* **91**, 1373–1378.
82 Shih YF, Hsiao CK, Chen CJ, *et al.* (2001). An intervention trial on efficacy of atropine and multi-focal glasses in controlling myopia progression. *Acta Ophthalmol Scand.* **79**, 233–236.
83 Chua WH, Balakrishnan V, Tan D, Chan YH and Group AS (2003). Efficacy results from the atropine in the treatment of myopia (ATOM) study. In *2003 Annual Meeting Abstract and Program Planner.* Abstract 3119. Accessed at www.arvo.org (Association for Research in Vision and Ophthalmology).
84 Marr JE, Halliwell-Ewen J, Fisher B, Soler L and Ainsworth JR (2001). Associations of high myopia in childhood. *Eye* **15**, 70–74.
85 Ainsworth JR and Marr JE (2000). Myopia in young children. *Ophthalmic Physiol Opt.* **20S**, 1–2.
86 Logan NS, Gilmartin B, Marr JE, Stevenson MR and Ainsworth JR and (2002). Community-based study of the association of high myopia in children with ocular and systemic disease. *Optom Vis Sci.* **81**, 11–13.
87 Grosvenor T, Perrigan DM, Perrigan J and Maslovitz B (1987). Houston Myopia Control Study: A randomised clinical trial. Part 2. Final report of the patient care team. *Am J Optom Physiol Opt.* **64**, 482–498.
88 Saw S-M, Gazzard G, Au Eong KG and Tan DTH (2002). Myopia: Attempts to arrest progression. *Br J Ophthalmol.* **86**, 1306–1311.
89 Walline JJ, Mutti DO, Jones LA, *et al.* (2001). The contact lens and myopia progression (CLAMP) study: Design and baseline data. *Optom Vis Sci.* **78**, 223–233.
90 Bedrossian RH (1979). The effect of atropine on myopia. *Ophthalmology* **86**, 713–717.
91 McKanna JA and Casagrande VA (1981). Atropine affects lid-suture myopia development. Experimental studies of chronic atropinization in tree shrews. *Doc Ophthalmol Proc Ser.* **28**, 187–195.
92 Raviola E and Wiesel TN (1985). An animal model of myopia. *N Eng J Med.* **312**, 1609–1615.
93 Troilo D, Gottlieb MD and Wallman J (1987). Visual deprivation causes myopia in chicks with optic nerve section. *Curr Eye Res.* **6**, 993–999.
94 McBrien NA, Moghaddam HO, Cottriall CL, Leech EM and Cornell LM (1995). The effects of blockade of retinal cell action potentials on ocular growth, emmetropization and form deprivation myopia in young chicks. *Vis Res.* **35**, 1141–1152.
95 Wildsoet CF, Howland HC, Falconer S and Dick K (1993). Chromatic aberration and accommodation – their role in emmetropization in the chick. *Vis Res.* **33**, 1593–1606.
96 Stone RA, Lin T and Laties AM (1991). Muscarinic antagonist effects on experimental chick myopia. *Exp Eye Res.* **52**, 755–758.
97 McBrien NA, Moghaddam HO and Reeder AP (1993). Atropine reduces experimental myopia and eye enlargement via a nonaccommodative mechanism. *Invest Ophthalmol Vis Sci.* **34**, 205–215.
98 Goyal RK, Flier J and Bruzzone R (1989). Muscarinic receptor subtypes – physiology and clinical implications. *N Eng J Med.* **321**, 1022–1029.

99 Eglen RM and Watson N (1996). Selective muscarinic receptor agonists and antagonists *Pharmacol Toxicol.* **78**, 59–68.
100 McKinnon LA and Nathanson NM (1995). Differential expression of muscarinic receptor messenger-RNAS and their subtypes during development of embryonic chick heart and retina. *Life Sci.* **56**, 1022.
101 Pang IH, Matsumoto S, Tamm E and Desantis L (1994). Characterization of muscarinic receptor involvement in human ciliary muscle-cell function. *J Ocul Pharmacol.* **10**, 125–136.
102 Yin GC, Gentle NA and McBrien NA (2003). Is regulation of ocular growth in chick mediated via the M1 receptor? In *2003 Annual Meeting Abstract and Program Planner*. Abstract 4339. Accessed at www.arvo.org (Association for Research in Vision and Ophthalmology).
103 Tigges M, Iuvone PM, Fernandes A, *et al.* (1999). Effects of muscarinic cholinergic receptor antagonists on postnatal eye growth of rhesus monkeys. *Optom Vis Sci.* **76**, 397–407.
104 Stone RA, Lin T and Laties AM (1991). Muscarinic antagonist effects on experimental chick myopia. *Exp Eye Res.* **52**, 755–758.
105 Leech EM, Cottrial CL and McBrien NA (1995). Pirenzepine prevents form deprivation myopia in a dose dependent manner. *Ophthalmic Physiol Opt.* **15**, 351–356.
106 Cottrial CL and McBrien NA (1996). The M(1) muscarinic antagonist pirenzepine reduces myopia and eye enlargement in the tree shrew. *Invest Ophthalmol Vis Sci.* **37**, 1368–1397.
107 Bartlett JD, Niemann K, Houde B, Allred T and Edmondson MJ (2000). Safety and tolerability of pirenzepine ophthalmic gel in paediatric myopic patients. *Invest Ophthalmol Vis Sci.* **41S**, 303.
108 Quinn GE, Berlin JA, Young TL, Ziylan S and Stone RA (1995). Association of intraocular pressure and myopia in children. *Ophthalmology* **102**, 180–185.
109 Lee SMY and Edwards MH. In (2000)t raocular pressure in anisometropic children. *Optom Vis Sci.* **77**, 675–679.
110 Zadnik K, Mutti DO, Friedman NE, *et al.* (1999). Ocular predictors of the onset of juvenile myopia. *Invest Ophthalmol Vis Sci.* **40**, 1936–1943.

6

Binocular Vision Disorders: Aetiology, Pathophysiology and Clinical Characteristics

Alison Finlay

Binocular vision can be defined as the system of sensory motor co-operation between the eyes.[1] The prevalence of binocular vision or eye movement disorders within the general population is high. Epidemiological studies estimate that, by the age of 5 years, 5 per cent of the entire population have some sort of visuomotor abnormality.[2]

The majority of these abnormalities have no sinister implications, but a few do. In this chapter the normal development of binocular vision and eye movements is considered and the aetiology of primary concomitant and incomitant deviations is examined. The aim is to clarify which deficits can be treated in optometric practice and which should be referred to the hospital eye service as potentially indicative of other neurological or ocular pathology.

Normal development of binocular function

Acuity and binocular vision are processes of both cortical and behavioural development, dependent on the existence of the appropriate 'hard wiring' and adequate visual experience. The visual system is relatively advanced at birth, undergoes active development in the first year of life and remains malleable for the first decade.

Normal visual system at birth

The globe, orbit and visual pathway

Anteroposteriorly, the eye is 70 per cent of its adult length at birth, but only 50 per cent of its volume.[3,4] The soft tissue within the orbit is well developed, but with the changing shape of the globe some modification of the muscle insertions occurs relative to the limbus during the first year of life.[5] There is some capacity for fixation from birth, but bifoveal fixation is only possible after migration of photoreceptors leads to the development of a fovea. Full maturation of the fovea is not complete until 5 years of age.[6] Visual pathway myelination is complete by 2 years of age.[7]

Cortex

The visual cortex (V1) is the first area within the visual processing system to have binocular input into a single cell. The structures for binocularity are present at birth, but the connections are immature.

In V1 the cortex is subdivided into areas or columns of cells that normally are innervated binocularly by one or the other eye. For each individual column one eye has the dominant input, and the dominance alternates across adjacent columns. In cats these ocular dominance columns develop over the first 6 weeks,[8,9] thought to be equivalent to 6 months in humans. Beyond V1, or the striate cortex, visual input travels to V2 and a plethora of visual processing centres beyond. These areas can be grouped together and described as the pre-striate areas. Understanding of the normal development of pre-striate areas is still in its infancy,[10] but it has been implicated in the development of strabismic amblyopia.[11]

Eye movement control

Control of eye movements is dependent on cortical and subcortical pathways. Vestibular ocular reflexes (VORs), searching eye movements and the ability to fixate a patterned target are present from birth. Fine oculomotor control is dependent on numerous cortical and subcortical centres, illustrated in *Figure 6.1*, and so is dependent on maturation of the cortex, supranuclear pathways and brainstem.[12]

A young infant makes sequential small saccades to fixate an eccentric target, maturing to almost adult standards by 5 months of age. Smooth pursuit and head tracking are evident before 2 months of age,[13] but by 6 months have yet to reach full maturity.[14]

Visual and ocular motor responses

To isolate different aspects of the visual system is difficult, so the visual and ocular motor responses are generally considered as a unitary sensory–motor development,

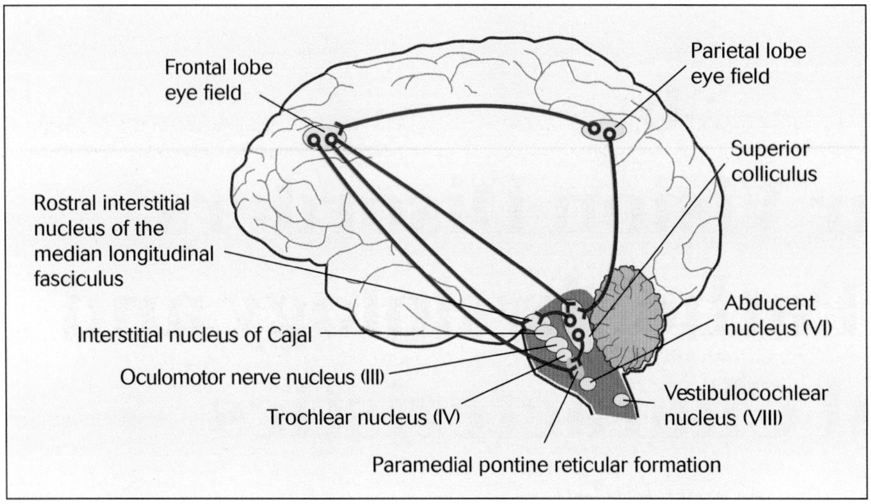

Figure 6.1
Higher order ocular motor control centres for saccadic eye movements (schematic)

although recent evidence suggests that the development of the two systems is distinct.[15] Being able to fixate an object and follow it accurately with a smooth eye movement is normally achieved by 6 weeks of age.

Some evidence indicates that subcortical mechanisms have a dominant role in the early visual and ocular motor responses.[16] Optokinetic nystagmus (OKN) is a subcortical visuomotor reflex present within hours of birth, but when tested monocularly in the neonate the nasalward following movement is the more mature.[17]

OKN becomes symmetrical by the age of 5 months, a finding that has been linked to the establishment of cortical connections.

Binocular perception

Bifoveal binocular single vision is a prerequisite to normal binocular perception. Fusion and stereopsis develop at similar times, between 3 and 5 months of age.[18] The development is quite abrupt, being almost complete by the age of 6 months, possibly as a result of the maturation of cortical connections. Subtle improvements in stereoacuity have been reported up to 5 years of age.[19]

Accommodation and convergence

The ability to adjust both accommodation and convergence is limited at birth, but improves rapidly during the first 6 months of age,[20,21] and can be driven by fusion or stimulus blur. Most infants should be intermittently orthotropic from birth and constantly so by the age of 3–6 months,[22] which facilitates the development of bifoveal binocular single vision. Whether the development of an accurate near response is led by accommodation or convergence appears to vary between individuals, a factor that may have implications for the development of heterotropia and the development of the accommodative convergence/accommodation (AC/A) ratio.[23,24]

Abnormal development

Having summarised the normal development of the visuomotor system, in this section the effect of abnormal development on binocular vision is considered. Likely scenarios include constant or intermittent misalignment of the visual axes, amblyopia or nystagmus. Sensory motor factors that can cause a disruption in the development of binocular vision, and result in the development of amblyopia, fall into three broad categories:

- Form deprivation, such as anisometropia or partial unilateral cataract;
- Stimulus deprivation, such as ptosis or total cataract;
- Strabismus, which results in disturbed positional information.

The globe

If the fovea is involved, abnormal development of the retina affects binocular vision. When both eyes are affected, such as in Leber's amaurosis or rod monochromatism, failure of foveal differentiation is accompanied by nystagmus. Peripheral fusion may allow a substandard binocular vision to accompany monocular foveal defects, such as in toxoplasmosis.

A unilaterally blind eye results in a concomitant heterotropia. The direction of the heterotropia depends on the age of onset of the blindness.[25–31] Monocular blindness at birth can result in exotropia or esotropia, during infancy it results in esotropia and in late childhood or adulthood it results in exotropia. Onset of monocular blindness in childhood can result from ocular disease, the most renowned of which is retinoblastoma. A thorough fundus examination is essential in all children who present with concomitant esotropia.

Abnormal development of the anterior eye may result in congenital cataracts or corneal anomalies. Either leads to a partial or complete opacity within the ocular media. A complete opacity, if left untreated, leads to dense, early-onset stimulus-deprivation amblyopia, probably the most difficult form of amblyopia to treat successfully. If uniocular, a cataract rapidly results in the permanent loss of any potential for the development of binocular single vision. Early intervention (before 2 months of age) can have some success if followed by an extensive period of occlusion.

If asymmetric, ocular growth can affect binocular vision. Anisometropia or high astigmatism commonly results in amblyopia, especially if the refractive error is hypermetropic.

The orbit

Abnormal development of the orbit can have several forms. Examples include abnormalities to:

- The structure or positioning of the orbits themselves;
- The soft tissues of the orbit;
- The extraocular muscles or their insertions;
- The fascia or neuronal connections.

Orbital architecture

Malpositioning of the orbits, such as in craniofacial anomalies, may prevent the development of a binocular field of view and result in concomitant heterotropia. On a lesser scale, the natural variation in orbital position between healthy individuals can affect the heterophoria. Those with a wide interpupillary distance are more prone to exophoria. Distortion of the orbits can result in malpositioning of the orbital fascia, and hence incomitancy.

Soft tissue

Abnormalities of the soft tissues of the orbits include space-occupying lesions, which may be benign or malignant. Examples include haemangiomas, orbital myositis or rhabdomyosarcoma. All these can form mechanical obstructions to eye movements, and so produce an incomitant deviation. With the possibility that a space-occupying lesion could be malignant, all such tumours should be referred rapidly to the medical services.

Extraocular muscles

Abnormalities of the extraocular muscles take on many forms, some of which have been described only since the recent advent of magnetic resonance imaging. Defects include absence of an extraocular muscle,[32] the presence of an additional extraocular muscle[33] or heterotopic pulley positions.[34,35] The pulleys are structures within the orbit that modify the mechanical action of the extraocular muscles when the eye moves into eccentric positions of gaze. Abnormal pulley positions have been implicated in the apparent inferior oblique overactions that often accompany otherwise concomitant esotropia. Abnormal muscle insertions are a possible cause of the alphabet patterns (A and V pattern deviations, etc.), which appear clinically as an alteration in the horizontal deviation on upgaze and downgaze.

Orbital fascia

Abnormalities of the orbital fascia include defects of the superior oblique or the trochlear, which obstruct the smooth movement of the tendon through the pulley. Such defects result in Brown's syndrome. Possible aetiologies include a lump on the tendon itself, thickening of the vascular sheath that surrounds the muscle and reduced flexibility in the tendon itself. Other fascial abnormalities within the orbit include the adhesion syndromes, first described by Johnson.[36–38]

Typically, upgaze is restricted because of an attachment between the superior rectus and superior oblique, or abduction is restricted because of an attachment between the lateral rectus and inferior oblique. Strabismus fixus is cosmetically the most extreme defect of the orbital fascia, in which each eye is fixed permanently in adduction. Generalised fibrosis syndrome is the most severe form, in which all the extraocular muscles and their surrounding tissue is fibrotic. It tends to be familial and presents with bilateral ptosis and the eyes fixed in downgaze. There is little or no horizontal movement, usually no vertical movement and normally it is associated with a constant strabismus and amblyopia.

These conditions are present at birth and, without surgical intervention, stay static throughout life. They should be referred routinely if cosmetically poor or associated with an abnormal head posture. Children should be observed regularly to minimise the risk of amblyopia.

Nerve supply

Neurological misdirection of a motor nerve is the favoured explanation for Duane's retraction syndrome. The branch of the third nerve that serves the medial rectus sends an abnormal projection to the lateral rectus. The lateral rectus may or may not have an abducens input and may be underdeveloped or partially fibrotic. Horizontal eye movements are affected, the classification of which is shown in *Table 6.1*. The palpebral fissure narrows on adduction because of a retraction of the globe, and widens on abduction. There may be some vertical up- or downward drift on adduction.

A second form of congenital neurological misdirection results in Marcus Gunn jaw-winking syndrome. There is an abnormal connection between the supplies to the levator palpebrae superioris and the pterygoid muscles of the mandible. It is usually monocular, and the eyelid on the affected side elevates on opening the mouth or moving the jaw to one side. It normally has no effect on the development of binocular vision.

The visual pathway

As with all forms of blindness, a complete obstruction of the visual pathway from one eye leads to a concomitant heterotropia. Post-chiasmal deficits affect only one hemifield in each eye, with normal binocular vision developing in the intact hemifield. Delayed visual maturation[39,40] normally presents in a child of age 3–4 months, who fails to fixate or follow an object. The aetiology is unknown, but electrophysiological evidence suggests possible involvement from the visual pathway. Electroretinograms (ERG) are usually normal, but visual evoked potentials (VEPs), which assess cortical activity, are abnormal. The vision usually starts to improve by the age of 6 months, and develops to normal levels. There is commonly an exotropia at presentation, but normal binocular function develops alongside visual responses.

Cortex

The involvement of the visual cortex in visuomotor deficits is still being explored. There is much evidence that, in cats and primates at least, amblyopia results in defects of striate and pre-striate areas because of reduced visual responses in one or both eyes during the critical periods of development.[41] Evidence from human studies suggests our system behaves in a similar way.[42–45] The extent and region of developmental change varies with the type of amblyopia. Striate areas appear to be affected in early-onset conditions, such as congenital cataracts, whereas pre-striate areas seem to be affected predominantly in the later-onset conditions, such as anisometropic and strabismic amblyopia. The cortex is only just being investigated as the primary area involved in the aetiology of a visuomotor deficit. Abnormalities in the visual cortex may be implicated in congenital nystagmus, but this has yet to be validated. Acquired cortical anomalies can lead to pursuit deficits and the abnormal generation of saccades.

Albinism

Albinism deserves a mention on its own, as there are defects throughout the afferent visual system. It is a congenital condition characterised by a general loss of melanin. Oculocutaneous albinism results in the characteristic pallor of the skin and hair, and has a substantial effect on the visual system. At the ocular level the fovea fails to differentiate and there is increased light scatter, which results from the lack of pigment in the uvea. Along the visual pathway an increased number of fibres cross at the optic chiasm, so most of the neuronal input, both nasal and temporal, is to the contralateral visual cortex. Lack of binocular input to the cortex has an effect on the development of both striate and pre-striate areas.[45–51] Patients present with photophobia, nystagmus, poor acuity and little or no binocular function.

Eye movement control, subcortical systems

The brain stem

Supranuclear palsies

Within the brain stem many nuclei serve the ocular motor system. In the midbrain, at the

Table 6.1 Classifications of Duane's retraction syndrome

Brown's	
Type A	Limited abduction and less marked limitation of adduction
Type B	Limited abduction, normal adduction
Type C	Limit of adduction exceeds limit of abduction
Huber's	
Type 1	Marked limitation or absence of abduction with normal and/or slightly limited adduction
Type 2	Normal or mildly limited abduction with limited or absent adduction
Type 3	Limited or absent abduction and adduction

level of the third nerve nucleus, lies the vertical saccade generator and neural integrator, which controls fixation, and the vergence centre. Within the pons, at the level of the sixth nerve nucleus, lie the horizontal saccade generator and neural integrator, the vestibular nucleus and the pursuit centre. There are also extensive connections with the cerebellum. Disruption to any of these centres can result in a defect of eye movement.

Vestibular
A congenital defect of the vestibular system is unusual, but can result in nystagmus and a defective VOR. The VIIIth nerve, which carries the sensory input from the vestibular apparatus in the inner ear, can become damaged in meningitis. Despite the lack of a VOR, such patients cope remarkably well. An acquired defect of the vestibular input can result in a skew deviation. This is defined as a vertical deviation caused by defective supranuclear inputs, and it can be concomitant or incomitant in nature.

Midbrain
Defects of the dorsal midbrain have been implicated in a double elevator palsy and may be involved in spasmus nutans. Spasmus nutans is a vertical nystagmus accompanied by head nodding, seen in infants between the ages of 3 and 18 months. It tends to resolve spontaneously, but may last several years.

Saccadic system
Defects of saccade generation can lead to an inability to initiate saccades, as occurs in congenital ocular motor apraxia, or to inappropriate saccades, as in ocular flutter or opsoclonus. Infants with congenital ocular motor apraxia normally are characterised by the head thrusting that initiates the VOR to help them change their direction of gaze. Opsoclonus and ocular flutter are back-to-back saccades that have been associated with both brain stem and cerebellar dysfunction.

Neural integrator
Defects of the neural integrators, which control fixation in eccentric gaze, can result in gaze-evoked nystagmus.

The cerebellum
The cerebellum has a role in the generation of all types of eye movement, vestibular, saccadic and smooth pursuit. It is involved in the adaptive control of eye movements or, in other words, their calibration. A cerebellar defect tends to result in saccadic dysmetria (saccades of an inappropriate length to fixate the target of interest) or defective gain of smooth pursuit. Cerebellar defects often result in nystagmus. These supranuclear brain stem defects are, thankfully, rare.

Nuclear palsies
Isolated congenital defects of the ocular motor nuclei do occur, but tend to be associated with damage to the surrounding areas. A lesion that affects the third nerve nucleus is normally associated with a vertical gaze palsy because of the proximity to the vertical saccadic generator. A lesion to the VIth nerve nucleus is usually associated with a horizontal gaze palsy.

Moebius syndrome
Moebius syndrome is a congenital condition that affects the VIth, VIIth, IXth and XIIth nerves, usually bilaterally. It is thought to be caused by brain stem injury during development. The VIIth nerve palsy results in a typically inexpressive face, and the VIth nerve palsy results in an inability of the eye to abduct because of the effect on the lateral rectus, and may be accompanied by an ipsilateral horizontal gaze palsy. The condition is described further in Chapter 10.

Infranuclear deficits
Most palsies, congenital and acquired, occur because of damage to the infranuclear pathways.

Third nerve
Ocular motor nerve deficits rarely are isolated to a single muscle and a total defect of the inferior branch is virtually unheard of. A congenital third nerve lesion usually affects all the muscles supplied by the nerve, including the levator, although the effects may be partial. A congenital or acquired defect to the superior branch affects both the superior rectus and levator palpebrae superioris, which results in a defect of upgaze in abduction, accompanied by a partial ptosis. A complete third nerve palsy, whether congenital or acquired, may be followed by aberrant regeneration. How this happens is uncertain, but the eye movements are quite characteristic:

- The upper lid elevates on downgaze;
- On attempted upgaze the affected eye adducts;
- Retraction of the globe on attempted up or downgaze;
- The pupil constricts on adduction.

If this pattern of movements occurs without the history of a third nerve palsy, an intracranial tumour or aneurysm may be indicated.[47,52,53] A cyclic oculomotor palsy is a rare condition in which an oculomotor palsy intermittently turns into a spasm of the muscles supplied by the nerve.

Fourth nerve
The trochlear nerve supply to the superior oblique is unique among the cranial nerves in that it exits from the dorsal aspect of the brain stem, crossing over before travelling around the brainstem and forward towards the orbit. This long route and the narrow nerve mean that both congenital and acquired superior oblique palsies are common. Intermittent irritation of the nerve results in spasms of the muscle, known as superior oblique myokymia.[54,55]

Sixth nerve
The long route of the abducens nerve and its pathway over the petrous portion of the temporal bone make it prone to damage. Of all the ocular motor nerve palsies, a lateral rectus palsy is the most common acquired lesion, although it is rare as a congenital defect.[25]

Aetiology of infranuclear deficits
The cause of an acquired infranuclear lesion in a child is usually trauma or compression. The compression may be local, as in an aneurysm in the wall of a neighbouring vessel or an adjacent neoplasm, or it may be general, as in hydrocephalus. Raised intracranial pressure is most likely to affect the VIth nerve, whereas a local tumour, malignant or benign, may affect any nerve. Congenital palsies are normally benign,[1,45] but should be referred to the hospital eye service for confirmation. After this, they can be managed in the practice unless the child has problems maintaining binocularity, the deviation is cosmetically poor or the deviation causes the adaptation of a head posture. Failure to act early to relieve an abnormal head posture is thought to lead to permanent skeletal changes and facial asymmetry. An acquired palsy, in a child or adult, should always be referred for medical advice as an emergency.

Concomitant deviations

The level of the defect for most concomitant deviations is unclear. Many occur alongside hypermetropia or are associated with a high or low AC/A ratio. Whether the deviation or the associated accommodative imbalance comes first is still uncertain. Concomitant deviations can be associated with intracranial disease, although rarely. With recent-onset deviations, whatever the age of the patient, the possibility of sinister implications must be considered.

The most common classification of primary concomitant esotropic deviations describes the clinical picture and associated refractive findings, as shown in *Table 6.2*.

Table 6.2 Primary esotropia as classified by clinical presentation

Accommodative	*Non-accommodative*
Constant	Constant
partially accommodative	infantile esotropia
Intermittent	acquired non-accommodative
fully accommodative	esotropia associated with myopia
convergence excess	nystagmus blockage syndrome
	microtropia
	Intermittent
	near esotropia (convergence excess)
	distance esotropia (divergence weakness)
	non-specific
	cyclic esotropia

Primary esotropia

Aetiology and characteristics

The accommodative esotropias are associated with a hypermetropic refractive error and/or a defect in the AC/A ratio. Their main characteristic is that the angle of deviation reduces or disappears when the patient is wearing the appropriate refractive correction. These are considered at length in Chapter 7.

Non-accommodative esotropia

The non-accommodative types of esotropia have a normal AC/A ratio and normally are not associated with hypermetropia.

Infantile esotropia

The pathological processes involved in the onset of infantile esotropia still elude us.[1] Infantile esotropia has an onset before the age of 6 months. The deviation is usually large and is often alternating, in which case it is not associated with amblyopia. Such patients tend to cross fixate, using the right eye when looking to the left and the left eye when looking to the right. This can lead to an apparent underaction of the lateral recti, but tends to respond rapidly to alternating occlusion therapy.

Infantile esotropia is often associated with nystagmus (latent or manifest latent), a dissociated vertical deviation (DVD) and an asymmetrical monocular OKN.[56]

Latent or manifest latent nystagmus

Latent nystagmus is not present under normal binocular conditions, but becomes apparent on occlusion of either eye. Current literature suggests that most of these cases have a fine manifest nystagmus, the amplitude of which increases on occlusion of either eye; hence the more recent term of manifest latent nystagmus (MLN).[57]

Dissociated vertical deviation

When occluding or placing a neutral density filter in front of one eye, the eye behind the cover elevates and often extorts. The angle of the hyperdeviation tends to increase with increasing dissociation. On removal of the cover the eye tends to dip slightly below the primary position, and then incyclorotates to resume its original position.

Generally, the condition is associated with manifest infantile esotropia, in which there is little evidence of binocularity.[58] The upward movement usually occurs whichever eye is covered, but it is often asymmetrical. If one eye is occluded and the fixating eye is darkened gradually behind a neutral density wedge, the covered eye can be seen to move down towards the horizontal.[25]

The condition is usually asymptomatic, but in some the upward rotation of one eye occurs when the patient is tired, in which case surgery can be effective in improving the cosmesis. DVD is often accompanied by bilateral superior oblique overactions. A horizontal equivalent characterised by slow outward rotation of the eyes (dissociated horizontal deviation) has also been described, though this is rare.[59]

Optokinetic nystagmus

Monocular horizontal OKN is normally asymmetrical in the infant, but becomes symmetrical after the age of 2–3 months. In infantile esotropia the asymmetry of the OKN remains. It has been presumed that the absence of symmetry in the OKN indicates the absence of binocular vision,[12] but recent evidence has thrown this presumption into doubt.[60]

The condition usually remains stable, although the angle may steadily increase in the first few months after onset.[25] A binocular outcome of any sort is unlikely unless surgery is performed within the first year of life. Later surgery can be regarded as purely cosmetic.

Nystagmus blocking syndrome

Nystagmus blocking syndrome is an unusual form of esotropia. The patient has a congenital horizontal nystagmus, the amplitude of which reduces with increasing convergence. When patients are being attentive, the nystagmus decreases and the angle of the esotropia increases. When they are not concentrating on a visual stimulus, the angle of the esotropia decreases and the amplitude of the nystagmus increases.[25] The head is often turned to avoid bringing the eye out of adduction. Amblyopia frequently is found in the non-fixating eye.

Microtropia

Microtropia, which is generally an esotropia, is usually defined as a strabismus less than 10 prism dioptres in size.[61] There is foveal suppression and binocular function, which may be normal or abnormal. The following presentations, discussed below, have been differentiated:

- Monofixation syndrome;
- Without identity;
- With identity.

In all of these types of microtropia, heterophoria may or may not be visible on continued dissociation. On removal of the cover, recovery is to the microtropic angle. The patient is normally cosmetically excellent and asymptomatic, so intervention is not recommended.

Monofixation syndrome

In monofixation syndrome[62] there is central suppression in one eye, which may or may not be accompanied by a small angle heterotropia. Fusion with normal retinal correspondence is maintained parafoveally and in the periphery because of the enlargement of Panum's fusional area with increasing eccentricity.

Microtropia without identity

The microtropia is accompanied by harmonious abnormal retinal correspondence (ARC).[63] On occlusion of the fixating eye the deviating eye moves to take up fixation, whether fixation is central or eccentric.

Microtropia with identity

A microtropia in which the angle of the deviation equals the angle of anomaly (or ARC), which equals the angle of eccentricity.[64] On covering the fixating eye there is no movement of the non-fixating eye. This type of deviation can only be recognised by looking at the fixation point on the fundus.

Intermittent esotropia
By definition, an intermittent deviation does, at times, have normal binocular single vision. As such the potential for full binocularity is high and sensory adaptation is normally limited to suppression. Amblyopia normally only develops if there are other mitigating factors, such as anisometropia.

Near esotropia
Near esotropia is esotropia on near fixation with a reduced angle on distance fixation, becoming an esophoria or orthophoria. Where there is an accommodative element the AC/A ratio is high and the deviation may be controlled at near through positive addition lenses.

Distance esotropia
Primary distance esotropia is rare. It is usually associated with either a lateral rectus paresis, some other form of incomitancy or a spasm of accommodation or convergence.[25]

Cyclical esotropia
In cyclical esotropia the deviation is manifest for 1–2 days, and then disappears, without evidence of an esophoria.[25] It can occur in the absence of binocular single vision.[65,66] It normally has no known cause, but can be associated with neurological dysfunction. It commonly progresses to a constant esotropia over time.[25]

Primary exotropia
Primary infantile exotropia
Primary exotropia that lasts beyond the age of 3 months is much more unusual than primary infantile esotropia, but otherwise similar in its characteristics.[67]

Intermittent exotropia
Near exotropia
Near exotropia is exotropia on near fixation with a reduced angle on distance fixation, becoming an exophoria or orthophoria. In its purest form a near exotropia has a normal near point of convergence, but as the deviation is commonly associated with convergence insufficiency the near point of convergence may be remote.

Distance exotropia, true or simulated
The most common classification of primary concomitant exotropic deviations is shown in *Table 6.3*. There is normally exophoria or orthophoria on near fixation, with the angle increasing markedly on distance fixation. In some instances the deviation only becomes manifest on far-distance fixation (beyond 6m).

In true distance exotropia the AC/A ratio is normal if a steady fixation distance is maintained.

In simulated distance exotropia there is a large AC/A ratio. The angle of deviation on fixation of a near target increases if that target is viewed through positive lenses. Viewing the near target binocularly, through +3.00DS in front of each eye, the deviation equals or exceeds the angle measured on distance fixation when viewing without any additional lenses. A similar increase in the angle of deviation may be seen only after prolonged (approximately 45 minutes) uniocular occlusion.[1]

Table 6.3 Primary exotropia as classified by clinical presentation

Constant	*Intermittent*
Infantile exotropia	Near
Decompensated exophoria	Distance
	true
	simulated
	Non-specific

Summary

Whatever the characteristics of an eye movement disorder, whether incomitant or concomitant, it could potentially indicate a neurological pathology. Any recent-onset condition should be regarded with suspicion. Benign conditions are usually longstanding and stable, and are often best left without active intervention.

References
1 Von Noorden GK and Campos EC (2002). *Binocular Vision and Ocular Motility. Theory and Management of Strabismus* (St Louis: Mosby).
2 Graham PA (1974). Epidemiology of strabismus. *Br J Ophthalmol.* **58**, 224–231.
3 Larsen JS (1971). The sagittal growth of the eye. 1. Ultrasonic measurement of the depth of the anterior chamber from birth to puberty. *Acta Ophthalmol.* **49**, 239–262.
4 Gordon RA and Donzis PB (1985). Refractive development of the human eye. *Acta Ophthalmol.* **103**, 785–789.
5 Swan KC and Wilkins JH (1984). Extraocular muscle surgery in early infancy – anatomical factors. *J Pediatr Ophthalmol Strabismus* **21**, 44–49.
6 Hendrickson A (1992). A morphological comparison of foveal development in man and monkey. *Eye* **6**, 136–144.

7 Magoon EH and Robb RM (1981). Development of myelin in human optic nerve and tract. A light and electron microscopic study. *Acta Ophthalmol.* **99**, 655–659.
8 Le Vay S, Stryker MP and Shatz CJ (1978). Ocular dominance columns and their development in layer IV of the cat's visual cortex: A quantitative study. *J Comp Neurol.* **179**, 223–244.
9 Crowley JC and Katz LC (2002). Ocular dominance development revisited. *Curr Opin Neurobiol.* **12**, 104–109.
10 Batardiere A, Barone P, Knoblauch K, *et al.* (2002). Early specification of the hierarchical organization of visual cortical areas in the macaque monkey. *Cereb Cortex* **12**, 453–465.
11 Hess RF (2002). Sensory processing in human amblyopia: Snakes and ladders. In: *Amblyopia: A Multidisciplinary Approach*, p. 19–41. Eds Moseley M and Fielder A (Oxford: Butterworth–Heinemann).
12 Atkinson J (1984). Human visual development over the first 6 months of life. A review and a hypothesis. *Hum Neurobiol.* **3**, 61–74.
13 Von Hofsten C and Rosander K (1997). Development of smooth pursuit tracking in young infants. *Vis Res.* **37**, 1799–1810.
14 Jacobs M, Harris CM, Shawkat F and Taylor D (1997). Smooth pursuit development in infants. *Aust NZ J Ophthalmol.* **25**, 199–206.
15 Wright KW (1996). Clinical optokinetic nystagmus asymmetry in treated esotropes. *J Pediatr Ophthalmol Strabismus* **33**, 153–155.
16 Dubowitz LM, Mushin J, De VL and Arden GB (1986). Visual function in the newborn infant: Is it cortically mediated? *Lancet* **i**, 1139–1141.
17 Naegele JR and Held R (1982). The postnatal development of monocular optokinetic nystagmus in infants. *Vis Res.* **22**, 341–346.
18 Birch E and Petrig B (1996). FPL and VEP measures of fusion, stereopsis and stereoacuity in normal infants. *Vis Res.* **36**, 1321–1327.
19 Ciner EB, Schanel-Klitsch E and Herzberg C (1996). Stereoacuity development: 6 months to 5 years. A new tool for testing and screening. *Optom Vis Sci.* **73**, 43–48.
20 Banks MS (1980). The development of visual accommodation during early infancy. *Child Dev.* **51**, 646–666.
21 Aslin RN (1986). Dark vergence in human infants: implications for the development of binocular vision. *Acta Psychol.* **63**, 309–322.
22 Sondhi N, Archer SM and Helveston EM (1988). Development of normal ocular alignment. *J Pediatr Ophthalmol Strabismus* **25**, 210–211.
23 Turner J, Horwood A, Houston S and Riddell P (2002). Development of the response AC/A ratio over the first year of life. *Vis Res.* **42**, 2521–2532.
24 Moore A (1997). Inherited retinal dystrophies. In: *Paediatric Ophthalmology*, p. 557–598. Ed. Taylor D (Oxford: Blackwell Science).
25 Ansons AM and Davis H (2001). *Diagnosis and Management of Ocular Motility Disorders* (Oxford: Blackwell Science).
26 Gallie B and Moore A (1997). Retinoblastoma. In: *Paediatric Ophthalmology*, p. 519–536. Ed. Taylor D (Oxford: Blackwell Science).
27 Yamamoto M, Dogru M, Nakamura M, Shirabe H, Tsukahara Y and Sekiya Y (1998). Visual function following congenital cataract surgery. *Jpn J Ophthalmol.* **42**, 411–416.
28 Hertle RW, Quinn GE, Minguini N and Katowitz JA (1991). Visual loss in patients with craniofacial synostosis. *J Pediatr Ophthalmol Strabismus* **28**, 344–349.
29 Desa LCC and Good WV (1996). Craniofacial anomalies and strabismus. In: *Strabismus Management*, p. 117–135. Eds Good WV and Hoyt CS (Boston: Butterworth–Heinemann).
30 Carruthers JD (1988). Strabismus in craniofacial dysostosis. *Graefes Arch Clin Exp Ophthalmol.* **226**, 230–234.
31 Shields JA, Bakewell B, Augsburger JJ and Flanagan JC (1984). Classification and incidence of space-occupying lesions of the orbit. A survey of 645 biopsies. *Acta Ophthalmol.* **102**, 1606–1611.
32 Taylor RH and Kraft SP (1997). Aplasia of the inferior rectus muscle. A case report and review of the literature. *Ophthalmology* **104**, 415–418.
33 Lueder GT, Dunbar JA, Soltau JB, Lee BC and McDermott M (1998). Vertical strabismus resulting from an anomalous extraocular muscle. *J Am Assoc Pediatr Ophthalmol Strabismus* **2**, 126–128.
34 Clark RA, Miller JM and Demer JL (1997). Location and stability of rectus muscle pulleys. Muscle paths as a function of gaze. *Invest Ophthalmol Vis Sci.* **38**, 227–240.
35 Demer JL (2002). The orbital pulley system: A revolution in concepts of orbital anatomy. *Ann NY Acad Sci.* **956**, 17–32.
36 Johnson LV (1950). Adherence syndrome: Pseudoparalysis of the lateral or superior rectus muscle. *Acta Ophthalmol.* **44**, 870–878.
37 Gurwood AS and Terrigno CA (2000). Duane's retraction syndrome: Literature review. *Optometry.* **71**, 722–726.
38 Freedman HL and Kushner BJ (1997). Congenital ocular aberrant innervation – new concepts. *J Pediatr Ophthalmol Strabismus* **34**, 10–16.
39 Tresidder J, Fielder AR and Nicholson J (1990). Delayed visual maturation: Ophthalmic and neurodevelopmental aspects. *Dev Med Child Neurol.* **32**, 872–881.
40 Kraemer M and Sjostrom A (1998). Lack of short-latency potentials in the VEP reflects immature extra geniculate visual function in delayed visual maturation (DVM). *Doc Ophthalmol.* **97**, 189–201.
41 Horton JC and Hocking DR (1998). Effect of early monocular enucleation upon ocular dominance columns and cytochrome oxidase activity in monkey and human visual cortex. *Vis Neurosci.* **15**, 289–303.
42 Anderson SJ (2002). Funtional neuroimaging in amblyopia. In: *Amblyopia: A Multidisciplinary Approach*, p. 43–67. Eds Moseley M and Fielder A (Oxford: Butterworth–Heinemann).
43 Barnes GR, Hess RF, Dumoulin SO, Achtman RL and Pike GB (2001). The cortical deficit in humans with strabismic amblyopia. *J Physiol.* **533**, 281–297.
44 Meyer CH, Lapolice DJ and Freedman SF (2002). Foveal hypoplasia in oculocutaneous albinism demonstrated by optical coherence tomography. *Am J Ophthalmol.* **133**, 409–410.
45 Brodsky MC, Baker RS and Hamed LM (1996). *Pediatric Neuro-ophthalmology* (New York: Springer).
46 Morland AB, Hoffmann MB, Neveu M and Holder GE (2002). Abnormal visual projection in a human albino studied with functional magnetic resonance imaging and visual evoked potentials. *J Neurol Neurosurg Psychiatry* **72**, 523–526.
47 Leigh RJ and Zee DS (1999). *The Neurology of Eye Movements* (Oxford: Oxford University Press).
48 Wizov SS, Reinecke RD, Bocarnea M, Gottlob I and Wizow SS (2002). A comparative demographic and socioeconomic study of spasmus nutans and infantile nystagmus. *Am J Ophthalmol.* **133**, 256–262.
49 Harris CM (1997). Other eye movement disorders. In: *Paediatric Ophthalmology*, p. 897–924. Ed. Taylor D (Oxford: Blackwell Science).
50 Miller MT and Stromland K (1999). The Moebius sequence: A relook. *J Am Assoc Pediatr Ophthalmol Strabismus* **3**, 199–208.
51 Schumacher-Feero LA, Yoo KW, Solari FM and Biglan AW (1999). Third cranial nerve palsy in children. *Am J Ophthalmol.* **128**, 216–221.
52 Loewenfeld IE and Thompson HS (1975). Oculomotor paresis with cyclic spasms. A critical review of the literature and a new case. *Surv Ophthalmol.* **20**, 81–124.
53 Mansour AM and Reinecke RD (1986). Central trochlear palsy. *Surv Ophthalmol.* **30**, 279–297.
54 Leigh RJ, Tomsak RL, Seidman SH and Dell'Osso LF (1991). Superior oblique myokymia. Quantitative characteristics of the eye movements in three patients. *Acta Ophthalmol.* **109**, 1710–1713.
55 Tiffin PA, MacEwen CJ, Craig EA and Clayton G (1996). Acquired palsy of the oculomotor, trochlear and abducens nerves. *Eye* **10**, 377–384.
56 Schor CM, Fusaro RE, Wilson N and McKee SP (1997). Prediction of early-onset esotropia from components of the infantile squint syndrome. *Invest Ophthalmol Vis Sci.* **38**, 719–740.
57 Abadi RV and Scallan CJ (2000). Waveform characteristics of manifest latent nystagmus. *Invest Ophthalmol Vis Sci.* **41**, 3805–3817.
58 Neely DE, Helveston EM, Thuente DD and Plager DA (2001). Relationship of dissociated vertical deviation and the timing of initial surgery for congenital esotropia. *Ophthalmology* **108**, 487–490.
59 Wilson ME, Saunders RA and Berland JE (1995). Dissociated horizontal deviation and accommodative esotropia: Treatment options when an eso- and an exodeviation co-exist. *J Pediatr Ophthalmol Strabismus* **32**, 228–230.

60 Westall CA, Woodhouse JM and Brown VA (1989). OKN asymmetries and binocular function in amblyopia. *Ophthalmic Physiol Opt.* **9**, 269–276.
61 Houston CA, Cleary M, Dutton GN and McFadzean RM (1998). Clinical characteristics of microtropia – is microtropia a fixed phenomenon? *Br J Ophthalmol.* **82**, 219–224.
62 Parks MM (1969). The monofixation syndrome. *Trans Am Ophthalmol Soc.* **67**, 609–657.
63 Lang J (1983). Microtropia. *Int Ophthalmol.* **6**, 33–36.
64 Helveston EM and Von Noorden GK (1967), Microtropia. A newly defined entity. *Acta Ophthalmol.* **78**, 272–281.
65 Riordan-Eva P, Vickers SF, McCarry B and Lee JP (1993). Cyclic strabismus without binocular function. *J Pediatr Ophthalmol Strabismus* **30**, 106–108.
66 Pillai P and Dhand UK (1987). Cyclic esotropia with central nervous system disease: Report of two cases. *J Pediatr Ophthalmol Strabismus* **24**, 237–241.
67 Biglan AW, Davis JS, Cheng KP and Pettapiece MC (1996). Infantile exotropia. *J Pediatr Ophthalmol Strabismus* **33**, 79–84.

7
Binocular Vision Disorders: Clinical Investigation, Diagnosis and Management

Alison Finlay

Categories of binocular vision defect

This chapter considers the clinical investigation, diagnosis and management of visual defects that result from disruptions to the normal development of sensory motor co-operation between the eyes. Differential diagnosis is a pre-requisite to determining an appropriate management plan and prognosis. Broadly speaking, the management and prognosis vary depending on which of the following three categories the condition falls into:

- Visual defect that affects both eyes;
- Disruption to binocularity because of monocular visual loss or strabismus;
- Ocular motor defect with a latent or intermittent deviation and full binocular capability.

Visual defect that affects both eyes

Conditions that fall into this group include high ametropia, congenital idiopathic nystagmus and congenital or developmental retinal disorders. The best-possible vision should be achieved using an optical correction, and patients with nystagmus or retinal disorders should be referred to the hospital eye service to confirm the diagnosis and, where possible, treat any pathology. Ametropic amblyopia normally improves with wearing of the prescription.[1] Often little else can be done, although optical aids, such as magnifiers and telescopes, or tints for the photophobic, can be considered.

Disruption to binocularity because of monocular visual loss or strabismus

Patients in this group should be treated promptly. During infancy any pathology should be treated as early as possible or the deprived eye will not achieve a useful level of visual acuity.[2] These children require optimal refractive correction in each eye with the aim to achieve normal binocular single vision (BSV).

In all such patients, the treatment of amblyopia is of primary concern, and early intervention with spectacles and occlusion therapy is still the preferred course of action.[3] For patients who have a constant squint after optimal refractive correction, consider prismatic correction or referral for surgery.

Those patients with the potential to develop normal binocularity may derive a functional benefit,[4] and those with no binocular capabilities may improve cosmetically. The development of a sensory adaptation to a constant strabismus should be assessed, and treated only if it is appropriate.[5]

Ocular motor defect with a latent or intermittent deviation and full binocular capability

In this group of patients development of amblyopia is less likely. The more unusual eye movement disorders, such as gaze palsies or ocular motor apraxia, should be referred for hospital investigation.

Otherwise, having considered the potential involvement of any pathology and referred accordingly, these conditions can usually be dealt with in practice. An intermittent or decompensating concomitant deviation may be assisted by manipulation of the refractive correction, the use of prisms or exercises. An incomitant deviation may not need treatment, but an abnormal head posture may be cosmetically improved by surgery. Recently, some doubt has been cast upon the long-held belief that an abnormal head posture can result in skeletal malformations and facial asymmetry,[6] but referral is recommended until such time as this doubt becomes universally accepted. With all children, the visual condition should be considered in terms of the child as a whole.

The benefits of a small prescription should be considered carefully in a child with severe learning difficulties, and a child with physical disabilities may have many other difficulties to cope with, making amblyopia therapy low in their priorities.

The clinical procedures used to investigate binocular vision anomalies are discussed next, followed by a discussion of the diagnostic features and treatment options for the different conditions.

The text concentrates on the latter two patient groups listed above, those with treatable monocular visual loss, strabismus, an intermittent deviation or heterophoria.

Assessment

Observation
The first diagnostic tool is to observe the patient at the initial presentation. There may be strabismus, nystagmus, ptosis, abnormal head posture or head movements, unusual facial features or facial structure.[5]

History
As with so many clinical investigations, the history should not be undervalued as a diagnostic tool. With younger children, normally 'symptoms' are limited to observations made by the parents or teacher. Duration of the condition is an example of a critical piece of information that can affect prognosis.[3] A patient with a strabismus with onset prior to the critical period for the development of binocularity (3 months) has a poor prognosis of developing binocular function.[7]

The clinical picture of a condition with a much later onset may be similar, but the prognosis is very different. Consistency between the parent's observations and the clinical findings can indicate how good they are as an historian. Questions on general health, family history or a history of birth trauma may point to the aetiology, as discussed in Chapters 2 and 15. Previous ocular history can be of value in making management decisions. Amblyopia that has been treated extensively in the past is unlikely to respond readily to further treatment.[8]

Visual acuity
The normal development of and the methods used to assess visual acuity are considered in Chapters 1 and 3. In a baby, the ability to fixate and follow with each eye individually may be all that can be achieved in practice. This provides a qualitative observation of acuity, although it is of questionable value.[9] More quantitative techniques are available in specialised clinics.[10,11]

The aim with all patients is to use a standardised linear test type, so the method chosen should be as close an approximation to this as the child can reasonably achieve. Accurate results can be difficult with youngsters and interpretation of the responses often relies on the experience of the practitioner. Be wary of assuming a bad result is caused by poor co-operation. A child may behave badly to hide an apparent failure. An asymmetry in the responses tends to be easier to detect. If amblyopia is suspected, it is worth repeating the test through a 2 log unit neutral density filter.[12] If amblyopia is functional, a filter that reduces acuity by two lines in the good eye has no effect or may even enhance the acuity in the amblyopic eye.

Cover test
An appropriate target size is vital when examining youngsters who may have an accommodative-type deviation.[13] Detailed pictures are usually fine, but it may be essential to question the infant on a picture's features to ensure he or she is concentrating and for the deviation to become apparent.

An accommodative-type squint typically appears straight when fixating a non-accommodative target such as a pen light.[5] If a child is a poor fixator, this should be recorded in the notes, as small-angle deviations may be misdiagnosed because of unsteady fixation.[13]

Ocular motility
Ideally, an ocular motility test should be performed with the patient fixating a light. An accommodative-type deviation should have been noted when doing a cover test.

Very young infants tend to fixate readily and follow a light, and an advantage is that they allow observation of corneal reflections. This helps the examiner ensure that the fixation target is always within the limits of the facial contours, so any asymmetry in the reflections could indicate a deviation. Be aware though, that this can be deceptive because of parallax.[14] The cover test should always be performed in any direction of gaze in which there is the suspicion of a deviation.[5] In an incomitancy, watch out for different angles when either eye fixates, because of the difference between the primary and secondary angles.

In infants, the epicanthic folds often give the impression of an esotropia or an inferior oblique overaction. If the child allows it, pinch the top of the nose to lift the skin, which allows the entire palpebral aperture to be viewed. When investigating the alphabet patterns, control of the horizontal deviation may vary with accommodative effort. It can therefore be beneficial to repeat ocular motility in direct up- and downgaze by doing the cover test with an accommodative fixation target, while the patient is wearing glasses.[5]

Recording the results
Unless absolutely certain of the diagnosis, avoid trying to record motility disorders in terms of the paretic muscle. Instead, record how the deviation varies with angle of gaze.

Few incomitancies conform to the typical picture of a single muscle palsy, and many congenital defects are mechanical in origin rather than neurogenic. If an incomitancy is discovered, a Hess chart should be plotted wherever possible. This assists diagnosis and allows comparison at future visits, to ensure that the condition is non-progressive.[13] If the facilities to plot a Hess chart are not available, plot a diplopia chart.[13] This involves recording the approximate direction and amplitude of the separation of the diplopic images in the nine positions of gaze while the patient wears red and green goggles and views a spot light or, preferably, a bar light. Such a plot is shown in *Figure 7.1*. For both the Hess and diplopia charts, the patient must not suppress his or her deviating eye.[5]

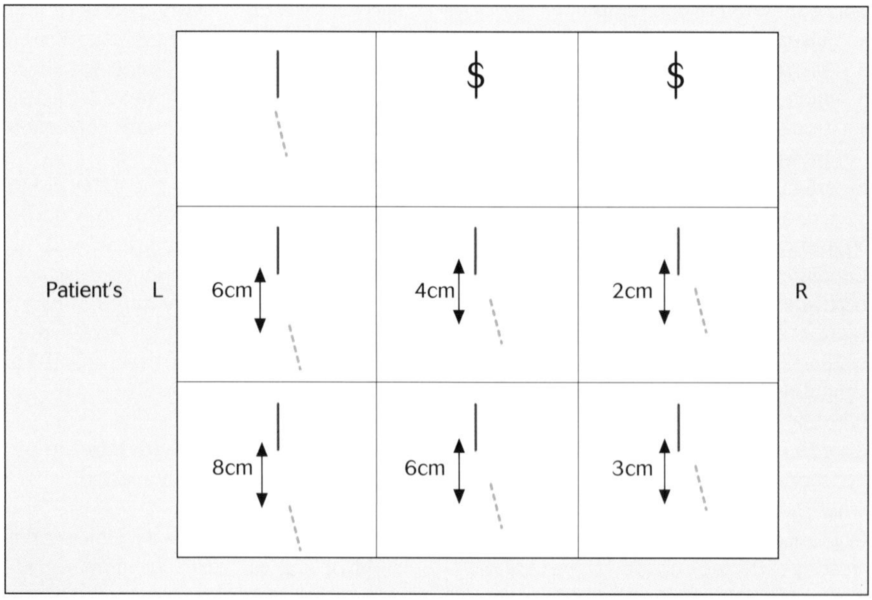

Figure 7.1
Diplopia chart of a patient with a right fourth nerve palsy. $ = where both targets are coincident

Measurement of the angle

Strabismus and dissociated heterophoria

Measurement of the angle is important to determine if the deviation changes in size over time. The parent of a child with an accommodative-type deviation can often become distressed, believing that, although the deviation is reduced when the child wears glasses, it is increased without glasses. For all but the smallest deviations the best method of assessment is probably neutralisation with a prism. With a large-angle deviation, prisms are not strictly additive,[15] but they give a repeatable approximation. With small-angle deviations (less than 6 prism dioptres), subjective methods of assessment, or estimation of the angle, may be more reliable.

Associated phoria

The term 'associated phoria' can be used to describe the size of prism needed to realign the nonius strips in the presence of a fixation disparity, and indicates the uncompensated element of a heterophoria.[16] Decompensation is likely to affect a child's performance in school, although there is no evidence of an increased incidence of associated phoria among dyslexics.[17]

Sensory status

Normal binocular single vision

Assessment of sensory status in the presence of heterophoria or an intermittent heterotropia refers to fusion, sensory and motor, and stereopsis.[5] The presence of motor fusion can be assessed objectively in infants as young as 6 months by looking at binocular recovery to a base-out prism.

The selection of prism power can vary between practitioners, but the 12 prism dioptre prism available in most trial cases is sufficient.[18] With larger prisms the child may need encouragement to overcome the prism, but it is most important to look for spontaneous recovery after its removal from in front of either eye.[13] The sequence of movements observed in the presence of normal fusional reserves is illustrated in *Figure 7.2*. A quantitative measure of motor fusion can be obtained with a prism bar or Risley rotating prism. A reduced base-in fusional reserve has been associated with a failure to emmetropise,[19] and reduced base-in and base-out fusional reserves have been associated with reading difficulties.[17]

Stereopsis can be demonstrated qualitatively with Lang's two-pen test[20] (*Figure 7.3*) or a more quantitative assessment can be obtained using one of the commercially available stereotests.

The TNO test uses random dots with red–green dissociation. It is arguably the most challenging, and has been favoured as a screening tool.[21] The Titmus test uses a polarising vectograph. It is easy to do and compelling for younger children, with the fly having a disparity in the region of 3000 seconds of arc,[22] but it has been criticised for its monocular clues. Lang and Frisby tests have the advantage of needing no glasses, and have been used with children less than 1 year of age.[23]

Abnormal binocular vision

In the presence of a manifest deviation, management decisions can be based on the presence of binocular functions, normal or abnormal. Post-surgically, residual infantile esotropias (onset before 6 months of age) rarely have anything more than the most tentative signs of binocularity.[7,24] Evidence of binocular single vision using Bagolini lenses or of stereopsis using the Lang's two-pen test is probably the most lightly ingrained form of binocular

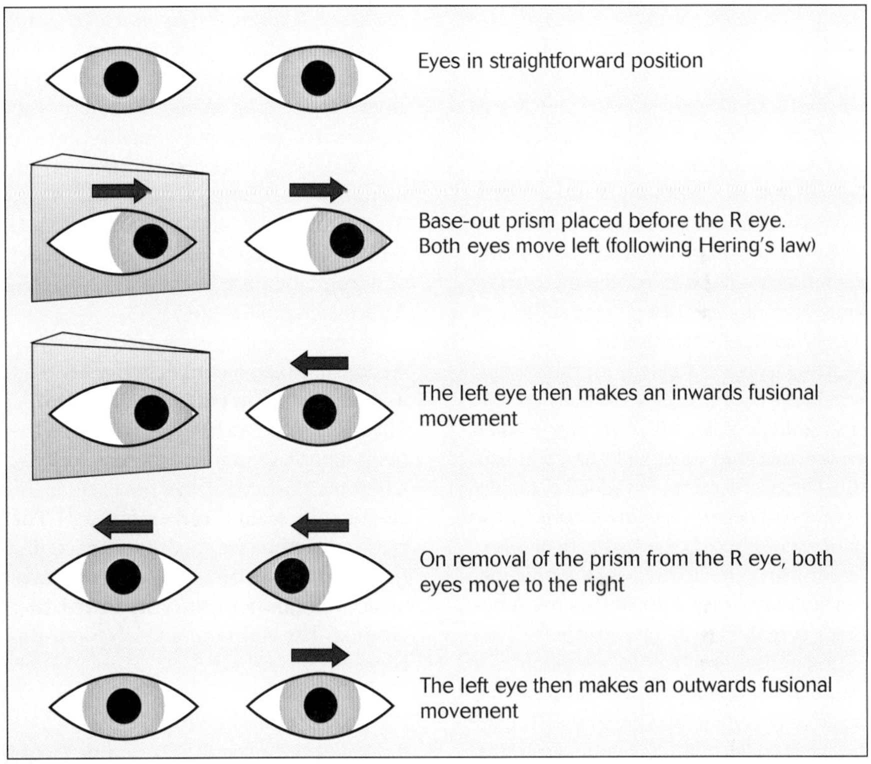

Figure 7.2
Base-out prism test

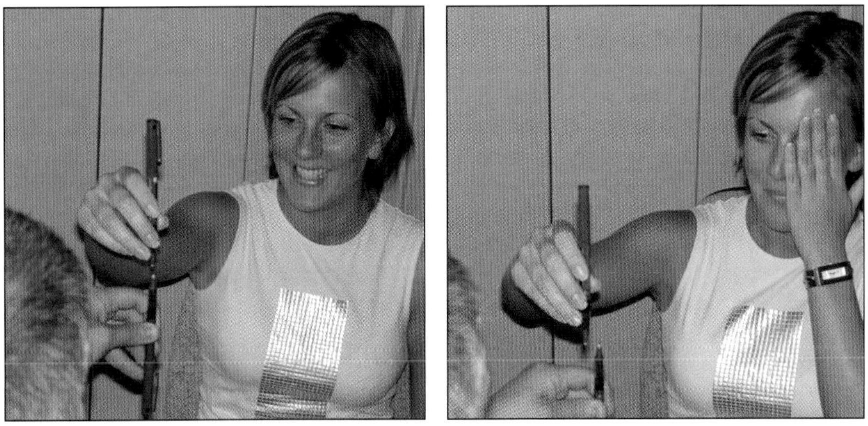

Figure 7.3
The Lang two-pen test. Accurate location of the patient's pen to the examiner's with both eyes open suggests good stereopsis as compared with the monocular situation. Equal binocular and monocular responses suggest an absence of binocular depth perception

vision demonstrable. The streaks crossing through the light in the presence of strabismus suggests harmonious abnormal retinal correspondence (ARC).[25]

Any form of abnormal BSV ingrained more deeply than this usually exists only in a deviation with an onset after the age of 6 months, but before the end of the critical period for cortical plasticity.[5] Well-ingrained harmonious ARC is rare in anything but a manifest deviation with a constant angle, usually less than 20 prism dioptres in size.[26]

In these cases simultaneous perception and fusion can often be demonstrated using Worth's four-dot test or with the Mallet unit. A sub-standard level of stereoacuity may also be demonstrated.[22] Normal retinal correspondence (NRC) in a patient with a constant manifest deviation can be demonstrated by artificially correcting the deviation, either with prisms or on a synoptophore. The presence of BSV after artificial correction of the deviation indicates an excellent prognosis for a functional result following surgery or other means of correction.[27]

The presence of deeply ingrained ARC provides a poor prognosis for normal BSV, but the angle of deviation is normally small and cosmetically acceptable, and is unlikely to change over time.[5] In addition, amblyopia is unlikely to become severe. These patients ought to be treated with caution, as any disruption to the anomalous binocularity may cause a previously asymptomatic condition to develop problems.

In lightly ingrained ARC the retinal correspondence can appear to change with the angle of deviation, and provides little control over the deviation. These cases, and those with no demonstrable binocular function, usually can be considered as cosmetic. Amblyopia can become dense, with acuity levels that drop to less than 6/60.

Near point of convergence

Normal binocular single vision

A simple pen-to-nose test can be used, but if there is any indication of a breakdown in convergence, a more appropriate target is indicated, such as the RAF rule. Assessment of convergence should always be objective as well as subjective. Many children suppress the diplopic image.

When convergence breaks, a record should be made of which eye diverges first and whether or not diplopia is recognised. Jump convergence or use of flipper prisms assesses rapid changes of vergence angle.[28] A remote near point of convergence, or slow changes in vergence angle, has been implicated in children with reading difficulties.[29]

Abnormal binocular vision

In esotropia, an angle of deviation that is maintained as the fixation point is brought closer to the nose could indicate ARC. An angle that reduces until the visual axes cross, and then becomes binocular, indicates NRC. An angle that reduces until the visual axes cross, and then one eye diverges, indicates an absence of any form of binocular function.[30]

Accommodation

Amplitudes of accommodation should be assessed monocularly and binocularly in any child with a manifest deviation or reading difficulties.[31] A reduced near point of accommodation binocularly, but not monocularly, in a child with normal BSV suggests a strain on the binocular system.[32] Accommodative facility can be assessed using flipper lenses and accommodative lag can be assessed using dynamic or monocular estimation method (MEM) retinoscopy.[33] Reduced amplitudes of accommodation have been associated with reading difficulties.[17]

Accommodative convergence to accommodation ratio (AC/A ratio)

The AC/A ratio can be measured using the heterophoria or gradient method, but the heterophoria method does not exclude the effects of proximal convergence.[34] The gradient method varies, dependent on distance of fixation and the range of lenses used, and opinions vary as to the best method. The ratio is considered normal between 3:1 and 4:1.[35]

Binocular visual acuity

Binocular visual acuity (BVA) represents the level of acuity that can be achieved while maintaining BSV. A child with an accommodative-type deviation should be asked to read down the letter chart. The point at which the deviation becomes manifest provides a measure of the limit of BVA.[13] On near fixation, bar reading is an analogous task.[13] A bar, approximately 1cm in width, is positioned between the reading text and the patient. While the patient is binocular the bar appears transparent, but as soon as the deviation becomes manifest or there is suppression of either eye, the bar blocks a portion of the print.

Refraction

All children of pre-school age with any suspicion of a visual defect should have a cycloplegic refraction,[36] as discussed in Chapter 4. If there is any evidence of an esotropia the full hypermetropic prescription should be issued, with no allowances made for the cycloplegia.[37] High hypermetropes may have ametropic amblyopia, in which case the full prescription should be recommended until acuity reaches normal levels.[22] Those who were uncorrected previously may, initially, find difficulty adapting to their full prescription, in which case the pre-cycloplegic refraction can be issued as a first step. Where there is no evidence of squint, a slight under-correction may allow for emmetropisation.[19,38]

Differential diagnosis and management

This section concentrates on concomitant deviations that can be treated in practice or by the orthoptist. Differential diagnosis of an incomitancy is most likely confirmed subsequent to referral to the hospital eye service.

Amblyopia

Inadequate visual stimulation in one or both eyes during the critical period of visual development results in a loss of visual responsiveness.[39] Intervention with spectacles and suitable occlusion therapy is still thought to be the most effective form of treatment,[40,41] although opinions vary as to the importance of age at the onset of treatment.[41,42]

Treatment

Understanding of the pathophysiology of amblyopia has increased greatly in the past two decades, as discussed in Chapter 6, but treatment regimes are still based largely on accumulated clinical experience. An initial improvement frequently occurs after correction of the refractive error, after which occlusion remains the preferred mode of treatment for unilateral amblyopia,[8,43] but opinions differ as to the best protocol.[12,44] There is no doubt that the maximum advisable duration of occlusion varies with the age of the patient. Factors that must be considered include:

- Inducing reversal amblyopia;
- Disruption to the development or maintenance of BSV;
- Inducing intractable diplopia;
- Psychological impact upon the child.

In young infants the visual system responds very quickly to any change in visual input and so occlusion therapy should be monitored closely. Maximum periods of occlusion according to age are shown in *Table 7.1*, but should only be advised in the presence of dense amblyopia and should not be undertaken for longer than 1 week, at least initially, without follow-up.[13]

Table 7.1 Maximum advisable periods of occlusion according to age

Age	*Occlusion period*
2–8 months	10 minutes daily
9–24 months	30 minutes daily
2–3 years	4 hours daily
3–6 years	Full time
6–8 years	5 hours daily (depending on density of suppression)

In older children, extended periods of occlusion can result in the breakdown of a heterophoria and the loss of suppression.[13]

In children of school age or older, loss of suppression can leave patients with diplopia for the rest of their lives.[5] Short periods of occlusion accompanied by intensive visual stimulation are thought to be as effective[46] at improving acuity and are less likely to affect binocularity. In strabismics the density of suppression should be measured before and during treatment.[13] This is done by asking the patient to fixate a pen torch light and finding the strength of neutral density filter that is needed in front of the non-amblyopic eye to induce diplopia.[46]

Occlusion can be total or partial. Total occlusion refers to the use of an opaque occluder in front of the normally fixating eye. Adhesive occluders are available commercially, or opaque contact lenses make a viable alternative. Partial occlusion is not completely opaque, but removes some form or light sense, dependent on its density.[13] This can be achieved using a light diffuser, such as Bangerter foils,[47] or penalisation, which is an optical way to create a form of partial occlusion. This can be achieved with drugs (atropine instilled into the fixating eye)[48] or lenses (modification of spectacle prescription in front of the fixating eye).[49] Partial occlusion is more appropriate if there is a fear of losing binocular control or changing the state of sensory adaptation.

Heterotropia

Intermittent heterotropia seen soon after birth is normal[50] and may result from changing orbital growth or development of binocular and visuomotor pathways. A constant deviation from birth or a deviation that persists beyond the first 4–6 months is abnormal.[51] Incomitant deviations and secondary deviations are covered in Chapter 6.

The principles of management vary according to whether the deviation is constant or intermittent. If constant, early surgical intervention to correct any squint has a good prognosis for a high level of binocular function and resolution of any abnormal head posture.[52,53]

Vertical

Primary concomitant vertical deviations are rare.[54] They are normally secondary to an incomitancy (either mechanical or neurogenic) or to abnormal skeletal or facial development. A longstanding neurogenic incomitance can appear concomitant because of the development of muscle sequelae.[5] Manipulation of the refractive correction does not help these patients. Where a strabismus is cosmetically poor, surgical intervention could be considered. Otherwise, a patient who is asymptomatic is best left untreated. A small-angle strabismus can be corrected with prisms if the patient has potential for normal BSV.

Heterotropia or a decompensating heterophoria should be corrected using the minimum prism to re-align the nonius strips when fixation disparity is assessed.[16] Patients with a longstanding vertical heterophoria can have remarkable vertical fusion ranges.[55]

Horizontal

Accommodative esotropia

In all accommodative-type esotropia deviations, a full hypermetropic prescription should be issued after cycloplegic refraction, with a recommendation for full-time wear.[5]

Constant, partially accommodative deviations may have an onset after the critical period for binocular vision, and so have potential for a functional result.[56] If, after 2–3 months of spectacle wear, the deviation fails to be controlled, any amblyopia should be treated and alternative methods of obtaining BSV considered.[41] If prismatic correction within the practice is feasible, this could provide a long-term solution.

Surgical intervention for the non-accommodative element of the deviation can be successful.[57] If the patient shows any interest in the potential for surgical intervention, or the size of the prism is cosmetically unsightly or mechanically cumbersome, recommend referral. These attempts to obtain BSV may fail, in which case the advantages of wearing the prescription should be reconsidered and the deviation regarded in terms of its cosmesis.[13] A child with large amplitudes of accommodation has little to gain visually from wearing a small hypermetropic correction.

For fully accommodative deviations, 2–3 months of full-time spectacle wear consolidates binocular function and may produce visual improvement in an amblyopic eye.[56] Subsequently, any remaining amblyopia should be treated with occlusion.[45] Once BSV is firmly established, the patient should be reviewed annually.[57] At 6–7 years of age, the child can be taught to control the deviation without spectacles.[13] Children with moderate or large refractive errors often appreciate the cosmetic advantage of learning to keep their eyes straight for the short periods of time they may be without their glasses, such as swimming. Those with low refractive errors may learn to cope with intermittent wear or may learn to dispense with their spectacles entirely.

Convergence excess-type near esotropia

Convergence excess is an esotropia on near fixation that is controlled to an esophoria or orthophoria on distance fixation, when wearing full refractive correction. These patients can normally control the deviation for near fixation by wearing a positive addition on top of their distance Rx.

If there is a residual near esotropia, repeat the cover test using a non-accommodative fixation target, such as a pen light. An angle of deviation that reduces indicates a refractive element to the deviation. Measure the AC/A ratio and repeat the near cover test again through +3.00 spheres. If the patient becomes binocular, repeat the near cover test with a reduced addition until the patient becomes manifest when fixating an N5 target. Increase again by +0.25D and prescribe this addition in bifocal form.[58] The segment should be executive or a large 'D-seg', and it should be fitted high to encourage its use on downgaze. Opinions differ as to whether the segment is best set on the lower pupil margin or bisecting the pupil.[5] Over time, and with training, the strength of the addition can be reduced and the need for the bifocal segment may be eliminated.[59]

The pathophysiology of the various types of primary constant esotropia are considered in Chapter 6. Any amblyopia should be treated as early as possible.[3] If there is a sensory adaptation in the form of harmonious ARC, any visual improvement after amblyopia therapy is likely to be maintained, and the angle of deviation normally remains stable. Microtropias, for example, often have a high standard of abnormal binocularity and good cosmesis[60] that could be affected adversely by treatment. If there is no demonstrable binocularity, the level of acuity needs careful monitoring until 7–8 years of age, and the deviation should be considered in terms of its cosmesis only. Such deviations tend to diverge with age, so cosmetic surgery usually aims to leave a residual esotropia.[61]

Intermittent cases normally have a high standard of binocular function when they are straight, but suppress the deviating eye when squinting. Amblyopia should be treated cautiously so as not to break down any heterophoria.[14] Anti-suppression exercises are generally ill-advised as, if control cannot be established, the patient can be left with intractable diplopia.[62] The prescription should be issued as maximum plus or minimum minus, but because the aetiology is not refractive, correction is unlikely to have much of an effect on the deviation. Prisms can be used to control the deviation. Once binocularity is established, exercises can improve fusional reserves so that, in time, the prisms can be discarded. If the deviation proves difficult to control, these patients may be helped by surgery.

Exotropia

The principles of the management of constant exotropia are similar to those for esotropia. Until the debate on the timing of therapy is resolved, treat any amblyopia as early as possible.[41] If normal binocular function can be established every attempt should be made to obtain BSV, although anti-suppression exercises should be used with caution.[63] Spectacle correction should be minimum plus, maximum minus.[64]

If a patient has high amplitudes of accommodation control may be established by using a negative addition on top of the Rx for near and distance viewing.[65] The minimum negative addition to achieve a BVA of 6/6 and bar reading to N5 is the ideal. As binocular function improves the aim is to reduce this addition.

The minimum power prism that can control the deviation is an alternative mode of treatment.

Where there is no capacity for BSV the deviation should be considered according to its appearance and referred for surgery if the cosmesis is poor.[66]

For intermittent exotropia, as with a constant deviation, any amblyopia is treated to obtain BSV for all distances of fixation. Near exotropia (convergence weakness) is often associated with convergence insufficiency, and can be controlled by exercising the near point.[14] Distance exotropia (divergence excess) can be associated with a high AC/A ratio (simulated) and is likely to benefit from negative addition lenses.[67]

Heterophoria and accommodative deficiencies

Decompensating heterophorias and accommodative deficiencies have been implicated in specific learning difficulties.[68] Any binocular anomalies should be treated before considering the diagnosis of Irlen syndrome.[69] Care should be taken to differentiate heterophoria from accommodative deficiencies. Treatment of esophoria and exophoria follows the same principles as an intermittent tropia. Prescribe maximum plus or minimum minus for the former and vice versa for the latter.

As with intermittent heterotropia, a positive addition for near may help a convergence excess-type esophoria and a negative addition for all viewing distances may help a divergence excess-type exophoria.[64] Normally, consider aiming to reduce the deviation until the associated phoria is eliminated on the Mallet unit, using refractive means before prisms.[65]

Exercising 'positive relative accommodation' or 'negative relative convergence' (accommodation in excess of the angle of convergence) helps an esophoria. Exercising 'negative relative accommodation' or 'positive relative convergence' (convergence in excess of accommodation) helps an exophoria. The aim is to improve fusional reserves and increase flexibility in the accommodation to the convergence relationship.[28]

Flipper lenses, flipper prisms and stereograms are ideal for this purpose. Exercising the near point can treat near exophoria, convergence insufficiency and accommodative deficiencies. Exercise should be frequent (several times a day), but only for a few minutes at a time.[70]

Initially, the patient should be seen every 1–2 weeks to monitor progress and ensure the exercises are being done correctly. These deviations often respond rapidly and effectively to treatment.

Some authorities consider decompensating heterophorias to have an effect on the development of fine motor dexterity and spatial awareness, specifically hand–eye co-ordination and balance. There is some evidence of a general developmental improvement of motor skills[71] after exercises, but the validity of the evidence has been disputed.[72]

Summary

The treatment of BV problems in children is a rewarding experience. The age of the child is critical to success,[41,69] with treatment regimes being more acceptable to younger children and, arguably, more effective. Rapid improvements in school performance can be seen after appropriate refractive correction and treatment for any decompensating heterophoria. Active therapy can involve numerous visits to practice in a short period of time, which are not covered by the General Ophthalmic Service.[70] With this proviso, optometrists should not fear the treatment of binocular vision anomalies in children, but should recognise their limitations and refer where necessary.

References

1 Werner DB and Scott WE (1985). Amblyopia case reports – bilateral hypermetropic ametropic amblyopia. *J Pediatr Ophthalmol Strabismus* **22**, 203–205.

2 Taylor D, Vaegan, Morris JA, Rodgers JE and Warland J (1979). Amblyopia in bilateral infantile and juvenile cataract. Relationship to timing of treatment. *Trans Ophthalmol Soc UK* **99**, 170–175.

3 Williams C, Northstone K, Harrad RA, Sparrow JM, Harvey I and ALSPAC Study Team (2002). Amblyopia treatment outcomes after screening before or at age 3 years: Follow up from randomised trial. *BMJ* **324**, 1549–1551.

4 Weakley DRJ (2001). The association between nonstrabismic anisometropia, amblyopia, and subnormal binocularity. *Ophthalmology* **108**, 163–171.

5 Von Noorden GK and Campos EC (2002). *Binocular Vision and Ocular Motility. Theory and Management of Strabismus.* St Louis: Mosby.

6 Velez FG, Clark RA and Demer JL (2000). Facial asymmetry in superior oblique muscle palsy and pulley heterotopy. *J Am Assoc Pediatr Ophthalmol Soc.* **4**, 233–239.

7 Rowe FJ (2000). Long-term postoperative stability in infantile esotropia. *Strabismus* **8**, 3–13.

8 Cleary M (2000). Efficacy of occlusion for strabismic amblyopia: can an optimal duration be identified? *Br J Ophthalmol* **84**, 572–578.

9 Atilla H, Oral D, Coskun S and Erkam N (2001). Poor correlation between 'fix-follow-maintain' monocular/binocular fixation pattern evaluation and presence of functional amblyopia. *Binocul Vis Strabismus Q.* **16**, 85–90.

10 Day S (1997). History, examination and further investigation. In: *Paediatric Ophthalmology*, p. 77–92. Ed. Taylor D. (Oxford: Blackwall Science).

11 Kriss T and Thompson D (1997). Visual electrophysiology. In: *Paediatric Ophthalmology*, p. 93–121. Ed. Taylor D. (Oxford: Blackwall Science).

12 Kushner BJ (1981). Functional amblyopia associated with organic ocular disease. *Am J Ophthalmol.* **91**, 39–45.

13 Ansons AM and Davis H (2001). *Diagnosis and Management of Ocular Motility Disorders.* Oxford: Blackwell Science.

14 Rowe FJ (1997). *Clinical Orthoptics.* (Oxford: Blackwell Science).

15 Thompson JT and Guyton DL (1983). Ophthalmic prisms. Measurement errors and how to minimize them. *Ophthalmology* **90**, 204–210.

16 Jenkins TC, Pickwell LD and Yekta AA (1989). Criteria for decompensation in binocular vision. *Ophthalmic Physiol Opt.* **9**, 121–125.

17 Evans BJ, Drasdo N and Richards IL (1994). Investigation of accommodative and binocular function in dyslexia. *Ophthalmic Physiol Opt.* **14**, 5–19.

18 Riddell PM, Horwood AM, Houston SM and Turner JE (1999). The response to prism deviations in human infants. *Curr Biol.* **9**, 1050–1052.

19 Grounds A (1996). Child visual development. In: *Pediatric Eye Care*, p. 43–74. Eds Barnard S and Edgar D. (Oxford: Blackwell Science).

20 Lang J (1983). [The two-pencil test for testing stereopsis]. *Klin Monatsbl Augenheilkd.* **182**, 576–581.

21 Tomac S and Altay Y (2000). Near stereoacuity: Development in preschool children; normative values and screening for binocular vision abnormalities; a study of 115 children. *Binocul Vis Strabismus Q.* **15**, 221–228.

22 Rutstein RP and Eskridge JB (1984). Stereopsis in small-angle strabismus. *Am J Optom Physiol Opt.* **61**, 491–498.

23 Broadbent H and Westall C (1990). An evaluation of techniques for measuring stereopsis in infants and young children. *Ophthalmic Physiol Opt.* **10**, 3–7.

24 Helveston EM, Neely DF, Stidham DB, *et al.* (1999). Results of early alignment of congenital esotropia. *Ophthalmology* **106**, 1716–1726.

25 Lambert SJ, Murray JM and Ryan JB (1987). Effect of target size on anomalous sensory responses in the Bagolini striated lens test. *Am J Optom Physiol Opt.* **64**, 179–185.

26 Rutstein RP, Daum KM and Eskridge JB (1989). Clinical characteristics of anomalous correspondence. *Optom Vis Sci.* **66**, 420–425.

27 Maruo T, Kubota N, Sakaue T and Usui C (2000). Esotropia surgery in children: Long term outcome regarding changes in binocular alignment; a study of 956 cases. *Binocul Vis Strabismus Q.* **15**, 213–220.

28 Evans BJ (1997). *Pickwell's Binocular Vision Anomalies. Investigation and Treatment.* (Oxford: Butterworth–Heinemann).

29 Evans BJ, Patel R, Wilkins AJ, *et al.* (1999). A review of the management of 323 consecutive patients seen in a specific learning difficulties clinic. *Ophthalmic Physiol Opt.* **19**, 454–466.

30 Moore D (1990). Back to basics: Assessment of binocular convergence in esotropia. *Br Orthoptic J*, **47**, 67.

31 Daum KM (1983). Accommodative dysfunction. *Doc Ophthalmol.* **55**, 177–198.

32 Garcia A, Cacho P, Lara F and Megias R (2000). The relation between accommodative facility and general binocular dysfunction. *Ophthalmic Physiol Opt.* **20**, 98–104.

33 Gallaway M and Scheiman M (1990). Assessment of accommodative facility using MEM retinoscopy. *J Am Optom Assoc.* **61**, 36–39.

34 Franceschetti AT and Burian HM (1970). Gradient accommodative convergence to accommodative ratio in families with and without esotropia. *Am J Ophthalmol.* **70**, 558–562.

35 Firth AY, Griffiths HJ and Leach CM (2001). Normal values for the stimulus accommodative convergence to accommodation (AC/A) ratio measured by the gradient method on the synoptophore. In: *Transactions of 26th Meeting of the European Strabismus Association, Barcelona, 2000*, p. 226–229. Ed. De Faber JT. (Buren: Aeolus Press).

36 Edgar D and Barnard S (1996). Refraction. In: *Pediatric Eye Care*, p. 151–167. Eds Barnard S and Edgar D. (Oxford: Blackwall Science).

37 Jensen H (1997). Refraction and refractive errors. In: *Paediatric Ophthalmology*. p. 57–74. Ed Taylor D. (Oxford: Blackwall Science).

38 Ingram RM, Gill LE and Lambert TW (2000). Effect of spectacles on changes of spherical hypermetropia in infants who did, and did not, have strabismus. *Br J Ophthalmol.* **84**, 324–326.

39 Kiorpes L (2002). Sensory processing: Animal models of amblyopia. In: *Amblyopia: A Multidisciplinary Approach*, p. 1–18. Eds Moseley M and Fielder A. (Oxford: Butterworth–Heinemann).

40 Simmers AJ, Gray LS, McGraw PV and Winn B (1999). Functional visual loss in amblyopia and the effect of occlusion therapy. *Invest Ophthalmol Vis Sci.* **40**, 2859–2871.

41 Flynn JT, Woodruff G, Thompson JR, *et al.* (1999). The therapy of amblyopia: An analysis comparing the results of amblyopia therapy utilizing two pooled data sets. *Trans Am Ophthalmol Soc.* **97**, 373–390 (discussion p. 390–395).

42 Edelman PM and Borchert MS (1997). Visual outcome in high hypermetropia. *J Am Assoc Pediatr Ophthalmol Soc.* **1**, 147–150.

43 Pandey PK, Chaudhuri Z, Kumar M, Satyabala K and Sharma P (2002). Effect of levodopa and carbidopa in human amblyopia. *J Pediatr Ophthalmol Strabismus* **39**, 81–89.

44 Mazow ML, Chuang A, Vital MC and Prager T (1999). 1999 Costenbader Lecture. Outcome study in amblyopia: Treatment and practice pattern variations. *J Am Assoc Pediatr Ophthalmol Soc.* **4**, 1–9.

45 Krumholtz I and Fitzgerald D (1999). Efficacy of treatment modalities in refractive amblyopia. *J Am Optom Assoc.* **70**, 399–404.

46 Leonards U and Sireteanu R (1993). Interocular suppression in normal and amblyopic subjects: The effect of unilateral attenuation with neutral density filters. *Percept Psychophys.* **54**, 65–74.

47 Lang J (1999). An efficient treatment and new criteria for cure of strabismic amblyopia: Reading and Bangerter foils. *Binocul Vis Strabismus Q.* **14**, 9–10.

48 Wallace DK (1999). Visual acuity after cycloplegia in children: Implications for atropine penalization. *J Am Assoc Pediatr Ophthalmol Soc.* **3**, 241–244.

49 France TD and France LW (1999). Optical penalization can improve vision after occlusion treatment. *J Am Assoc Pediatr Ophthalmol Soc.* **3**, 341–343.

50 Horwood AM (1993). Maternal observations of ocular alignment in infants. *J Pediatr Ophthalmol Strabismus* **30**, 100–105.

51 Horwood A and Williams B (2001). Does neonatal ocular misalignment predict later abnormality? *Eye* **15**, 485–491.

52 Shalev B and Repka MX (2000). Restoration of fusion in children with intracranial tumors and incomitant strabismus. *Ophthalmology* **107**, 1880–1883.

53 Kraft SP, O'Donoghue EP and Roarty JD (1992). Improvement of compensatory head postures after strabismus surgery. *Ophthalmology* **99**, 1301–1308.

54 Anderson JR (1957). *Ocular Vertical Deviations and the Treatment of Nystagmus.* (London: British Medical Association).

55 Brodsky MC, Baker RS and Hamed LM (1996). *Pediatric Neuro-Ophthalmology*. (New York: Springer).
56 Mulvihill A, Maccann A, Flitcroft I and O'Keefe M (2000). Outcome in refractive accommodative esotropia. *Br J Ophthalmol* **84**, 746–749.
57 Kraft SP (1998). Outcome criteria in strabismus surgery. *Can J Ophthalmol.* **33**, 237–239.
58 Raab EL (2001). Monitoring of controlled accommodative esotropia. *Trans Am Ophthalmol Soc.* **99**, 225–228 (discussion p. 228–231).
59 Von Noorden GK, Morris J and Edelman P (1978). Efficacy of bifocals in the treatment of accommodative esotropia. *Am J Ophthalmol.* **85**, 830–834.
60 Ludwig IH, Parks MM and Getson PR (1989). Long-term results of bifocal therapy for accommodative esotropia. *J Pediatr Ophthalmol Strabismus* **26**, 264–270.
61 Hahn E, Cadera W and Orton RB (1991). Factors associated with binocular single vision in microtropia/monofixation syndrome. *Can J Ophthalmol.* **26**, 12–17.
62 Scheiman M and Ciner E (1987). Surgical success rates in acquired, comitant, partially accommodative and nonaccommodative esotropia. *J Am Optom Assoc.* **58**, 556–561.
63 Brown S, Atkins I, Doyle M, *et al.* (1983). Symptom-producing diplopia. *Am Orthoptic J.* **33**, 105–110.
64 Scheiman M and Wick B (1994). *Clinical Management of Binocular Vision: Heterophoric, Accommodative, and Eye Movement Disorders*. (Philadelphia: JB Lippincott Co).
65 Mallett R (1988). The management of binocular vision anomalies. In: *Optometry*, p. 270–284. Eds Edwards K and Llewellyn R. (London: Butterworths).
66 Schworm HD and Rudolph G (2000). Comitant strabismus. *Curr Opin Ophthalmol.* **11**, 310–317.
67 Kushner BJ (1999). Does overcorrecting minus lens therapy for intermittent exotropia cause myopia? *Arch Ophthalmol.* **117**, 638–642.
68 Evans BJ, Patel R, Wilkins AJ, *et al.* (1999). A review of the management of 323 consecutive patients seen in a specific learning difficulties clinic. *Ophthalmic Physiol Opt.* **19**, 454–466.
69 Scott L, McWhinnie H, Taylor L, *et al.* (2002). Coloured overlays in schools: Orthoptic and optometric findings. *Ophthalmic Physiol Opt.* **22**, 156–165.
70 Wick B (1990). Vision therapy for preschool children. In: *Principles and Practice of Pediatric Optometry*, p. 274–292. Eds Rosenbloom AA and Morgan MW. (Philadelphia: JB Lippincott Co).
71 Adler P (1997). Understanding vision training. *Optometry Today*, 38–39.
72 Jennings J (2000). Behavioural optometry: A critical review. *Optom Pract.* **1**, 67–78.

Chapter 8
Paediatric Eye Disorders: Genetics

Richard Armstrong

The way in which genes control the manufacture of proteins and, thereby, determine the biochemical and physiological processes that take place within cells has been a major focus for research in recent decades. A review of this subject is given in Appendix 2.

Alterations or mutations of a gene can result in either failure to make the protein or the production of an altered form of the protein – a process that ultimately may result in disease.

A significant number of genes are now implicated in ocular disease.[1] These genes, however, exhibit different patterns of inheritance depending on whether they are dominant or recessive and whether they are located on an autosome or on a sex chromosome. In some cases, the genes are not even located within the nucleus of the cell; these genes exhibit a quite different pattern termed 'mitochondrial inheritance'. Depending on the type of inheritance, there are characteristic distributions of disease phenotypes among the individuals of succeeding generations. The first objective of this chapter is to describe these patterns of inheritance and to illustrate them with examples drawn from a variety of ocular diseases.

Autosomal dominant inheritance

Autosomal dominant inheritance is easy to identify through examination of individuals or 'phenotypes' in different generations, as these should demonstrate clearly the characteristics associated with the defective gene. As shown in *Figure 8.1*, an individual acquires two distinct alleles of each gene from its respective parents for most inheritable traits and, in most cases, may be termed heterozygote for these traits. In the case of autosomal dominance, one allele is expressed largely at the expense of the other, and hence its effects are observed readily in the phenotype of the offspring.

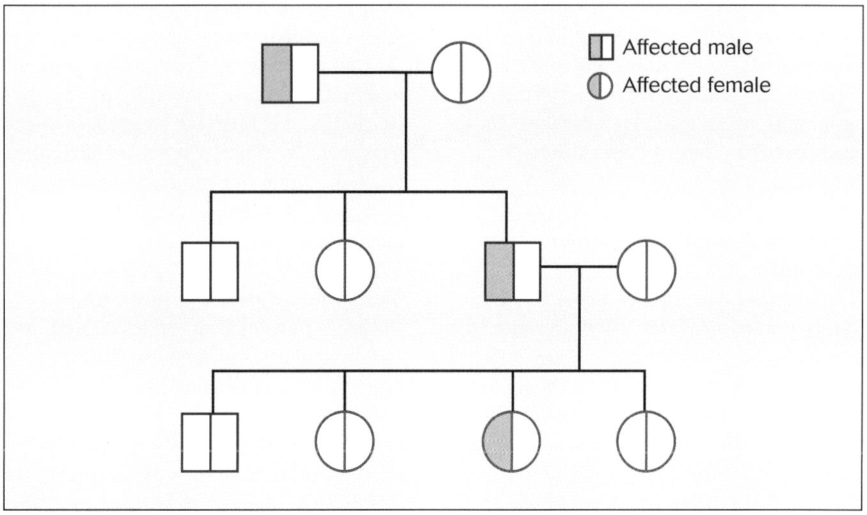

Figure 8.1
Autosomal dominant inheritance in three generations of a family

An important concept related to autosomal dominant inheritance is the degree of 'penetrance', that is, whether or not an individual who possesses the gene expresses the corresponding phenotype. Hence, in normal circumstances, if an individual inherits an autosomal dominant gene from one of its parents, the chance of expressing that gene is 100 per cent. For some autosomal dominant genes, however, the chance of expressing the gene may be considerably less than 100 per cent because of lack of penetrance. Various ocular diseases are associated with autosomal dominant genes and are described in the following sections.

Developmental abnormalities

The development of the eye is dependent on the co-ordinated action of several genes. One of the most important in the control of this process, and which is inherited as an autosomal dominant gene, is the PAX6 gene located on chromosome 11.[2] This gene is involved in the interaction between the optic cup and the overlying ectoderm. Mutations of the gene can cause aniridia, which results from a failure of forwards growth of the rim of the optic vesicle. Patients with aniridia often have reduced visual acuity and may also experience various degrees of photophobia. The disorder may also affect the trabeculae and, ultimately, could be a cause of secondary glaucoma.

Differentiation of the retina from the optic cup is also controlled by a number of genes. An important gene in this group is the 'Mi' gene, which encodes for a protein expressed in the melanocytes of the pigment epithelium. Mutations of the Mi gene result in microphthalmos, a general failure of the eye to develop. However, there are various degrees of this condition – the less severe types are fully compatible with vision. The pattern of inheritance of microphthalmos depends on the type,[3] but autosomal dominant forms are particularly common.

Autosomal dominant corneal dystrophy

The corneal dystrophies are a complex group of disorders that result in reduced corneal clarity in both eyes. Many different types have been described, the majority of which are quite rare. Most of the corneal dystrophies described to date exhibit autosomal dominant inheritance. Corneal dystrophy can affect any layer of the cornea and varying degrees of opacity may be present; opacities located near or along the visual axis are the most common. The most prevalent types are, first, anterior dystrophy (also known as the Reis–Bückler type), which develops in the first decade of life and is associated with a gene on chromosome 5.[4] There is intermittent pain caused by the presence of recurrent corneal erosions. Second, lattice dystrophy develops during the first year of life and is characterised by the appearance of distinct opaque 'lines' in the anterior stroma. This type has been associated with a mutation of the keratoepithelin gene.[5] Third is granular dystrophy, in which milky white spots appear in the superficial stroma along the visual axis. A number of the corneal dystrophies are associated with genes located at the same genetic site or 'locus', which suggests that they may be variants of the same disease.

Congenital cataract

Autosomal dominance is the most common pattern of inheritance of familial congenital cataract, and the genes involved possess a high degree of penetrance.[6] Cataract is often classified according to the location of the opacity. Hence, anterior polar cataract has been linked to a gene on the long arm of chromosome 17 and posterior polar cataract to genes on chromosomes 1 and 16. Zonular pulverulent cataract has been linked to a number of genes located to chromosomes 1, 2, 13 and 16. The locus on chromosome 1 is particularly interesting as this is the site of the connexin-50 gene, which codes for the intercellular channels in the lens. The intercellular channels between lens fibre cells allow the cells to share molecules and, consequently, disruption of this means of communication could be an important factor in the development of cataract. Caerulean cataract is linked to two genes, one of which is located on chromosome 17, while the other was mapped to a region of chromosome 22 that contains the β-crystallin gene. In addition, progressive juvenile-onset punctate cataract is linked to a region of chromosome 2 in which the γ-crystallin genes cluster. Congenital cataract is also linked to a gene in the α-crystallin region on chromosome 21.

Autosomal dominant glaucoma

Various patterns of inheritance are observed in association with the different types of glaucoma. Hereditary factors are believed to be important in 13–25 per cent of cases of primary open-angle glaucoma.[7,8] Both autosomal dominant and recessive patterns of inheritance are observed, with considerable variation in the clinical expression of the disease in different families and in the degree of penetrance. In types of glaucoma characterised by normal intraocular pressure (IOP), the hereditary aspects are even more unclear. Most cases of this type are sporadic or are found in families in which other members of the family may have elevated IOP. One type of this disorder is clearly genetic, with an autosomal dominant pattern of inheritance and a young age-of-onset.[9]

A number of major genetic loci are associated with glaucoma. Five of them, designated GLC1A to GLC1E, are associated with forms of primary open-angle glaucoma and two, designated GLC3A and GLC3B with congenital glaucoma. In addition, a number of loci are implicated in the secondary glaucomas (GLC2).

The first of these genes to be mapped to a specific chromosome site was GLC1A, which is associated with autosomal dominant juvenile-onset glaucoma located on chromosome 1. This location contains the gene for the trabecular meshwork-induced glucocorticoid response protein (TIGR), subsequently accepted as the protein myocilin. Individuals with this type of glaucoma demonstrate a number of single substitution mutations in the third exon (e.g., a glycine to valine substitution at codon 357 and a tyrosine to histidine at codon 430). Substitution mutations are associated with the replacement of only a single nucleotide within the DNA, and thereby leave the remaining nucleotide sequence undisturbed (see Appendix 2). Mutations of this type generally result in minor protein modification. More marked disturbances in the protein, however, may be associated with 'stop mutations', which result in truncated proteins of little normal function. Stop mutations, located at codon 361 of the TIGR gene, have also been observed in two families with juvenile onset open-angle glaucoma to date. By contrast, to date no single gene has been associated with the remaining GLC1 loci, although possible candidate genes have been reported.

Autosomal dominant retinitis pigmentosa

Retinitis pigmentosa (RP) is characterised by a degeneration of the retina that affects both eyes, and results in the deposition of pigment, attenuation of retinal blood vessels and a pale optic disc. An annular scotoma develops, which spreads to the periphery and towards the macula until, ultimately, a very small central visual field remains. Initially, the pathological changes affect the photoreceptor cells of the retina, and usually the rods before the cones. The outer segment is the first part of the photoreceptor to be affected, which is followed by degeneration of the inner segment and gradual depigmentation of the pigment epithelial cells. This deposition of pigment results in the characteristic 'bone spicule' appearance of the pigment. There is a decrease in mean cell counts in all cell layers of the retina, with the outer nuclear layer being the worst affected. Nevertheless, the ganglion cell layer and the nerve fibre layer are often preserved until the later stages of the disease. The degree of optic disc pallor may be dependent on the degree of degeneration of the ganglion cell layer. Later in the disease, central visual acuity often deteriorates, which may be associated with the development of cystoid macular swelling and other pathological changes at the macular area.

RP is associated with several different genes that exhibit various inheritance patterns. Autosomal dominant forms of retinitis pigmentosa (ADRP), however, account for approximately 20 per cent of cases. In a significant proportion of these cases, the disease is associated with mutations of the photoreceptor protein rhodopsin.[10] It is likely that these mutations result in abnormal forms of rhodopsin, which then cause the photoreceptor cells to die.[11] Several other genes are also implicated in ADRP, including the gene for peripherin-retinal degeneration slow protein (peripherin/rds) located on chromosome 6. Peripherin/rds is a membrane protein found in the discs of photoreceptor cells. In normal discs, this protein associates with a second protein called Rom-1 to form a complex. A mutation of the peripherin/rds gene in mice results in abnormal protein-folding and the inability of peripherin/rds to associate with Rom-1.[12] The result is that the photoreceptor cells fail to develop outer segments. More than 30 mutations have now been identified in the peripherin/rds gene in various retinal disorders, including ADRP and the macular degenerations.

Retinoblastoma

Retinoblastoma is both the most common tumour of the eye to affect children and the most common tumour of the retina (see Chapter 9). It occurs throughout the world, with no apparent racial or gender bias, and has a prevalence in the UK of 1/23,000 births. The incidence of retinoblastoma is dependent on age – most cases are diagnosed in children less than 3 years of age. The tumour can be observed at birth and in some premature infants, but the disease is very rare in adults.

An indication of the presence of retinoblastoma is often an abnormal pupil, with leucocoria observed in about 90 per cent of cases – the pupil appears white, pink or greyish yellow because of the reflection of the tumour. In 35 per cent of cases there is strabismus, while rare cases may exhibit a dilated fixed pupil, hyphaema (blood in the anterior chamber) or heterochromia.

Retinoblastoma arises as a result of mutations in a gene carried either by the germline or somatic cells. When a germinal mutation occurs, every cell of the offspring carries one mutant allele of the retinoblastoma gene. Hence, multiple primary retinoblastoma always develops from a germinal mutation and is an inheritable disease. In the majority of these familial cases, the disease exhibits autosomal dominant inheritance, but with 'incomplete penetrance' (i.e., 5–10 per cent of children who inherit the retinoblastoma gene do not develop the disease). Of the individuals who do, 25–35 per cent develop a unilateral and 60–75 per cent a bilateral tumour. In addition, there are rare families, called 'low penetrance pedigrees', in which individuals can transmit the mutant gene, but are not affected themselves.

Dominant optic atrophy

Optic atrophy is caused by damage to the retinal ganglion cells or their processes that results in cell death. As a consequence, the number of glial cells increases at the affected sites (gliosis) and the number of blood vessels at the optic disk decreases, which results in disk pallor. Optic atrophy can be caused by a variety of problems that affect the retinal ganglion cells, and so hereditary factors are only one of many causes.

The most common optic atrophy linked to hereditary factors is autosomal dominant optic atrophy (ADOA). This disorder is characterised by a slowly developing visual loss in individuals 4–8 years of age. There is a moderate reduction in visual acuity, colour vision is affected and there is temporal disk pallor with thinning of the papillomacular bundle – the patient often becomes legally blind by middle age. In many families, the disorder is linked to a gene on chromosome 3, but there is extreme variation in the expression of the disease in different patients. In addition, some families do not show linkage to the gene on chromosome 3 and it is likely that several other genes could be involved.

Congenital nystagmus

Nystagmus is associated with many causes, which include disease of the semicircular canals of the inner ear, the nuclei of the eighth cranial nerve, the vestibular nuclei and the cerebellum. Congenital nystagmus is similar to acquired vestibular nystagmus in having a slow and fast phase, with the movement usually being horizontal. The development of the condition, which may be present at birth or appear within the first 6 months of life, is usually associated with reduced visual acuity. The disorder is inherited as an autosomal dominant gene and, in many families, is located on chromosome 6. There is considerable variation in the expression of the disease, however, including in the degree of visual acuity, ocular alignment and type of nystagmus present.

Marfan's syndrome

Marfan's syndrome is an example of an autosomal dominant disorder with widespread abnormalities that affect the skeleton, eye and cardiovascular system. Affected individuals have long arms and digits (arachnodactyly) and also have a high arched palate. In these patients, a disorder affects the elastic fibres of connective tissue and causes disorganisation of collagen, which makes the patients vulnerable to thrombosis and to the development of aneurysms on the aorta. The suspensory ligaments of the lens are also affected, so that the lens becomes dislocated into the vitreous. Retinal degeneration is also frequent in these patients and there may be secondary glaucoma.

Marfan's syndrome has been shown to be associated with mutations of the fibrillin genes on chromosome 15. At least two genes are involved – fibrillin 1 (FBN1), which is the main protein of elastic tissue and is present in the suspensory ligaments of the lens, and fibrillin 2 (FBN2), which is present in cartilage and tissues rich in elastin. As in many ocular genetic disorders, there is variability in expression of the disease in different patients because of differences in the mutations present. The prognosis of the condition often depends on the degree of cardiovascular involvement, since the root of the aorta tends to develop aneurysms, and collapse of the mitral valves may also .

Autosomal recessive inheritance

A number of genes associated with ocular disease show a quite different inheritance pattern to that of autosomal dominance. Unlike autosomal dominant inheritance, which is associated with a marked manifestation of the phenotype, those individuals who inherit a single autosomal recessive allele are unlikely to demonstrate any sign of the disease. Nevertheless, as demonstrated in *Figure 8.2*, individuals who inherit two similar defective alleles from their parents become homozygous for the recessive character, and thereby demonstrate the phenotypic characteristics associated with the defective gene. As recessive genes are not expressed in heterozygous individuals, large families or potentially inter-related human populations are required to study the phenotypic manifestation of recessive genes.

Autosomal recessive albinism
Oculocutaneous albinism, which affects both the skin and eye, is inherited as an autosomal recessive gene.[13] In some milder forms, the pigmentation of the skin and hair may be normal, but lighter in colour compared with unaffected siblings. The disorder results from a failure of the synthesis of melanin from the amino acid tyrosine because of an enzyme deficiency. The degree of pigmentation may be highly variable between patients, but the fundus normally appears pale. Vision is often poor and pendular nystagmus is a common associated condition.

Autosomal recessive corneal dystrophy
In contrast to the autosomal dominant forms, macular corneal dystrophy is an autosomal recessive disorder that develops within the first decade of life and has been mapped to chromosome 22.[14] Initially, there is a superficial clouding of the cornea, which then spreads to affect its whole thickness. By early middle age, vision is usually severely affected.

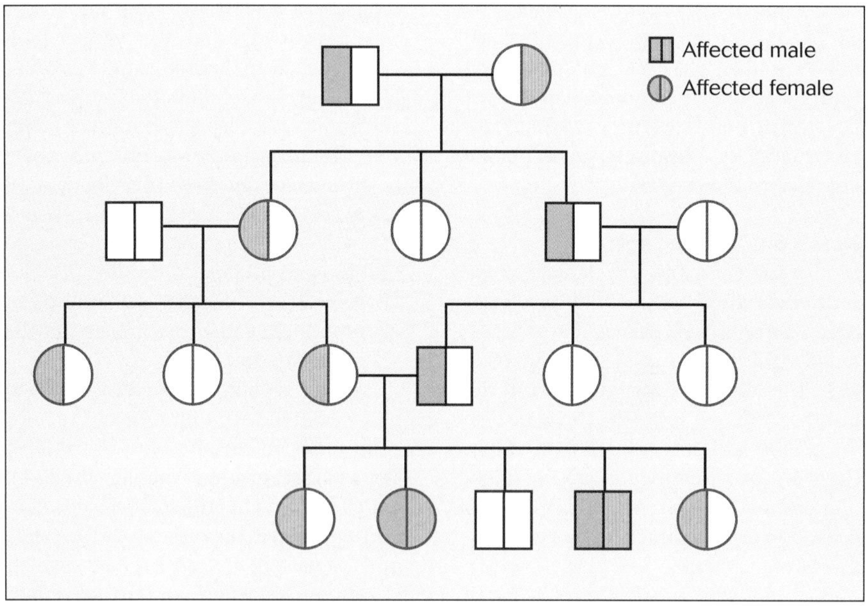

Figure 8.2
Autosomal recessive inheritance in four generations of a family. Notice that marriage of cousins in the third generation was necessary to reveal the phenotype of the recessive gene in the fourth generation

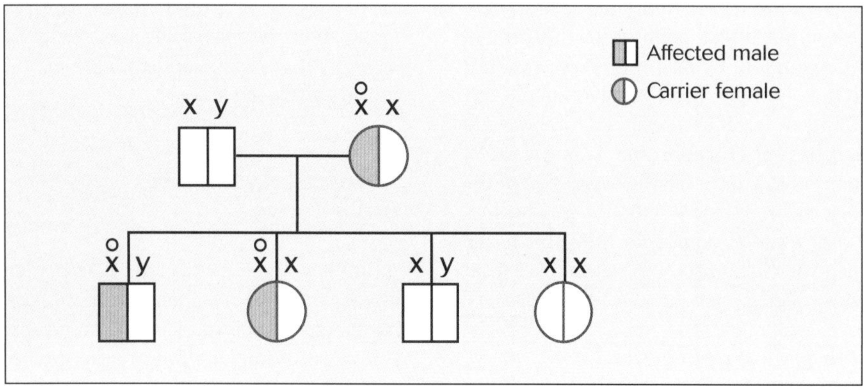

Figure 8.3
Sex-linked inheritance in two generations of a family. Notice that an X-linked recessive gene (X°) may be passed to male and female offspring, but only the male is likely to manifest the disease because of the lack of dominant genes on the Y chromosome to mask its effects

Autosomal recessive glaucoma
Both gene loci associated with congenital glaucoma (GLC3A and GLC3B) exhibit an autosomal recessive pattern of inheritance. Both have a disease onset of less than 3 years of age. GLC3A has been located to a region of chromosome 2, a likely candidate gene being CVP1B1 (the gene for cytochrome P4501B1), while GLC3B has been located to the long arm of chromosome 1.

Autosomal recessive retinitis pigmentosa
Autosomal recessive retinitis pigmentosa (ARRP) is believed to be the most common of the familial forms of RP. As in ADRP, some forms of ARRP are linked to mutations of the rhodopsin gene. ARRP has also been linked to at least nine different genes, however, including the gamma-aminobutyric acid (GABA) receptor gene on chromosome 6,[15] the phosphodiesterase-β subunit gene,[16] the cyclic GMP-gated channel and the Stargardt's disease (STGD) gene (ABCR) located on chromosome 1.[17]

Stargardt's disease
Stargardt's disease is a macular dystrophy (MD) with a juvenile onset and an autosomal recessive pattern of inheritance. This disease, which accounts for up to 7 per cent of human retinal degenerative diseases, is characterised by a progressive loss of central vision, atrophy of the macular region of the retina and pigment epithelium layer, and the presence of orange–yellow flecks on the fundus. Stargardt's disease is linked to mutations of the ABCR gene on chromosome 1, which is also implicated in some forms of RP.[18]

Sex-linked (X) inheritance

Some ocular diseases exhibit inheritance patterns associated with gender, often termed sex linkage. Defective genes and their associated modified phenotypes may manifest more frequently in male members of a pedigree or family under study (*Figure 8.3*). Such an imbalance in phenotype manifestation occurs because females have two copies of the X chromosome and, therefore, two copies of all the X chromosome genes, while the male has only one complete X chromosome. Should a defective gene that shows recessive inheritance occur on the male X chromosome, the lack of a sound partner on the Y chromosome often results in manifestation of the defective gene – an exception to the principle that recessive genes are not manifest in a single dose.

Colour blindness

Of the several forms of colour blindness (see Chapter 2), some can be linked to gene defects. The most common form is anomalous trichromatism, in which there is a 'weakness' in the response to one of the primary colours and the patient, as a result, shows impaired discrimination between certain combinations of colours. Of these types, red–green colour blindness is an X-linked disorder and therefore significantly more common in males than in females.

Sex-linked ocular albinism

Some forms of albinism affect the eye alone and are termed ocular albinism. This type of albinism is inherited as a sex-linked recessive gene termed OA1, a membrane-bound protein believed to be involved in the development of melanosomes. A large number of gene deletions and missense mutations have now been identified in the OA1 gene.[19] Nystagmus, iris transillumination and foveal hypoplasia may all be associated with this disorder. Treatment, including tinted lenses or contact lenses, is often necessary to protect the eye. Refractive errors and strabismus may also require correction.

Sex-linked retinitis pigmentosa

Sex-linked forms of retinitis pigmentosa (XRP) are the least common form of the disease, but the most severe in terms of onset and progression.[20] The majority of cases are linked to the RPGR gene on chromosome 21.[21] The RPGR gene is believed to code for a protein localised within the golgi complex of the cell, which may be involved in cellular transport.[22]

Sex-linked juvenile retinoschisis

Sex-linked juvenile retinoschisis is a degeneration of the periphery of the retina, which usually originates in the plexiform layer and affects the superior temporal quadrant. The gene responsible for this disorder has been located to the 'p' arm of the X chromosome, a region that contains a gene sequence implicated in cell-to-cell interactions and in cell adhesion processes.

Mitochondrial inheritance

Another form of sex-linked inheritance exhibited by some ocular diseases is associated with the female line of inheritance (*Figure 8.4*). Such forms of inheritance are associated with genes that code for mitochondria (cellular organelles responsible for intracellular energy conversion). Mitochondria have their own DNA, which (compared with the more familiar nuclear DNA) demonstrates a unique form, mutation rate and inheritance pattern.

Human beings inherit their mitochondrial DNA, and therefore any defective genes, by acquisition of mitochondria from the female egg during fertilisation. Ocular diseases associated with mitochondrial dysfunction demonstrate one further characteristic, which correlates with the unique nature of mitochondrial DNA and its inheritance. The autonomous nature of mitochondria, particularly their potentially different rates of replication and absence of obvious DNA segregation, results in the nearly random incorporation of mitochondria and associated DNA within developing eggs. Consequently, individuals born to a mother with a mitochondrial genetic defect may show considerable phenotypic variation, which ranges from individuals with more or less normal mitochondrial function and little obvious disease to those with few effective mitochondria and, therefore, more marked disease.

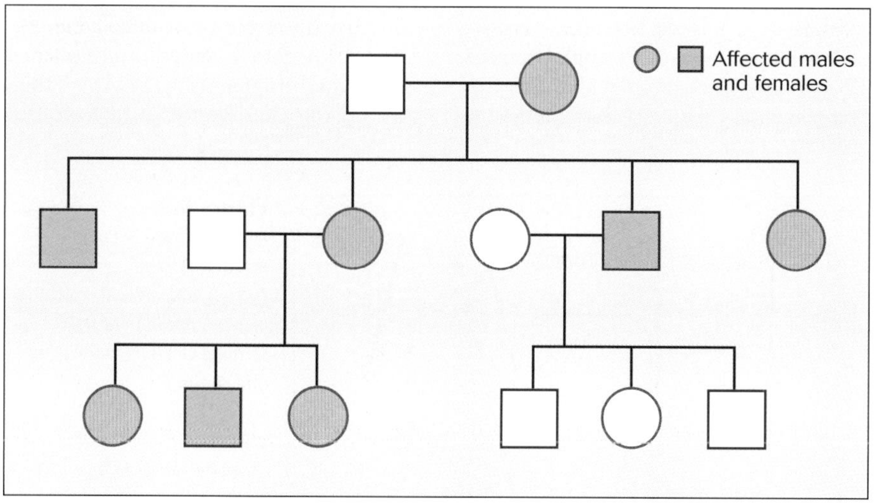

Figure 8.4

Mitochondrial inheritance in three generations of a family. Notice that, although affected males and females may be in the family, the gene is passed on only when an affected female is involved in the pairing

Leber's optic atrophy

Leber's optic neuropathy is a bilateral condition that affects young adults and is characterised by a severe and progressive visual loss. A notable feature is the presence of mitochondrial inheritance[23] and, therefore, the disorder is inherited maternally. In most cases of mitochondrial inheritance, males and females are affected equally, but Leber's optic atrophy is an exception, with young men being affected predominantly. Different mutations of the mitochondrial DNA may be present, and so various degrees of optic atrophy occur.

Retinitis pigmentosa

In addition to sex-linked forms of RP, some cases have been linked to mitochondrial inheritance with point mutations in the ATPase 6 gene of the mitochondrial DNA.[23]

Summary of patterns of inheritance

Virtually all of the known types of inheritance are exhibited by ocular disease (*Table 8.1*). Many individual disorders, such as glaucoma or RP, are complex and may be linked to several different genes that exhibit different patterns of inheritance. Even if an ocular disease is caused by a single gene, there may be variable expression of the disease attributable to variations in the type of mutation present. Studies of the patterns of inheritance of ocular diseases in affected families are a vital first step in locating genes to particular sites on chromosomes. However, development of the techniques of molecular genetics has allowed genes to be located more accurately to particular sites on chromosomes, enabled the DNA to be extracted, cloned within 'vectors' such as bacterial cells and then studied in detail. These studies, which have culminated in the publication of the results of the Human Genome Project, will have a profound impact on many aspects of ocular disease, and are discussed in the final part of this chapter.

Table 8.1 Summary of the patterns of inheritance of the ocular diseases

Type of disorder	*Subtype*	*Inheritance*
Developmental	Aniridia	AD[4]
	Congenital microphthalmos (dominant form)	AD[5]
	Congenital microphthalmos (recessive form)	AR[5]
	Congenital microphthalmos (sex-linked form)	X[5]
Pigment	Oculocutaneous albinism	AR[15]
	Sex-linked albinism	XR[21]
Corneal dystrophy	Reis–Bückler's	AD[6]
	Lattice	AD[7]
	Macular	AR[16]
Cataract	Zonular pulverulent	AD[8]
	Congenital	AD[8]
	Polymorphic	AD[8]
	Cerulean	AD[8]
Glaucoma	Primary open-angle glaucoma	AD[11]
	Congenital glaucoma	AR
Retinitis pigmentosa	ADRP	AD[12–14]
	ARRP	AR[17–19]
	Sex-linked form	X[22–24]
Stargardt's disease	–	AR[20]
Malignant disease	Retinoblastoma	AD
Optic atrophy	Dominant form	AD
	Mitochondrial maternal	M[25]
Nystagmus	Congenital	AD
Marfan's syndrome	–	AD
Colour blindness	Red–green	X-linked
Retinoschisis	Juvenile type	X-linked

AD, autosomal dominant; AR, autosomal recessive; M, mitochondrial inheritance.

Advances in methodology

Until recently there was little information about the exact locations of the genes that cause disease, what type of gene defect was present or the processes by which the defective gene may cause the disease. To obtain this information, recent developments in molecular genetics, most specifically expressed in the Human Genome Project, have been necessary. Hence, the objective of the final sections of this chapter is to describe these recent developments and the impact that they are likely to have on the diagnosis, scientific understanding and future treatment of ocular disease.

Hybridisation

Two techniques of molecular genetics are particularly important in the analysis of the human genome. The first technique is called 'hybridisation' (*Figure 8.5*). As described previously, DNA consists of two strands of nucleotides helically wound around each other and weakly joined by chemical bonds between the respective bases. The two strands are joined in a very precise way, such that an adenine-containing nucleotide on one strand always binds to a thymine nucleotide on the second strand and, correspondingly, a cytosine to a guanine nucleotide. Hence, if one strand of DNA has the sequence AGC, the opposite or complementary strand must be TCG. If DNA is extracted from cells and heated gently, the chemical bonds between the strands are broken and the two strands separate. Conversely, if the strands are allowed to cool they rejoin. Once the two strands are separated, however, it is possible to join or 'hybridise' a single strand of DNA to any piece of DNA that has the complimentary sequence. For example, if a piece of single-stranded DNA is added to a preparation that contains several pieces of single-stranded DNA with different nucleotide sequences, hybridisation takes place only if there is a sequence complementary to that of the original strand. Consequently, this technique can be used to identify whether a particular piece of DNA is present in a mixed preparation of DNA fragments.

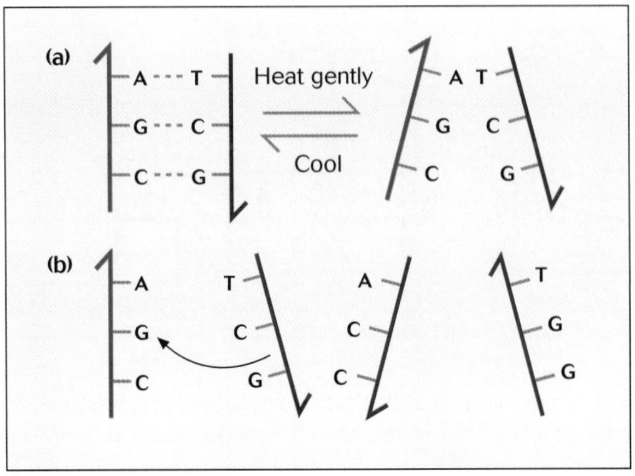

Figure 8.5
Hybridisation between strands of DNA.
(a) Separation and rejoining of the complementary strands of DNA by heating and cooling.
(b) Identification of the presence of a particular strand of DNA in a mixed preparation using hybridisation

Restriction enzymes

A second major advance was the discovery of a special class of enzymes, mainly isolated from bacteria, called 'restriction enzymes'. Each type of restriction enzyme 'recognises' a particular sequence of nucleotides and cuts the DNA at a defined point within that sequence. For example, the restriction enzyme 'PstI' recognises the DNA sequence CTCGAC and cuts it between the adenine-containing and the cytosine-containing nucleotides.

Hence, we have methods to break the DNA molecule into pieces so that it can be studied more readily and a particular piece of DNA identified. The development of these methods is extremely important because they enable a human gene to be isolated from the human genome and grown or 'cloned' inside a bacterial cell.

Cloning a human gene

The human genome is too complex to study in its entirety. Characterisation of ocular disease therefore requires the human genome to be broken up into smaller fragments so that an individual element can be isolated and studied. Hence, DNA is extracted from cells by homogenisation and then isolated and purified (*Figure 8.6*). Restriction enzymes, which cut the DNA in a specific way, are added to the preparation and split the original DNA into a series of fragments. Individual fragments of DNA are then incorporated into 'vectors', which are usu-

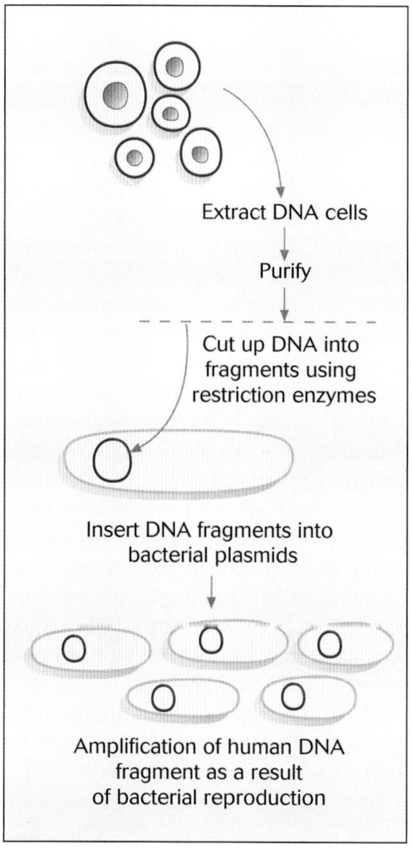

Figure 8.6
Cloning a human gene inside bacterial cells

which has a code matching that of the mRNA, is often synthesised for the detailed study of gene sequences.

As a consequence of breaking up the genome with restriction enzymes and the cloning of the DNA fragments, thousands of transformed cells result, many, if not all, of which play host to different DNA sequences. Identification of the cells that contain a particular sequence is carried out by a process called 'probing'. Essentially, this involves the hybridisation of single-stranded DNA with a defined sequence, marked or tagged so as to make it visible, to single-stranded DNA extracted and prepared from the transformed cells. Once identified, the order of nucleotides along the DNA can be established by 'sequencing'. This process involves separation of radioactive cDNA sequences by gel electrophoresis to produce a pattern that can be converted into a coding sequence. A comparison of the genetic material from normal subjects with that from patients with a specific disease enables the presence of changes in the DNA caused by gene mutations to be identified. One problem in this approach, however, is that only relatively short portions of DNA can be sequenced at a time. Since many genes involved in ocular disease may be 20,000 nucleotides long, more complex methods may be required to sequence the whole gene.

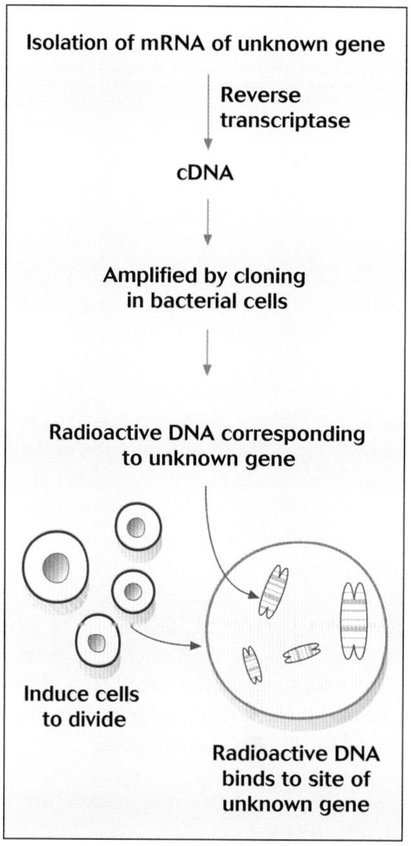

Figure 8.7
Establishing the location of a gene by 'in situ *hybridisation*'

ally bacterial plasmids or viruses. These 'vectors' have the capacity to transport the DNA fragments into other living cells that are particularly suited for storage and culture in the laboratory. Growth and reproduction of the transformed cells in culture results in a large number of copies of the original DNA fragment, such that after further extraction and purification it can be studied in detail.

Most of the DNA extracted from human cells has little relevance to ocular disease. The DNA of a gene consists of a number of exons that provide the code for the appropriate protein, separated by DNA sequences called introns, which do not. During protein synthesis, the DNA sequence of the gene is used as a template or code to manufacture a single-stranded nucleic acid called messenger RNA (mRNA). This process, called 'transcription', incorporates the DNA code represented by the exons only. Hence, to study the exons directly, the mRNA that corresponds to the DNA of interest is isolated and purified. RNA is degraded readily by enzymes, however, which makes it less useful than DNA to study gene defects. Hence, biologically more stable double-stranded DNA, called complementary DNA (cDNA),

Locating genes within the human genome

A combination of methods, which includes mapping, sequencing and cloning, is used to locate a particular gene in the human genome.

In situ hybridisation

The principal method used to determine the location of a gene within the human genome is called *in situ* hybridisation and was developed in the early 1980s (*Figure 8.7*). First, the mRNA, which codes for the gene and the chromosomal location of which is to be mapped, is isolated from the genome. An enzyme called reverse transcriptase is used to synthesise cDNA, which has a code corresponding to that of the mRNA. The cDNA is produced in large quantities by cloning in bacterial cells, as described above. A radioactive preparation of cDNA is added to cells that have been induced to divide so that their chromosomes, and therefore their unique banding patterns, are visible. The labelled cDNA has a base sequence corresponding to that of the particular part of the DNA that contains the gene in question and binds tightly to it, and thus reveals its chromosomal location.

Linkage analysis

If no information is available as to the DNA sequence of a disease-causing gene, in certain circumstances the gene can be located to a specific site by a technique called 'linkage analysis'. To understand linkage analysis requires knowledge of the events that take place in the cells to give rise to the sex cells (see Appendix 2). Each cell contains two complete sets of chromosomes, one set inherited from each of our parents. The sperm and eggs, however, only contain one complete set of chromosomes produced by a process of cell division called 'meiosis', during which the number of chromosomes is halved. During meiosis, each maternal chromosome pairs with the corresponding paternal chromosome, and the two exchange genes by 'crossing-over'. The consequence of this process of crossing-over is that some of the sex cells produced have chromosomes with genes from both parents. Such sex cells are said to contain 'recombinants'. Whether or not recombinants of a particular pair of parental genes occur depends on how close the genes are on the chromosome. If two genes are at either ends of the chromosome, it is almost certain that a cross-over point occurs between them. If two genes are very close together (i.e., side-by-side on the same chromosome), it is much less likely for recombinants to form as a cross-over point has to occur precisely between the two genes. As a consequence, both genes end up in the same sex cell and are inherited by the same individual.

To carry out linkage analysis requires a gene for which the mRNA sequence is established already and which is located adjacent to the unknown gene on the same chromosome, so close that it is unlikely to be separated from it at meiosis. Such a gene may be identified by examination of individuals in the family from different generations and by identifying characters that are shown only by individuals who have the disease and hence who carry the unknown gene. Once such a gene has been identified, it can be located by *in situ* hybridisation, as described previously. Examination of the DNA in regions of the chromosome close to this gene may then reveal the disease-causing gene.

Locations for genes responsible for ocular disease

As a result of the application of these methods, the genes associated with several ocular diseases have been identified and located to particular chromosomes (*Table 8.2*). Some of these disorders have relatively simple patterns of inheritance and are associated with a single defective gene. For example, the hereditary form of retinoblastoma is associated with a single gene located on chromosome 13 at a position designated 13q14 (i.e., the gene is located on the 'q' arm of the chromosome within band 14).[24,25] However, the majority of ocular diseases exhibit more complex patterns of inheritance (i.e., different gene defects may be present in different families with the same disease). For example, cataract is associated with at least seven different genes,[26,27] diabetic retinopathy with at least three genes and primary open-angle glaucoma with at least 10 different genes.[28–30] The retinal dystrophies are a particularly complex group of disorders in which at least 66 different genes have been implicated,[31] while RP itself, an important member of this group, may be associated with at least 22 genes. Further complexity arises because different mutations of the same gene may be present. For example, in a large survey of cases of retinoblastoma, several different types of point mutation were identified in different families.[32]

The 'Human Genome Project'

The human genetic programme is a library of instructions of how to make all the proteins necessary for life. Its individual elements, the genes, are arranged along the chromosomes (i.e., the genetic library is arranged in 23 separate 'volumes'). If this library was understood completely we would know the nucleotide sequence of each chromosome and the sequence and location of each of the genes. The Human Genome Project to provide a complete nucleotide sequence and expression map of the genome was discussed as early as 1985,[33] and the initial programme began in 1990. By June 2000, 90 per cent of the genome had been mapped and the process was completed and published early in 2001. Progress in sequencing the human genome relied on rapid progress in molecular genetics, technological advances and the appearance of private sector companies.

The human genetic programme comprises 3.2 billion base pairs[34] or nucleotides that code for approximately 30,000 genes – far fewer than originally predicted. One of the first conclusions of the project was that all human beings are remarkably similar; in fact, 99.9 per cent similar at the

Table 8.2 Locations within the human genome of the genes associated with a selection of ocular diseases and syndromes

Disorder	*Pattern of inheritance*	*Number of major genes*	*Gene locations (where known)*
Aniridia	AD	1	11p13
Anophthalmia	AD	1	14q22
Cataract	AD	7	1p, 2q33–35, 13 Cen, 17q24,17p12–13, 19q13.3–13.4, 22q, 21q22.3
Congenital juvenile retinoschisis	XR	1	X22.1–22.2
Congenital microphthalmos	AD, AR, X	3	14q32(AR type)
Congenital nystagmus	AD	1	6p12
Congenital stationary night blindness	XR	1	Xp11.23
Corneal dystrophies	AD, AR	7	1p35–36.1, 5p, 5q, 12q, 17q, 20q11, 16q22
Diabetic retinopathy	Unclear	3	7q21.3–22.1, 7q35
Duane's syndrome	AD	1	8q13–21.2
Marfan's syndrome	AD	1	15
Ocular albinism	X, AR	2	Xp22.3–22.2
Optic atrophy	AD, M	2	3q28–29 (AD type)
Primary open-angle glaucoma	AD, AR	10	1p36, 1q21–23, 2p21, 2cen-q13, 3q21–24, 8q23, 10p14–15
Ptosis	AD	1	1p32–34.1
Retinitis pigmentosa	AD, AR, X	22	1p12.1–12.3, 3q21–24, 4p16, 6p, 6q, Xp21.1
Retinoblastoma	AD	1	13q14
Stargardt's disease	AR	1	1p21–22

AD, autosomal dominant; AR, autosomal recessive; X, X-linked; M, mitochondrial inheritance. Each of the 23 individual chromosomes in the human genome is composed of a 'p' arm (p) and a 'q' arm (q) separated by a constriction called the centromere (cen). A gene location is defined by chromosome number, whether the gene is on the 'p' or 'q' arm, and the position of the gene in relation to the black-and-white bands unique to each chromosome.

genetic level, with the remaining 0.1 per cent being responsible for all human variation.[35] The full implications of the Human Genome Project, however, are still unclear. It provides a complete catalogue of genes and therefore will be extremely valuable in the study of disease susceptibility,[36] and in the cell biology of gene interactions. Most authors emphasise the particular importance of the project to the fundamental study of disease, including improved diagnosis, more specific screening and better treatment.[37] Nevertheless, there is a complexity of legal, ethical and social concerns about the use and abuse of the potential information from the genome project, as well as scientific concerns regarding the availability for study of data that result from the filing of patents.[38] In the future, all health professionals will need to be knowledgeable about the new genetics so that patients can be offered the most appropriate guidance and care.

Implications for ocular disease

Classification of disease

Increased knowledge of ocular genetics is likely to lead to a reclassification of some disorders – especially if they are determined by several genes. For example, RP is a member of a heterogeneous group of retinal degenerative diseases that includes congenital stationary night blindness (CSNB), MD, cone–rod dystrophy (CRD) and age-related macular degeneration (AMD).[39] A significant proportion of these cases may be linked to defective genes (see above). One of the major consequences of recent genetic research is the recognition that different disorders may be linked to mutations of the same gene. For example, mutations of the rhodopsin gene have been linked to RP and CSNB, the peripherin/RDS gene with RP and MD and the Stargardt's disease gene with RP, CRD and possibly AMD. In addition, considerable genetic heterogeneity has been discovered within RP itself, with several gene defects present, some of which may be associated with different clinical and pathological features. The consequence of this research is the likelihood that the retinal dystrophies and other types of genetic disorder could be reclassified, based on genetic data, with the relationships between RP and other disorders emphasised.

Diagnosis of genetic disease

Genetic screening that can identify the various mutations in defective genes will have important consequences for the genetic counselling of a number of ocular diseases. For example, identification of mutations in the genes associated with familial glaucoma could potentially aid early diagnosis and be important for the optimal application of existing therapies.[40] The majority of ocular diseases, like glaucoma, for example, are complex and different gene defects may be present in different families with the same disease. Although the identification of specific gene defects should aid diagnosis, the degree of heterogeneity present in some ocular diseases may make genetic counselling in individual cases particularly complex.

Understanding disease processes

Studies of the physiological function of the proteins coded by defective genes should provide a much greater understanding of the basic mechanisms that cause individual disorders. Although defects in the genes associated with many ocular diseases are now identified, how these mutations may result in disease processes has not been established clearly. Nevertheless, in a few cases it is possible to speculate about the basic mechanism of the disease process once the function of the protein coded by the defective gene is known.

The gene for retinoblastoma codes for a protein, called RB protein, involved in regulation of the cell cycle that leads to cell division.[41] The most common mutation observed in this gene is a substitution of a single nucleotide (i.e., a thymine nucleotide for a cytosine nucleotide). This mutation converts the code for the amino acid arginine into a code that instructs the cell to terminate protein synthesis.[42] Such a mutation results in the production of shortened or truncated versions of the RB protein. Hence, abnormal forms of RB protein could disrupt the cell cycle and result in cell proliferation.

Several of the genes associated with cataract may have a direct influence on lens transparency, such as the connexin-50 gene on chromosome 1 and the α-, β- and γ-crystallin genes on chromosomes 21,[26] 22,[43] and 2,[44] respectively.

An important gene associated with primary open-angle glaucoma is the gene for the protein myocilin located on chromosome 1,[28] which codes for the TIGR protein. TIGR is a cytoskeletal protein involved in the development of the organelle that, in ciliated epithelial cells, organises microtubules. Hence, it is possible that defects in TIGR protein may lead to abnormalities in the ciliated epithelium that lines the trabecular meshwork and, therefore, to an inhibition of the drainage of aqueous.

Some cases of insulin-dependent diabetes with retinopathy have been associated with the paraoxinase gene (PON1) on chromosome 7. Serum paraoxinase binds to high-density lipoproteins and thus prevents their oxidation. Hence, an inhibition of this process could be an important factor in the development of diabetic retinopathy.

Treatment of genetic disorders

Increased understanding of the basic pathological processes that underlie genetic disorders may lead to improvements in conventional treatments. For example, in certain forms of glaucoma, increased knowledge of how defects in TIGR protein may lead to abnormalities in the ciliated epithelium that lines the trabecular meshwork could lead directly to better treatments in paediatric science. In addition, identification of the locations and defects in disease genes, and further development of the techniques of molecular biology, make gene therapy for some ocular diseases a future possibility.

References

1 Armstrong RA (1999). Ocular disease and the new genetics. *Ophthalmic Physiol Opt.* **19**, 193–195.

2 Drechsler M and Royer-Pokova B (1996). A line element is present at the site of a 300-kB deletion starting in intron-10 of the PAX6 gene in a case of familial aniridia. *Hum Genet.* **98**, 297–303.

3 Bessant DAR, Khaliq S, Hameed A, *et al.* (1996). A locus for autosomal recessive congenital microphthalmia maps to chromosome 14q32. *Am J Hum Genet.* **62**, 1113–1116.

4 Small KW, Mullen L, Barletta J, *et al.* (1996). Mapping of Reis–Bückler's corneal dystrophy to chromosome 5q. *Am J Ophthalmol.* **121**, 384–390.

5 Meins M, Kohlias M, Richard G and Gal A (1998). Lattice corneal dystrophy type 1: Clinical and molecular genetic analysis in a large family. *Klin Monat Augenheil.* **212**, 154–158.

6 Armstrong RA and Smith SN (2000). The genetics of cataract. *Optom Today* **Nov 17th**, 33–35.

7 Becker B, Kolkar AE and Roth FD (1960). Glaucoma family study. *Am J Ophthalmol.* **50**, 557–567.

8 Kellerman L and Posner A (1955). The value of heredity in the detection and study of glaucoma. *Am J Ophthalmol.* **40**, 681–685.

9 Bennett SR, Alward WL and Folberg R (1989). An autosomal dominant form of low-tension glaucoma. *Am J Ophthalmol.* **108**, 238–244.

10 Gal A, Apfelsted-Sylla E, Janecke AR and Zrenner E (1997). Rhodopsin mutations in inherited dystrophies and dysfunctions. *Prog Ret Eye Res.* **16**, 51–79.

11 Lewin AS, Dreuser KA and Hanswirth WW (1998). Ribozyme rescue of photoreceptor cells in a transgenic rat model of autosomal dominant retinitis pigmentosa. *Nature Med.* **4**, 967–971.

12 Goldberg AFX, Loewen JR and Molday RA (1998). Cysteine residues of photoreceptor peripherin/RDS: Role in subunit assembly and autosomal dominant retinitis pigmentosa. *Biochemistry* **37**, 680–685.

13 Morell A, Spritz RA, Ho L, *et al.* (1997). Apparent digenic inheritance of Waardenburg syndrome type 2 (WS2) and autosomal recessive ocular albinism (AROA). *Hum Mol Genet.* **6**, 659–664.

14 Liu NP, Baldwin C, Lennon F, *et al.* (1998). Coexistence of macular corneal dystrophy types I and II in a single sibship. *Br J Ophthalmol.* **82**, 241–244.

15 Ruiz A, Borrego S, Marcos I and Antinolo G (1998). A major locus for autosomal recessive retinitis pigmentosa on 6q determined by homozygosity mapping of chromosomal regions that contain gamma-aminobutyric acid receptor clusters. *Am J Hum Genet.* **62**, 1452–1459.

16 Saga M, Mashima Y and Akeo K (1998). A novel homozygous Lle535Asn mutation in the rod cGMP phosphodiesterase beta subunit gene in two brothers of a Japanese family with autosomal recessive retinitis pigmentosa. *Curr Eye Res.* **17**, 332–335.

17 Cremers FPM, van de Pol DJA and van Driel M (1998). Autosomal recessive retinitis pigmentosa and cone–rod dystrophy caused by splice site mutations in the Stargardt's disease gene ABCR. *Hum Genet.* **7**, 355–362.

18 Armstrong RA (2000). The ROD photoreceptor ABCR gene and its significance in ocular disease. *Optician* **220**, 19–24.

19 Schnur RE, Gao M, Wick PA and Keller M (1998). OA1 mutations and deletions in X-linked ocular albinism. *Am J Hum Genet.* **62**, 800–809.

20 Capeans C, Blanco MJ and Lareu MV (1998). Analysis in a large family with X-linked retinitis pigmentosa: Phenotype–genotype correlation. *Clin Genet.* **54**, 26–32.

21 Weleber RG, Butter MS and Murphey WH (1997). X-linked retinitis pigmentosa associated with a two base pair insertion in codon 99 of the RP3 gene RPGR. *Arch Ophthalmol.* **115**, 1429–1435.

22 Yan D, Swain PK and Breur D (1998). Biochemical characterisation and subcellular localisation of the mouse retinitis pigmentosa GTPase regulator (mRpgr). *J Biol Chem.* **273**, 19656–19663.

23 Graeber MB and Muller U (1998). Recent developments in the molecular genetics of mitochondrial disorders. *J Neurol Sci.* **153**, 251–263.

24 Benedict WF, Srivatsan ES, Mark C, Banerjee A, Sparkes RS and Murphree AL (1987). Complete or partial homozygosity of chromosome 13 in primary retinoblastoma. *Cancer Res.* **47**, 4189–4191.

25 Toguchida J, McGee TL, Paterson JC, *et al.* (1993). Complete genomic sequence of the human retinoblastoma susceptibility gene. *Genomics* **17**, 535–543.

26 Litt M, Kramer P, La Morticella DM, Murphey W, Lovrien EW and Welaber RG (1998). Autosomal dominant congenital cataract associated with a missense mutation in the human alpha crystallin gene CRYAA. *Hum Mol Genet.* **7**, 471–474.

27 Martin ME, Fargion S, Brissot P, Pellat B and Beaumont C (1998). A point mutation in the bulge of the iron-responsive element of the L-ferritin gene in two families with hereditary hyperferritinemia–cataract syndrome. *Blood* **91**, 319–323.

28 Angius A, De Gioia E, Loi A, *et al.* (1998). A novel mutation in the GLCIA gene causes juvenile open-angle glaucoma in four families from the Italian region of Puglia. *Arch Ophthalmol.* **116**, 793–797.

29 Graff C, Jerndal T and Wadelius C (1997). Fine mapping of the gene for autosomal dominant juvenile onset glaucoma with iridogoniodysgenesis in 6p25-tel. *Hum Genet.* **101**,130–134.

30 Nishimura DY, Swiderski RE, Alward WLM, *et al.* (1998). The forkhead transcription factor gene FKHL7 is responsible for glaucoma phenotypes which map to 6p25. *Nature Genet.* **19**, 140–147.

31 Inglehearn CF (1998). Molecular genetics of human retinal dystrophies. *Eye* **12**, 571–579.

32 Blanquet V, Turleau C, Gross-Morand MS, Beaufort CS, Doz F and Besmond C (1995). Spectrum of germline mutations in the RB1 gene: A study of 232 patients with hereditary and non-hereditary retinoblastoma. *Hum Mol Genet.* **4**, 383–388.

33 Le Paslier D and Bernot A (2001). Human Genome Project: After fifteen years of effort. *M S-Med Sci.* **17**, 294–298.

34 Semsarian C and Seidman CE (2001). Molecular medicine in the 21st century. *Int Med J.* **31**, 53–59.

35 Collins FS and Mansoura MK (2001). The Human Genome Project: Revealing the shared inheritance of all humankind. *Cancer* **91**, 221–225.

36 Schimpf MD and Domino SE (2001). Implications of the Human Genome Project for obstetrics and gynecology. *Obst Gyn Surv.* **56**, 437–443.

37 Greene RA, Jenkins TM and Wapner R (2001). The new genetic era in reproductive medicine: Possibilities, probabilities and problems. *Int J Fertil Womens Med.* **46**, 169–183.

38 Gilbert PX and Walter C (2001). Patents and the human genome project: New claims for old? *Trends Biotechnol.* **19**, 49–52

39 Armstrong RA and Smith SN (1999). Retinitis pigmentosa and the new genetics. *Optom Today* **Dec 17th**, 26–32.

40 Stone EM, Fingert JH, Alward WLM, *et al.* (1997). Identification of a gene that causes primary open angle glaucoma. *Science* **275**, 668–670.

41 Stahl A, Levy N, Wadzynska T, Sussan JM, Jourdanfonta D and Saracco JB (1994). The genetics of retinoblastoma. *Ann Genet.* **37**, 172–178.

42 Hogg A, Bia B, Onadim Z and Cowell JK (1993). Molecular mechanisms of oncogenic mutations in tumors from patients with bilateral and unilateral retinoblastoma. *Proc Natl Acad Sci USA* **90**, 7351–7355.

43 Litt M, Carrero-Valenzuela R, *et al.* (1997) Autosomal dominant cerulean cataract is associated with a chain termination mutation in the human beta-crystallin gene CRYBB2. *Hum Mol Genet.* **6**, 665–668.

44 Rogaev EI, Rogaeva EA, Korovaitseva GI, *et al.* (1996). Linkage of polymorphic congenital cataract to the gamma-crystallin gene locus on human chromosome 2q33-35. *Hum Mol Genet.* **5**, 699–703.

9

Paediatric Eye Disorders: Cataract, Retinopathy and Visual Dysfunction

Susmito Biswas and Christopher Lloyd

Childhood cataract
Retinopathy of prematurity
Retinoblastoma
Abnormal visual development

Childhood cataract

Cataract affects approximately three in every 10,000 children in the UK. The successful management of paediatric cataract (*Figure 9.1*) falls under five headings:

- Assessment of cataract morphology and/or severity;
- Timing of surgical intervention;
- Optical correction;
- Acuity measurement and amblyopia therapy;
- Management of complications.

Assessment of cataract morphology and/or severity

The paediatric ophthalmologist who examines a child with a cataract should first of all determine the morphology of the cataract and its severity.[1] This requires a slit-lamp examination. The hand-held slit lamp is a very useful tool for use in younger children. Anterior polar cataracts are central superficial opacities located on the anterior lens capsule. Surgical intervention is rarely needed, but these opacities can be associated with anisometropic amblyopia, and occasionally progress. Nuclear cataracts (*Figure 9.1*) involve the nucleus of the crystalline lens (central fetal or embryonic). They are usually visually significant[2] and must be recognised in early infancy to ensure the appropriate intervention (usually surgical).

Sutural cataracts are opacities of the Y-shaped sutures of the fetal nucleus. These are less amblyogenic and may or may not require intervention. Lamellar cataracts are cataracts of the cortex around the lens nucleus and usually carry a good visual prognosis. Often they do not require intervention until later in childhood.

Posterior lenticonus, a congenital abnormality of the posterior capsule, leads to a posterior opacity and refractive changes related to the increased curvature of the posterior lens surface. This may be minimal in infancy, but later in childhood it may progress to a dense opacity that requires surgical removal. Posterior subcapsular cataracts can occur after the use of systemic corticosteroids or external beam radiation. They may also occur following trauma. Persistent hyperplastic primary vitreous (PHPV) is usually unilateral and associated with persistence of the primitive fetal vascular system. Affected eyes are usually microphthalmic. The opacity varies in its severity, but is usually significant. There is an association with glaucoma in affected eyes.

Timing of surgical intervention

If a cataract causes significant visual problems, surgical removal is indicated. Visually significant cataracts in a neonate should be removed within the critical peri-

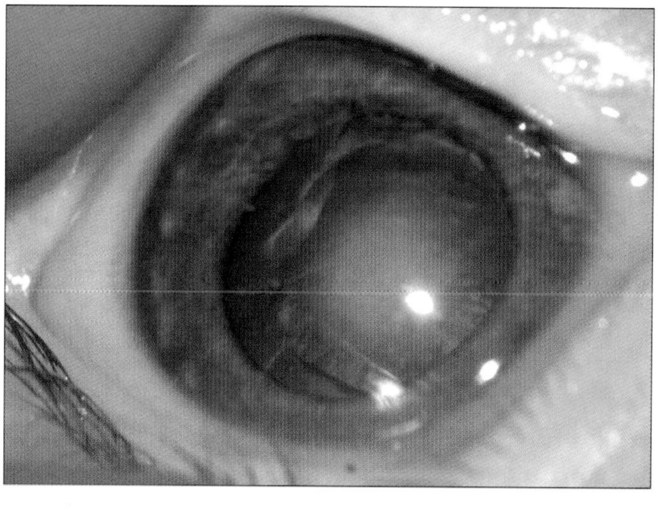

Figure 9.1
A nuclear (highly amblyogenic) congenital cataract

od for visual development to avoid irreversible deprivation amblyopia. Children with lamellar cataracts or milder posterior lenticonus cataracts may be managed conservatively or by operative intervention deferred until later in life.

Modern microsurgical techniques that combine small-incision surgery and capsulorrhexis have improved the management of paediatric cataracts dramatically. Intraocular lenses are becoming a common method of optical rehabilitation, although most paediatric ophthalmologists continue to perform lensectomy followed by contact lens correction in the infant born with dense congenital cataract.

Implantation of an intraocular lens in a young infant is technically more difficult than in an older child or adult. Even when such surgery is carried out successfully the re-operation rate is very high.[3] This is usually because of the consequences of re-proliferation of lens epithelial cells and/or capsular opacification. Despite this, encouraging results have been reported,[1,3,4] and some authors have even suggested that there is a protective effect against the onset of aphakic glaucoma, although this claim is probably premature.

Optical correction

Early optical correction of such children is critical. In those children who have lensectomy, the fitting of contact lenses should occur within days of surgery. Aphakic glasses are provided as a back up for when contact lenses are not used. In some families with inherited cataract, the main carer may be visually impaired. It is difficult for such individuals to manage contact lens insertion and removal, and in this situation the prescription of aphakic spectacles for permanent wear is sensible.

If an intraocular lens is to be implanted, a decision has to be made as to the power of the intraocular lens used. In our unit, keratometry and biometry are carried out under anaesthesia immediately prior to the cataract operation. However, the infant eye is in a period of rapid ocular growth and emmetropisation. The post-operative refraction required must take this into account. Infants less than 4 months of age are therefore left 8–9D undercorrected (i.e., hypermetropic) to allow for the subsequent rapid axial elongation and corneal curvature changes that occur over the next year. This overcorrection is modified in older children whose eyes have undergone the majority of expected growth. Children of 5 years and older are left with only 1D of overcorrection (to allow for the small amount of axial elongation that occurs in late childhood at around puberty).

Acuity measurement and amblyopia therapy

It is essential to monitor acuity development regularly in each eye separately and to tailor amblyopia treatment accordingly. Children born with unilateral congenital cataract need long-term 'aggressive' occlusion therapy (6–8 hours daily) if a good result is to be achieved in the affected eye.[1]

Children with bilateral cataracts often exhibit strabismus with associated amblyopia, which is treated with low levels of part time occlusion. A significant proportion of children born with unilateral congenital cataract achieve a good outcome in the affected eye (visual acuity better than 6/24) if surgery is carried out early, but this outcome is very dependent on compliance with occlusion and optical correction.

Children with bilateral cataracts do well (6/18 or better) if they have early surgery, comply with optical correction and avoid major complications, such as glaucoma.[1]

Management of complications

Aphakic (open-angle) glaucoma may occur in the early post-operative period or as late as decades after surgery.[5] Late-onset aphakic glaucoma occurs in approximately one-third of children who undergo infantile surgery for cataracts.

Pupil-block glaucoma is seen in neonates, usually soon after lensectomy. This is caused by the formation of a post-operative pupillary membrane or as a result of acute prolapse of the residual vitreous body into the anterior chamber, when a peripheral iridectomy has not been performed at the initial lensectomy. Treatment is by surgical vitrectomy and peripheral iridectomy. The prognosis is good if the eye is treated early before the formation of anterior synechiae.

Strabismus is very common in children with untreated cataracts and also in those who have undergone cataract surgery. It reflects the suboptimal binocular functions present in such children. Esotropia is seen more commonly than exotropia.

Nystagmus affects at least 50 per cent of children and is associated with deprivation amblyopia, late surgery and poorer acuity outcomes. Latent nystagmus is very common and thus the binocular acuity of a child with cataracts is often markedly better than their monocular acuity. Pupil irregularities are often seen and may be iatrogenic.

Intervention is needed if a vitreous strand extends to the incision site and causes peaking of the pupil. Such vitreous wicks can predispose to infection, uveitis and retinal detachment. Retinal detachment is a serious and, fortunately, relatively rare complication (approximately 2 per cent), but can occur many years after cataract surgery.

Capsular fibrosis and secondary membranes result from residual lens material left after surgery. Management involves anterior segment revision. The horizontally mounted yttrium–aluminium–garnet (YAG) laser can be used to clear the visual axis in older children under general anaesthesia.

Surgical intervention is usually required in infants who have had procedures that spare the posterior capsule, as the capsular fibrosis formed is very thick and not cleared easily with the laser.

Post-operative intraocular infection (endophthalmitis) is a very rare, but potentially devastating, complication (0.07–0.4 per cent).[6] Prompt treatment with intraocular antibiotics is necessary to save visual function in affected eyes.

Retinopathy of prematurity

Retinopathy of prematurity (ROP), previously known as retrolental fibroplasia, was first described in 1942 in infants born prematurely[7] and exposed to oxygen therapy. It has become clear that many other factors play a role in the pathogenesis of this condition and that oxidative insult is only part of the story.

In addition to gestational age and low birth weight, a number of other risk factors for the development of this condition are really markers of a sick neonate (e.g., unstable haemodynamic state or respiratory distress).

Severe disease is confined mainly to infants with a birth weight less than 1250g and less than 30 weeks gestational age. Detailed screening protocols have been drawn up and implemented in neonatal units to ensure infants at risk of developing severe ROP are not missed[8] (for a more detailed review of these, see Chapter 14). ROP affects the immature retinal vessels at the interface of the preterm infant's fundus between vascularised and non-vascularised retina.

ROP is divided into five stages. In stage one a demarcation line separates vascularised and non-vascularised retina. This demarcation may become elevated to form a ridge in stage two ROP. If there is no progression beyond this, infants who reach these stages usually show spontaneous regression and do not require treatment.

In stage three the demarcation line has evidence of neovascularisation. If this involves more than five contiguous or more than eight cumulative clock hours in the presence of 'plus' disease (dilation and tortuosity of posterior pole vessels), treatment is indicated. This usually involves laser treatment to the avascular retina. Cryotherapy used to be the mainstay of treatment, but is technically more difficult to apply and is less well tolerated than laser, but remains helpful in some situations. Stage four disease is typified by a subtotal retinal detachment. In stage five disease, there is a funnel-shaped complete retinal detachment. Treatment of stage four and stage five disease has not yet been shown to offer a significant benefit to affected children.

Children who have been treated successfully require long-term follow-up. They are at significant risk of developing strabismus, refractive error, anisometropia and amblyopia. Retinal vessels may have a dragged appearance and folds may exist across the macula, which limits vision in children with regressed ROP.

Many children affected by ROP also suffer neurological problems related to cerebral intraventricular haemorrhage and periventricular leukomalacia. Cortical visual impairment is a common problem in this group.

Retinoblastoma

Retinoblastoma (*Figures 9.2* and *9.3*) is the most common malignant ocular tumour of childhood. It arises from primitive retinal cells and, thus, usually presents in children under the age of 4 years. It is, fortunately, rare and affects approximately one in every 20,000 children. If left untreated it is almost always fatal.

Modern treatment modalities result in a survival rate of over 90 per cent in developed countries. Close collaboration between ophthalmologists and oncologists in a centre that specialises in the management of retinoblastoma is needed for the best outcomes. Modern treatment has moved away from external beam radiotherapy (which may predispose treated children to secondary tumours) and towards a combination of chemotherapy and focal localised treatment.

Approximately 44 per cent of all cases of retinoblastoma are hereditary cases with a germ-line mutation in the RB1 gene (i.e., mutation present in virtually every cell in the body). This gene has been shown to have a role as a tumour suppressor. Studies of retinoblastoma tumours show that both hereditary and non-hereditary tumours develop because of the loss of the last normal allele of this gene.

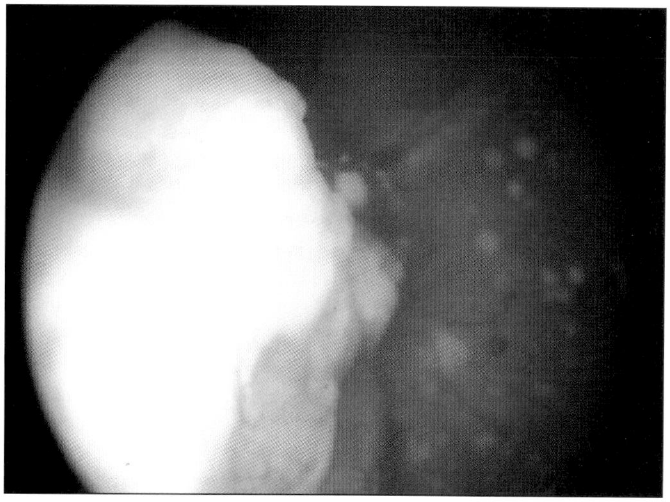

Figure 9.2
A large endophytic retinoblastoma with vitreous seeding (Retcam image). (Courtesy of Mr H Willshaw)

Knudson noted that children with bilateral retinoblastoma presented at a younger age than those with non-hereditary retinoblastoma. This resulted in the 'two-hit' hypothesis,[9] and has improved the understanding of tumour formation in general.

A single second mutation, or 'second hit', of the RB1 gene in the primitive retinal cells of a child predisposed by a previous germ-line mutation, 'first hit', in RB1 is a relatively likely occurrence. Thus, hereditary retinoblastomas, in which the child inherits a germ-line mutation of one of the RB1 alleles, are often multiple and present early. The chance that two mutational events will occur in the same retinal cell is relatively remote, and thus non-hereditary tumours are usually single and present later in childhood.

Retinoblastomas are malignant neuroblastic tumours characterised on histological examination by cellular rosette formation in some areas. They are usually pale or creamy lesions on clinical examination. These thus form part of the differential diagnosis of leucokoria.

Strabismus is also a common presenting sign. All children with constant unilateral strabismus should have a fundus examination to rule out retinal pathology. Children with more advanced disease may present with a painful red eye or signs that mimic orbital cellulitis. Calcification is pathognomonic and helps in diagnosis because this calcification shows up on both ultrasound and computed tomography (CT) scan.

There are two main growth patterns. Endophytic tumours grow forwards into the vitreous cavity, while exophytic tumours grow into the subretinal space and cause a retinal detachment. Diffuse infiltrating retinoblastoma is a rarer form of tumour that presents in an older age group and mimics posterior uveitis.

The management of children with retinoblastoma should include an oncological assessment and investigations to rule out metastatic spread of the tumour. Genetic counselling is also very important. Enucleation of the eye is often necessary when there is a large tumour confined to

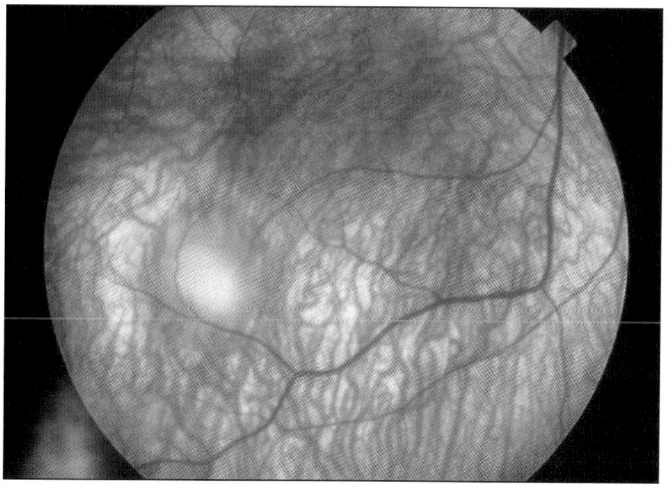

Figure 9.3
A very small intraretinal retinoblastoma. (Courtesy of J Kanski, Clinical Ophthalmology, *5th edition, Butterworth–Heinemann)*

the eye, which is commonly the situation in unilateral tumours. A long piece of optic nerve should also be obtained at surgery to ensure a clear margin of resection free of any tumour that may be invading the nerve. An orbital implant is usually placed at the time of the enucleation to facilitate subsequent good cosmetic rehabilitation.

Bilateral tumours typically present with one severely affected eye (which may require enucleation) and a fellow eye with smaller tumour(s). Smaller tumours may be treated by a combination of systemic chemotherapy and focal treatment. The focal treatment may take the form of irradiation using an episcleral radioactive plaque, cryotherapy or laser coagulation. There is still a place for external beam irradiation, particularly if there is orbital recurrence or histological involvement of the cut end of the optic nerve. However, the significant complications associated with this treatment, which include cosmetic deformity (it retards orbital growth) and secondary tumour formation (usually osteosarcoma).

The prognosis for most children affected by retinoblastoma is now very good with a 3 year survival of over 95 per cent in both unilateral and bilateral cases.[10] Careful screening combined with genetic testing of families at risk is essential.

Abnormal visual development

The terms 'critical' and 'sensitive' are often used to describe the period of eye and brain maturation during which external factors can influence visual development. However, we prefer to use the term 'critical period' to describe the very early time span in infancy (approximately 10–16 weeks) during which abnormal circumstances can cause irreversible change. This period varies for different visual modalities and is longer for crude visual functions, such as form perception and movement. It is shortest for complex visual modalities, such as high spatial frequency, contrast sensitivity and binocularity. Thus, the first (relatively crude) modality developed is the most robust and, therefore, the last to be lost. The sensitive period, about 7–8 years of age, is the longer time frame during which the developing visual system can be manipulated and/or modified by experience before complete maturation, namely by means of occlusion or optical correction. This is described fully in Chapter 1. The critical period for the development of vision has been demonstrated clearly in animals[2] and subsequently in children who have undergone treatment of congenital cataract.[1] This period for the development of normal vision in the presence of dense bilateral congenital cataract seems to be between 10 and 12 weeks (i.e., if the visual axis is not cleared and a focused image restored in both eyes by 10–12 weeks of age, irreversible changes occur in the lateral geniculate nuclei and visual cortex of the developing afferent visual system).

This period is probably slightly longer (16 weeks) in children with unilateral congenital cataract, although the best results appear to be in those who have surgery earlier than this.[1] There appears to be a less sensitive 'pre-cortical' period of approximately 6 weeks during which insults to the developing visual system, which would lead to amblyopia in older infants, leave the young baby without a long-term problem. Thus, birth-related neonatal macular haemorrhage[11] that resolves within 6 weeks does not lead to irreversible amblyopia. This pre-cortical period allows some preparation for congenital cataract surgery in very young infants.

The visual system retains some plasticity until at least 8 years of age, although this plasticity decreases with maturity. Few ophthalmologists would treat well-established amblyopia that presents in a child 10 years of age. Sometimes anisometropic amblyopia can be improved at such a late stage, but this is the exception rather than the rule.

Classification of amblyopia

Amblyopia can be classified into four different subgroups:

- Strabismic;
- Anisometropic;
- Deprivational;
- Ametropic.

Strabismic

The most common subgroup of amblyopia is strabismic amblyopia caused by ocular misalignment. It is usually associated with an esotropia, but can occasionally occur with exotropia.

Anisometropic

The next most common form of amblyopia is anisometropic amblyopia. Hypermetropic anisometropia is the most common and usually requires a difference of refraction between the two eyes of more than 1D. Myopic anisometropia typically requires a greater difference in refraction of 3D or more to cause amblyopia, but can be a very potent causative factor. Astigmatic differences can lead to meridional amblyopia.

Deprivational

Deprivational amblyopia is much rarer and is usually caused by cataract. However, ptosis, periocular haemangioma, corneal opacity and vitreous abnormalities may also lead to deprivational amblyopia. Strabismus and refractive error often coexist and complicate the clinical picture. Bilateral amblyopia is very rare, except in this circumstance. Deprivational amblyopia is seen in children who present late with congenital cataract

Ametropic

Ametropic amblyopia occurs in children with uncorrected large (bilateral) refractive errors. Correction of such refractive errors leads to gradual visual recovery, but this may take some months.

Management of amblyopia

Amblyopia is seen in between 2 and 5 per cent of the population and the mainstay of treatment is occlusion therapy (after correction of any coexistent refractive error). It is essential that the occlusion therapy be monitored and carried out in association with appropriate orthoptic supervision.

Occlusion amblyopia (amblyopia in the eye being occluded as a result of over-zealous occlusion) can occur in rare circumstances. It is usually reversed readily, but its occurrence emphasises that children who have a patch must be monitored appropriately. In general, compliance with occlusion remains more of a problem.[12] A guide to occlusion in general optometric practice is given in Chapter 7.

Alternatives to patching include optical and pharmacological penalisation. Atropine 1 per cent eye drops can be used to cause cycloplegia in the fixing eye. This has been shown to be an effective alternative to occlusion, but is probably less effective when the interocular difference in vision is great.

Non-organic visual loss and/or functional visual impairment

Non-organic visual loss (NOVL) is the term used to describe a disturbance of the afferent visual system that cannot be attributed to demonstrable pathology. It may present with apparent loss of vision, blurring, headaches or ocular pain. Sometimes facial ticks or lid twitching are a feature. NOVL is common during pre-pubertal years.

Social conflict, either at school or in the home, often appears to be a causative factor. It has been estimated to comprise approximately 1 per cent of new referrals to a major UK paediatric ophthalmic unit.[13] There is a gender bias towards girls (3:2) and a cluster in the group 8–13 years of age. The level of claimed visual loss is usually moderate (6/12–6/36). Most referrals are instigated after a visit to an optometrist. Typically, the majority of affected children can be shown to have 6/6 acuity or normal stereoacuity at the first visit to hospital. A comprehensive orthoptic assessment, which includes the use of neutralising lenses and prisms, is usually enough to make the diagnosis without further invasive investigations. A small number of children require further tests that may involve electrodiagnostics and neuroimaging.

The visual prognosis in NOVL is usually excellent, but it should be remembered that it is a diagnosis of exclusion and can only be made when normal visual function has been confirmed in the absence of other pathology. Once the non-organic nature of the problem has been demonstrated to the parents of the child, they should be reassured that this is a normal reaction to stress – in much the same way that headaches and tummy aches often are. This should also be discussed in an appropriate manner with the child and further reassurance proffered.

Non-accidental injury and the eye

Non-accidental injury is an area of great medical controversy as a result of several high-profile trials that have involved allegations of shaken-baby syndrome. It is estimated that up to 2 per cent of children in the UK suffer significant physical abuse and/or non-accidental injury and that 4 per cent of children who present to an ophthalmic casualty department have suffered some form of non-accidental injury.[14] Periocular and ocular tissues are often important markers of such injury. Direct blunt trauma to the eye can cause periocular bruising, hyphaema, lens dislocation, cataract and retinal damage.

Young infants who are subjected to abusive shaking or shaking-impact injuries may develop intracranial injuries (most commonly subdural bleeding), typically in association with retinal bleeding and other fundus signs.[15]

Retinal haemorrhages of different morphologies (nerve fibre layer, intraretinal, pre-retinal and, rarely, subretinal) may be seen (*Figure 9.4*).

Vitreous haemorrhage, retinoschisis, perimacular folds and retinal detachment may occur in more severe cases. The correlation with intracranial damage is not invariable. Between 20 and 30 per cent of children who present with subdural bleeding related to non-accidental injury do not exhibit retinal haemorrhages. Similarly, rare cases of retinal haemorrhages occur without concurrent intracranial bleeding. This can cause difficulties in the diagnosis of non-accidental injury, particularly if there are no other signs of abuse, such as long bone fractures, rib injuries, bruising or mouth and/or facial injuries. It is essential that other causes of retinal and/or intracranial bleeding are looked for and ruled out before making the potentially devastating diagnosis of non-accidental injury.

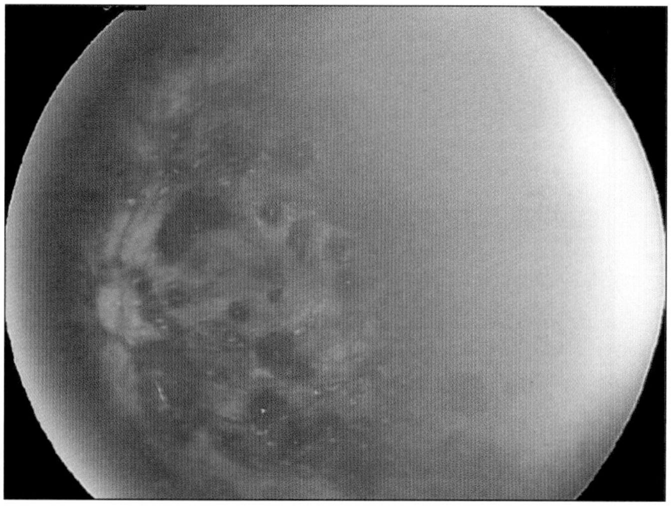

Figure 9.4
Fundus appearance of an infant after a non-accidental head injury. Multiple pre-retinal and nerve fibre layer haemorrhages are evident (Retcam image). (Courtesy of Mr H Willshaw)

Retinal haemorrhages may provide a clue as to the timing of an inflicted injury. Superficial retinal haemorrhages absorb very rapidly, usually within a few days. If found to be present these indicate that the causative injury was relatively recent.

Other types of haemorrhages, such as intraretinal or pre-retinal haemorrhages, may take much longer to disappear (up to 3 months) and are thus less helpful. Haemorrhages are seen mostly at the posterior pole in the clinical situation. Pathological studies have demonstrated that haemorrhages at the peripheral retina are also common.

The pathogenesis of the retinal haemorrhages observed in shaken-baby syndrome is not well understood. Most paediatric ophthalmologists feel that there are two probable mechanisms.

Firstly, tractional forces exerted upon the vitreoretinal interface and/or retinal blood vessels during the inflicted waves of acceleration and deceleration lead to vessel damage and retinal bleeding. This fits particularly well with those infants found to have significant peripheral retinal bleeding, perimacular folds and optic nerve sheath haemorrhages.

Secondly, intraocular venous hypertension, related to raised intracranial pressure or raised intrathoracic pressure, causes mainly posterior pole bleeding. This is a contentious issue because some pathologists who work in this area have put forward the hypothesis that a relatively minor injury to the brain stem of a very young infant (caused by a less vigorous shake than previously thought) can result in a respiratory arrest, profound hypoxia, hypoxic ischaemic encephalopathy and associated massive brain swelling. This profound hypoxia has been postulated to cause damage to the cellular walls of small blood vessels, which leads to leakage and thus the subdural and retinal bleeding observed in these infants.

This hypothesis does not account adequately for all of the ophthalmic manifestations observed in many abused children, including perimacular folds, retinoschisis and retinal detachment. Neither does it account for the retinal findings seen in those children with subdural bleeding and retinal haemorrhages who have not experienced an episode of profound hypoxia.

There still remains some uncertainty in this area and further research is needed.

References

1 Taylor D (1998). Congenital cataract: The history, the nature and the practice. *Eye* **12**, 9–36.
2 Wiesel T and Hubel D (1963). Effects of visual deprivation on morphology and physiology of cells in the cat's lateral geniculate body. *J Neurophysiol.* **96**, 578–585.
3 Lambert SR (1999). Management of monocular congenital cataracts. *Eye* **13**, 474–479.
4 Lambert SR, Lynn M, Drews-Botsch C, *et al.* (2001). A comparison of grating acuity, strabismus and reoperation outcomes among aphakic and pseudophakic children after unilateral cataract surgery during infancy. *JAAPOS* **5**, 70–75.
5 Robb R and Peterson RA (1992). Outcome of treatment for bilateral congenital cataracts. *Trans Am Ophthalmol Soc.* **90**, 183–200.
6 Good WV, Hing S, Irvine AR, Hoyt CS and Taylor DSI (1990). Postoperative endophthalmitis in children following cataract surgery. *J Paediatr Ophthalmol Strabismus* **27**, 283–284.
7 Terry TL (1945). Retrolental fibroplasia in premature infants. *Arch Ophthalmol.* **33**, 203–208.
8 Royal College of Ophthalmologists and British Association of Perinatal Medicine (1995). *Retinopathy of Prematurity: Guidelines for Screening and Treatment.* Report of a Joint Working Party. (London: Royal College of Ophthalmologists and British Association of Perinatal Medicine).
9 Knudson AG (1971). Mutation and cancer: Statistical study of retinoblastoma. *Proc Natl Acad Science USA* **68**, 820–823.
10 Sanders BM, Draper GJ and Kingston JE (1988). Retinoblastoma in Great Britain 1969–80, incidence, treatment, and survival. *Br J Ophthalmol.* **72**, 576–583.
11 Von Noorden G and Khodadoust A (1973). Retinal haemorrhages in newborns and organic amblyopia. *Arch Ophthalmol.* **89**, 91–93.
12 Woodruff G, Hiscox F, Thompson JR and Smith LK (1994). Factors affecting the outcome of children treated for amblyopia. *Eye* **8**, 627–631.
13 Bain KE, Beatty S and Lloyd C (2000). Non-organic visual loss in children. *Eye* **14**, 770–772.
14 Olver JM and Hague S (1989). Children presenting to an ophthalmic casualty department. *Eye* **3**, 415–419.
15 The Ophthalmology Child Abuse Working Party (1999). Child abuse and the eye. *Eye* **13**, 3–10.

10
Paediatric Eye Disorders: Congenital and Neuromuscular Conditions

Susmito Biswas and Christopher Lloyd

In this chapter an overview of paediatric eye disorders of interest and importance to the optometrist is provided. Though many of the conditions discussed are unlikely to be met in general optometric practice, it can be argued that they are still of significance to the optometrist as they may express themselves in a way that overlaps somewhat with the more common conditions that present, and appropriate management is essential. Some clinical signs are associated with both rare and common paediatric ocular syndromes and disorders. They may also be the root cause of ocular difficulties later in life, which may be more likely to present to an optometrist.

Strabismus syndromes

Duane's retraction syndrome

Alexander Duane described the main components of Duane's retraction syndrome (DURS), which is usually a unilateral motility disorder, in 1905.[1] However, the most popular classification system in use for DURS is that devised by Huber,[2] who characterised three types:

- Type 1 – marked limitation of abduction, minimally affected adduction, retraction of the globe on adduction accompanied by narrowing of the palpebral fissure;
- Type 2 – adduction limited more than abduction, exotropia of the affected eye, with narrowing of the palpebral fissure on attempted adduction;
- Type 3 – combined limitation or absence of abduction and adduction with narrowing of the palpebral fissure on attempted adduction.

DURS is infrequently bilateral, and can be of a different type in each eye. Co-contraction of the horizontal recti with variable co-contraction of the vertical recti causes globe retraction and palpebral fissure narrowing. Upshoots or downshoots of the affected eye are often seen in adduction, sometimes attributed to the leash effect of the horizontal rectus muscles slipping around the globe as the eye moves into adduction.

DURS is thought to be caused by an insult between the fourth and tenth week of embryogenesis. Abnormalities of the VIth cranial nerve nucleus have been demonstrated,[3] although supranuclear, brainstem or more peripheral lesions have been suggested also.

DURS has a greater prevalence in females and left eyes (more than 70 per cent in unilateral cases).[4] Esotropia is often present, but may be masked by a head turn to the affected side. Children otherwise exhibit orthotropia, or less frequently exotropia in the primary position. Amblyopia may occur from strabismus or anisometropia. An adopted head posture may maintain binocular single vision, avoid amblyopia and achieve normal stereoacuity. It is important to distinguish typical DURS from VIth cranial nerve palsy. Orbital diseases and various neuromuscular disorders may also mimic DURS (pseudo-Duane's syndrome).

DURS is usually observed in otherwise healthy children, but may also be seen in a variety of syndromes (e.g., Goldenhar syndrome).[5] Other extraocular associations may be observed, including skin, musculoskeletal and external and internal ear disorders.[6] Associated ocular features seen in DURS include nystagmus, epibulbar dermoids, colobomas, anisocoria and ptosis, Marcus Gunn jaw winking, crocodile tears, microphthalmos and optic disc anomalies.[7] The indications for surgical intervention in DURS are significant manifest squint, marked abnormal head posture, cosmetically unacceptable vertical eye movements or marked globe retraction. Typical DURS responds well to recession procedures.[8] Vertical eye movements are often managed by recession of the ipsilateral lateral rectus. Amblyopia and refractive error are managed in the usual way.

Moebius syndrome (congenital facial diplegia)

Moebius syndrome is defined as congenital bilateral or unilateral VIIth cranial nerve palsies, and is often associated with other cranial nerve palsies (Vth, VIth or IXth, Xth and XIIth).[9] Significant limb abnormalities may coexist, including absent pectoralis major muscle (Poland anomaly).[10] Autism and neurodevelopmental delay have been described in association.[11] It is thought that a vascular insult during embryogenesis interrupts the blood supply to the brainstem or the region of the facial nerve nucleus.[12] This can be through a variety of external factors,[13] but most cases appear to be sporadic. It may also be familial or associated with chromosomal abnormalities.[14]

Moebius syndrome is characterised by incomplete eyelid closure, which risks corneal exposure and ulceration.[15] This may be further exacerbated by the loss of corneal sensation and aberrant lacrimation. However, there is usually a protective Bell's phenomenon. Bilateral or unilateral limitation of abduction is present in the majority of cases because of the VIth nerve involvement. A 'V' pattern esotropia is observed commonly and vertical strabismus may be associated. There are often deficits in both adduction and abduction. A clinical picture that resembles DURS may occur. Occasionally, affected children may present with a very large angle exotropia, with greater limitation of adduction than abduction. Compound hypermetropic astigmatism is a frequent finding. Amblyopia is a risk because of the presence of manifest squint and astigmatism.

Management of the ocular disease involves assessment of eyelid function and corneal clarity. Artificial tear supplementation is usually necessary and lateral tarsorrhaphies may be required for severe exposure. Appropriate refractive correction is mandatory. Strabismus surgery typically comprises large bilateral medial rectus recessions, possibly combined with traction sutures.

Congenital fibrosis of the extraocular muscles syndrome

There are three main varieties of congenital fibrosis of the extraocular muscles syndrome, referred to as CFEOM1, 2 or 3. The classic features of CFEOM1, the most common form of CFEOM, are:

- Fibrosis of some or all of the extraocular muscles;
- Fibrosis of Tenon's capsule;
- Adhesions between Tenon's capsule, muscles and the globe;
- Inelasticity and fragility of the conjunctiva;
- No elevation or depression of either eye;
- Little or no horizontal movement;
- Eyes fixed in a downwards gaze (infraduction) 20–30° below the horizontal;
- Bilateral ptosis;
- Chin elevation and backwards head tilt;
- The condition is present at birth.

In addition to infraduction, there may be an eso- or exodeviation. Residual eye movements are often abnormal. Forced duction tests reveal a marked resistance to passive movement.[16] This disorder is autosomal dominant with complete penetrance. The putative gene for CFEOM1 lies within chromosome 12 (12p11.2-q12).[17] There is evidence of a primary innervational anomaly that affects the superior division of the IIIrd cranial nerve and its corresponding alpha motoneurons in the midbrain.[18] The extraocular muscles are abnormal, with normal striated muscle replaced by fibrous collagenous tissue. These muscle changes are likely to be secondary to lack of normal innervation. Phenotypic variation is not uncommon within families with classic CFEOM1.[19]

CFEOM2 is autosomal recessive.[20] Typically, there is congenital non-progressive bilateral ptosis and marked exotropia in the range 50–90 prism dioptres, with the eyes fixed in extreme abduction. In addition, the eyes may be hyper- or hypotropic. More rarely, the eyes may be in a neutral primary position with minimal residual downgaze. Voluntary globe movements are absent or consist of minimal residual abduction. Individuals with marked ptosis may develop severe amblyopia because of obstruction of the visual axis. Genetic analysis has revealed mutations in ARIX.[21] ARIX is a gene that encodes a homeodomain transcription factor, previously shown to be required for development of the IIIrd and IVth cranial nerves in other vertebrates.

CFEOM3 is a dominantly inherited, non-progressive congenital disorder. It is uncertain if the disorder is fully penetrant. The clinical features are variable with clinical overlap between CFEOM1 and CFEOM2.[22] Severely affected individuals have eyes fixed in hypo- and exotropia with marked restriction of ocular motility and ptosis. Phenotypic variability is demonstrable within families. Once again, severely affected individuals have dense amblyopia related to the ptosis, strabismus and compound myopic astigmatism. The putative gene for CFEOM3 lies on the long arm of chromosome 16 (16q24.2-q24.3).

It is important to distinguish CFEOM from other acquired disorders that result in ocular muscle fibrosis, including orbital inflammatory disease, trauma or infection, acquired restrictive esotropia associated with myopia, and disorders such as myasthenia gravis, mitochondrial cytopathies and myotonic dystrophy.

The management of these disorders is to treat any amblyopia and refractive error as required. Muscle surgery is reserved for those with cosmetically or functionally poor head posture. This usually comprises large muscle recession procedures combined with traction sutures. Ptosis surgery is often required and usually consists of a brow suspension procedure.

Double elevator palsy

Double elevator palsy (DEP) is a rare motility disorder that consists of an apparent paralysis of the superior rectus muscle and ipsilateral inferior oblique. This results in an inability to elevate the eye above the midline in both adduction and abduction. The disorder may be unilateral or bilateral, and congenital or acquired. In the primary position the eye may be hypotropic if the uninvolved eye is used for fixation. If the involved eye is used for fixation, the uninvolved eye may be hypertropic. In contrast, some cases of DEP may not have a deviation in the primary position. A true or pseudo-ptosis may accompany this disorder.

The aetiology of this disorder is unknown, although there have been suggestions that in a 'true' congenital DEP the lesion is supranuclear.[23] Support for this comes from observing an intact Bell's phenomenon, negative forced-duction tests and the presence of normal vertical saccadic velocities up to the primary position.[24] Other aetiologies include a primary inferior rectus restriction associated with a positive forced-duction test, or a superior rectus disorder. Magnetic resonance imaging of the superior rectus muscle in DEP demonstrates a decreased muscle volume, which suggests hypoplasia or paralysis.[25] Indeed, congenital absence of the superior rectus can give rise to a DEP-like motility disorder despite a normally functioning inferior oblique. Neuro-imaging may be necessary in cases of acquired DEP, as pineocytoma has been observed in an affected 8-year-old girl.[26]

The management of this disorder is conservative if there is no vertical deviation or significant head posture in the primary position. If there is a significant vertical deviation or chin-up posture, muscle surgery may be carried out. This may consist of an inferior rectus muscle recession with or without upwards translocation of the horizontal recti to the superior rectus insertion. Alternatively, a horizontal recti translocation alone may be performed. A persistent ptosis may be corrected after squint surgery (true ptosis).

Neuromuscular disorders

Disorders in this category include myasthenia gravis, myotonic dystrophy, mitochondrial cytopathy and congenital or juvenile myopathies. These often present with ophthalmoplegia and ptosis.

Congenital myasthenia may be transient, resolving in 1–12 weeks, because of cross-placental transmission of acetylcholine-receptor (AchR) antibodies from a myasthenic mother. About 12 per cent of such infants are affected in this way.[27]

Severe neonatal deformities or increased risk of stillbirth may occur.[28] Other congenital myasthenic syndromes include post-synaptic disorders that affect the AchR (which are autosomal dominantly or autosomal recessively inherited) or acetylcholinesterase deficiency.

Myotonic dystrophy is autosomal dominant through expansion of a repeat CTG nucleotide sequence within the gene-encoding myotonin-protein kinase.[29] It can present congenitally or in infancy. In the severe neonatal form, transmission of the disease is nearly always from the mother.[30] Mitochondrial cytopathies are inherited through the maternal line. A progressive external ophthalmoplegia and ptosis occur in the first decade of life.[31] Other abnormalities in this group of disorders include cardiac conduction defects, pigmentary retinopathy,[32] cerebellar ataxia, myoclonus, epilepsy and diabetes. Muscle biopsy shows characteristic pathological changes (ragged red fibres).[33]

Normal and abnormal ocular development

The eye develops through a programmed sequence of inductive events and regional specification. Many excellent reviews on this subject have been published,[34] and for a discussion of ocular embryology, see Appendix 1. The early developmental stages are summarised next.

Initially, an evagination of neural ectoderm in the region of the diencephalon, known as the optic pit, develops into the optic vesicle, which contacts the overlying surface ectoderm and induces the development of the lens placode. This separates from the surface ectoderm to form the lens vesicle, which eventually differentiates into the mature lens. Meanwhile, the optic vesicle invaginates to form the optic cup, a double-layered structure. The inner layer forms the prospective neural retina. The outer layer forms the prospective retinal pigment epithelium. The narrow medial end of the optic cup, the optic stalk, eventually develops into the optic nerve. These structures mature to form the functional eye, with neural connections developing between the retina and the optic tectum.

The development and pattern of the vertebrate eye is under control from a variety of regulatory proteins known as transcription factors. Transcription factors act by modulating the expression of genes involved in eye morphogenesis. The combination of transcription factors produced by cells or a region confers that region's identity. One of these is PAX6, a 'master regulator' of ocular development, which shows strong evolutionary conservation (i.e., it is present across vertebrates and invertebrates). PAX6 belongs to a group of homeobox transcription factors that contain paired DNA binding domains, each of which consists of 128 amino acids.[35] It is expressed widely in the embryonic head ectoderm, optic vesicle and lens placode. PAX6 modifies the transcriptional activity of genes by directly binding the enhancer or promoter DNA sequences of these genes. For example, PAX6 can bind to a variety of crystallin (lens protein) gene-promoter sequences to increase their expression.[36] This DNA binding can be modulated through PAX6 protein–protein interaction (e.g., co-operatively binding with SOX2, another transcription factor, which increases the binding affinity of this new protein complex to the crystallin promoter).[37] Finally, intramolecular interaction between the PAX6 binding domains can modify its activity, and provides a further level of control of gene expression.[38] Within the developing retina, PAX6 is an upstream regulator of a variety of basic helix–loop–helix transcription factors involved in the differentiation of retinal progenitor cells into photoreceptors and interneurones.[39] Expression of PAX6, like that of other transcription factors, is not restricted to the developing eye, but also occurs in the mature eye, particularly in the corneal epithelium and limbal region.

For a full discussion of the role of PAX6 and other molecular regulators of ocular development, see the many excellent reviews on this subject.[40] Homozygous mutations of PAX6 in mice result in the total absence of eyes (anophthalmia). The development of the eye ceases at the optic vesicle stage because of a failure of the lens placode to develop. Other malformations of the head are also present. In humans, heterozygous mutations in PAX6 cause aniridia (see below). Other whole-eye disorders can be caused by other PAX6 mutations (e.g., microphthalmos; see www.hgu.mrc.ac.uk/Softdata/PAX6/).

Anterior segment dysgenesis

Anterior segment dysgenesis involves congenital disorders of the structures at the front of the eye (i.e., the cornea, iris, anterior chamber angle and lens). An important category within this group of disorders is the Axenfeld–Rieger syndrome. A confusing array of terminology is used to describe this group of autosomal disorders (e.g., Axenfeld anomaly, Rieger anomaly and syndrome, iridogoniodysgenesis anomaly and syndrome and familial glaucoma iridogoniodysplasia). The clinical characteristics of the Axenfeld–Rieger anomaly are the presence of a prominent Schwalbe's line (posterior embryotoxon).[41] This appears as a prominent white ring 1mm from the corneal periphery.

The Axenfeld anomaly is characterised by strands of iris stromal tissue that bridge the iridocorneal angle and insert into the posterior embryotoxon. The iris appearance is otherwise normal. In the Rieger anomaly, the iris abnormalities include stromal hypoplasia, full thickness holes (polycoria) and corectopia, whereby the pupil is displaced towards abnormal thickened material in the iridocorneal angle. Isolated posterior embryotoxon is not associated with a risk of glaucoma.[41] Other features of the Axenfeld–Rieger syndrome are associated with a 50 per cent risk of glaucoma, often observed when a high iris insertion is found.[42] This condition is genetically heterogeneous. In the Rieger syndrome, ocular findings are found in association with midfacial hypoplasia, dental anomalies (peg-like teeth) and redundant peri-umbilical skin. Mutations in PITX2, a paired-like homeodomain transcription factor gene located on chromosome 4q25, have been found.[43] Iridogoniodysgenesis syndrome and Peter's anomaly, which have similar extraocular manifestations as the Rieger syndrome, have also been described in association with PITX2 mutations.[44] In this context, these other phenotypes should fall under the Axenfeld–Rieger umbrella.

In the Rieger anomaly, ocular findings are isolated and not associated with midfacial hypoplasia, dental or jaw anomalies, or excess peri-umbilical skin. Similarly, the iridogoniodysgenesis anomaly and iridogoniodysplasia are not associated with any systemic manifestations. In general, these are associated with mutations or deletions and/or duplications in the FOXC1 transcription factor gene located on chromosome 6p25.[45] The Rieger syndrome has also been described in families with deletions on chromosome 13q14, although no gene has been identified at this locus.[46]

Glaucoma associated with this condition may be congenital or developmental. Trabecular dysgenesis with a high iris insertion is observed in congenital cases. Infants present with buphthalmos, hazy corneas and Haab's striae. The management of this is as per primary congenital glaucoma (i.e., goniotomy or trabeculotomy). Children otherwise require frequent intraocular pressure checks in the clinic. In children who develop glaucoma when older, anti-glaucoma medication may achieve good control, but surgery is often required (i.e., enhanced trabeculectomy). Children need to have their refractive errors and anisometropia managed appropriately, in addition to amblyopia monitoring and treatment.

Peter's anomaly

Peter's anomaly is not a disease entity in its own right, but a description of a central corneal opacity of varying degrees. The disorder may be unilateral or bilateral. A defect in the posterior cornea that involves Descemet's membrane underlies this opacity and may extend into the corneal stroma. This defect may be visible on high-frequency ultrasound biomicroscopy of the cornea.[47] Iridocorneal and lenticular corneal adhesions may also be present. In addition, there may be coexisting cataract and glaucoma. Peter's anomaly is observed commonly with other ocular disorders, and may represent part of a whole-eye malformation syndrome.[48]

A number of systemic malformation syndromes are associated with Peter's anomaly, such as Peter's plus syndrome, fetal alcohol syndrome or Pfeiffer's syndrome.[49] Patients with Peter's anomaly often have associated midline defects (e.g., pituitary dysfunction or cleft palate).[50] The disorder is genetically heterogeneous and inheritance patterns suggest both autosomal dominant and autosomal recessive transmission. In addition to a variety of chromosomal anomalies, mutations in the PAX6,[51] CYP1B1 and FOXE3 genes[52] have been documented.

Surgical management of this condition is difficult. Associated ocular abnormalities determine the visual prognosis. Penetrating keratoplasty to prevent deprivation amblyopia has been advocated in bilateral cases, with surgery performed on the worst-seeing eye. The long-term success rate of this procedure is around 36 per cent, but this is reduced when coexisting glaucoma or cataract requires lensectomy.[53]

Sclerocornea

Sclerocornea is a bilateral congenital disorder of the cornea that presents with varying, and often asymmetric, degrees of corneal opacification and vascularisation. In some instances the cornea may be totally opaque, while in others there may be peripheral involvement only. In some instances the opacification may be central or sectoral in one eye, but more extensive in the fellow eye. The cornea may be small in diameter, with a flat curvature that results in significant hypermetropia.[54] The corneal opacity results from disorganisation of collagen fibres of variable diameters and irregularly arranged lamellae.[54] Descemet's membrane may be absent. Glaucoma secondary to trabecular dysgenesis may coexist.

Sclerocornea may be sporadic or inherited as an autosomal recessive or dominant disorder. A variety of malformation syndromes may be associated with it (e.g., Mietens–Weber syndrome[55] and Rothmund–Thompson syndrome[56]). Children with extensive sclerocornea present with poor visual behaviour and nystagmus. Lesser degrees of sclerocornea may not affect vision, although significant refractive error may be present.

Primary trabecular dysgenesis (primary congenital glaucoma)

Primary trabecular dysgenesis is a rare disorder that gives rise to congenital glaucoma. It is autosomal recessive and associated with mutations in the CYP1B1 gene.[57] Infants present in the first year of life with buphthalmos (*Figure 10.1*), photophobia and tearing, progressive refractive myopic shift, enlarged corneal diameters, Haab's striae, corneal clouding and progressive optic disc cupping. Gonioscopy reveals a poorly differentiated trabecular meshwork with a pale gelatinous appearance (so-called Barkan's membrane). The iris has a high insertion into the iridocorneal angle. There may be prominent iris vessels that enter the angle and variable degrees of iris stromal hypoplasia. This disorder is usually bilateral, but may be asymmetric. Infants who present at or shortly after birth have a poorer prognosis.

The management of this condition is primarily through angle surgery (goniotomy or trabeculotomy). The success rates of these operations are high (>90 per cent) in experienced hands, but patients do have a life-long risk of relapse.[58] In those who fail to have their glaucoma controlled through angle surgery, enhanced trabeculectomy procedures may be undertaken. Myopia is common in these children and, as the condition may be asymmetric, anisometropia is not unusual. Thus careful monitoring of amblyopia combined with refractive correction is mandatory.

Whole-eye disorders

Aniridia

Aniridia is a whole-eye disorder that involves the anterior segment, retina and optic nerve. The underlying gene defect is in PAX6 (see above).[59] This gene is expressed in the adult corneal epithelium and conjunctiva and also in the developing cornea, lens and retina;[60] hence the range of ocular defects observed. Iris abnormalities range from total or near absence of the iris (a stump of iris tissue is usually present) to more subtle iris stromal hypoplasia and loss of the iris sphincter pupillae muscle. A progressive keratopathy may be present because of the lack of normal corneal limbal stem cells. A vascular pannus is commonly observed on the margins of the cornea. Cataracts are often seen and may range from insignificant anterior polar to dense nuclear cataracts. A major concern is developmental glaucoma, which appears to result from a progressive closure of the angle from the residual iris stump, although trabeculodysgenesis may be present.[61] The risk of glaucoma is between 50 and 70 per cent.[62] Foveal hypoplasia and/or optic nerve hypoplasia is observed commonly, and is usually the main cause of poor visual acuity. Nystagmus is seen alongside this.

Familial aniridia is autosomal dominant with high penetrance. An important syndrome associated with aniridia is the WAGR [Wilms' tumour (nephroblastoma), aniridia, genital abnormalities and mental retardation (developmental delay)] syndrome. This occurs sporadically and is caused by a contiguous gene deletion at chromosomal position 11p13 that involves both PAX6 and the WT1 gene responsible for Wilms' tumour. Renal ultrasound screening for Wilms' tumour in spontaneously occurring aniridia on a 3 monthly basis until 5 years of age has

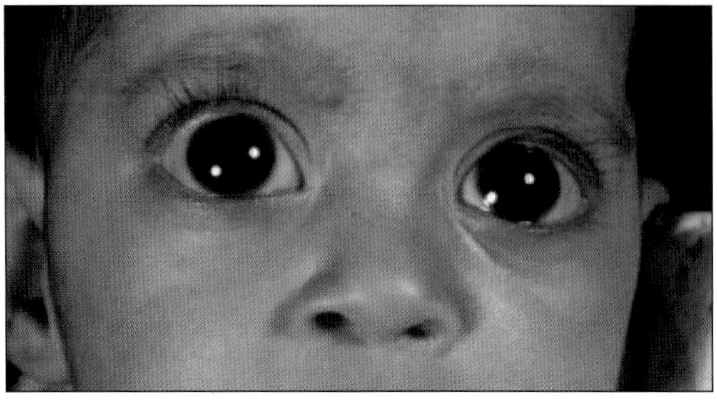

Figure 10.1 *Bilateral buphthalmos (enlarged globes) in primary congenital glaucoma*

been recommended.[63] Alternatively, cytogenetic studies may distinguish between children at risk of developing Wilms' tumour and those who simply have aniridia through isolated PAX6 mutations.[64]

Microphthalmos and coloboma

Microphthalmos can be unilateral or bilateral. Simple microphthalmos refers to a small eye (total axial length two standard deviations below age-matched means[65]), with no other ocular abnormalities, while complicated microphthalmos refers to eyes in which there are other ocular abnormalities such as coloboma or cataract. Anophthalmia usually refers to an extreme form of microphthalmos, in which intraocular structures are visible on histopathological sectioning. True anophthalmia, in which there is no evidence of ocular tissue histologically, is extremely rare. The cornea may be small (microcornea) and the shape oval because of differences between the horizontal and vertical dimensions.

Microphthalmos may arise through a variety of genetic mechanisms. Over 100 of the described monogenic entities are associated with microphthalmos, including autosomal dominant microphthalmos, X-linked Lenz microphthalmia and Goltz syndrome.[66] Examples of chromosomal anomalies associated with microphthalmos and coloboma include trisomy 18, trisomy 13 and trisomy 22 (cat-eye syndrome). Sporadic associations with other ocular malformations include dermoids, persistent fetal vasculature and anterior polar cataract, among others. Sporadic systemic congenital abnormalities, such as Goldenhar's syndrome, VATER (vertebral anomalies, anal atresia, tracheo-oesophageal fistula, ear abnormalities and radial limb defects) syndrome and the CHARGE (coloboma, heart defects, choanal atresia, retarded growth, genital abnormalities, and ear defects) association are also associated with microphthalmos. A variety of prenatal insults in early pregnancy, such as retinoic acid, alcohol and anticonvulsant agents, as well as maternal pyrexia, have been associated with sporadic microphthalmos.[67]

Microphthalmos and coloboma commonly are associated with orbital cysts of various sizes. These cysts are often contiguous with a defect in the posterior aspect of the eye. Anteriorly located orbital cysts are apparent clinically as a bulging of the lower eyelid, and occasionally displace the globe in the opposite direction. Posteriorly located cysts may escape detection until growth causes proptosis. These cysts may be evident on ultrasonography or radiological imaging.

In microphthalmos, a careful gestational history from the mother may disclose evidence of exposure to teratogens in early pregnancy, maternal diabetes or febrile illness. A family history may reveal other affected members in autosomal dominant disease, or a history of consanguinity in autosomal recessive disease. The pattern of any associated ocular or systemic abnormality may suggest a particular monogenic, chromosomal or sporadic non-hereditary disorder. Often genetic consultation is required to help make an overall diagnosis.

A uveoretinal coloboma is shown in *Figure 10.2*.

Albinism

The influence on binocular vision development is discussed in Chapter 6. There are several forms of albinism, which include oculocutaneous albinism (OCA; *Figure 10.3*), ocular albinism (OA), Hermansky–Pudlak syndrome (HPS) and Chediak–Higashi syndrome (CHS). All exhibit a range of ocular abnormalities that include reduced visual acuity, nystagmus, photophobia, iris transillumination, foveal hypoplasia, pale fundus and an abnormal decussation of nerve fibres at the optic chiasm. Many other syndromes are associated with hypopigmentation (e.g., Prader–Willi syndrome, Angelman syndrome, Waardenberg syndromes and piebaldism).[68] Some of these syndromes are associated with true albinism, while others are associated with skin hypopigmentation only.

OCA exists as three main autosomal recessive forms, types 1, 2 and 3. Type 1 OCA (OCA1 or tyrosinase-negative albinism) is caused by mutations in the gene that encodes the enzyme tyrosinase, which catalyses the first step in melanin synthesis. Mutations result in complete or partial inhibition of the enzyme. Different mutations give rise to a variety of subtypes [e.g., OCA1a, OCA 1b (yellow OCA)[69], OCA1-MP (minimal pigment OCA)[70] and OCA1-TP (temperature dependent OCA)[71]]. Where there is no tyrosinase function, as in OCA1a, individuals have 'snowy white' hair and skin and absent ocular pigmentation. With partial enzyme activity, as in OCA1b, there is some pigment accumulation in hair and irides with increasing age.

Type 2 OCA (OCA2 or tyrosinase-positive OCA) results from mutations of the P

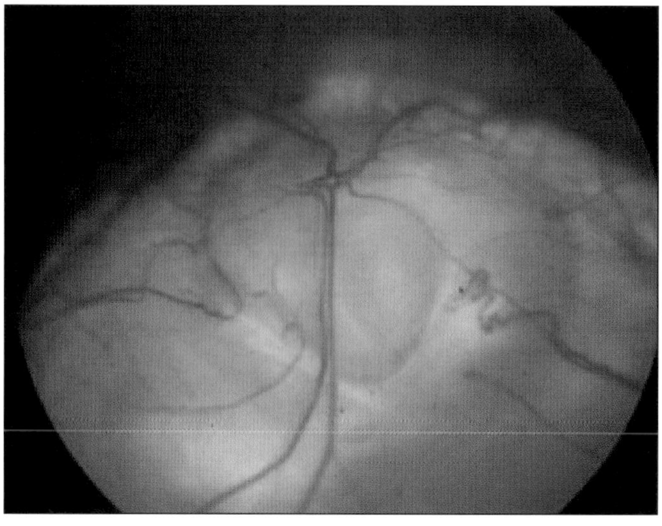

Figure 10.2
A large uveoretinal coloboma that involves the optic disc

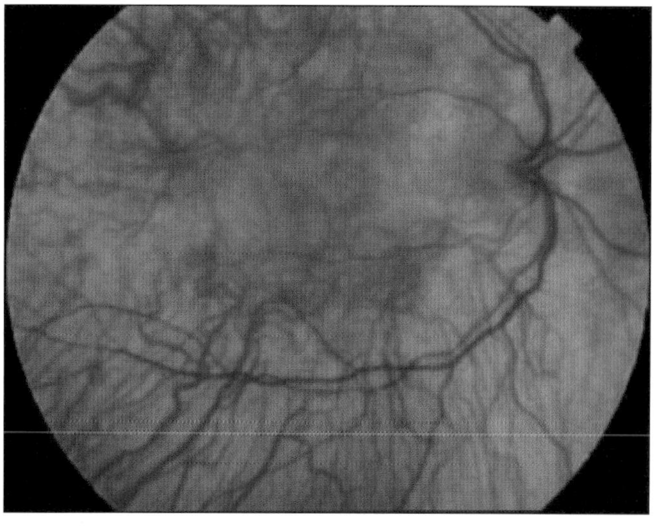

Figure 10.3
Foveal hypoplasia, optic nerve hypoplasia and hypopigmentation of the fundus in oculocutaneous albinism

gene, the human equivalent of the mouse p (pink-eye dilution) gene, on chromosome 15q11–12.[72] This gene encodes a transmembrane polypeptide that may be involved in the transport of tyrosine. This form of OCA is particularly common in African and African–American blacks. The expression of the disorder may vary according to the racial background of the individual. Individuals may accumulate hair pigmentation and pigmented naevi or freckles, but the skin does not tan. The ocular features of OCA1 and OCA2 are identical, but may be less obvious in some individuals with OCA2. The incidence of OCA2 in Prader–Willi and Angelman syndromes is 1 per cent through hemizygosity of mutant alleles of the P gene.[73]

Type 3 OCA (OCA3 or Brown OCA) is found only in African or African– American blacks. Individuals have light brown skin and hair, moderate tanning, blue–grey irides that transilluminate and nystagmus. The disorder has been associated with mutations in the gene that encodes tyrosinase-related protein-1 (TRP-1), which regulates the production of eumelanin.[74] OA is X-linked recessive.[75] The ocular features predominate with little evidence of abnormal pigmentation in the skin or hair. Individuals with OA often have a fair complexion compared with their unaffected siblings. The ocular features are similar to those of OCA, with nystagmus, reduced visual acuity, iris transillumination, posterior embryotoxon, foveal hypoplasia and a pale hypopigmented fundus. Carrier females (heterozygotes) may also have iris transillumination and a 'mud-splattered' fundus appearance. Skin biopsies in affected individuals and carrier female heterozygotes show macromelanosomes.[76]

HPS and CHS are important differential diagnoses in albinism. HPS is particularly common in Puerto Ricans and consists of albinism, abnormal platelet aggregation and abnormal tissue ceroid accumulation.[77] The albinism in HPS may be variable, but there is a history of bruising and excessive bleeding. CHS is characterised by dysfunction of leukocyte degranulation, which results in an increased susceptibility to infection, in addition to albinism. These frequent infections can lead to death in childhood.[77]

Similar ocular features are found among the different forms of albinism, but may vary in severity. Iris transillumination is an important diagnostic feature, but may be observed in non-albinos. Foveal hypoplasia is a consistent diagnostic feature, but is not unique to albinism.[78] At ophthalmoscopy the foveal pit is absent and vessels may be seen to course over the central macula. As a result, visual acuity is reduced. More than 60 per cent of individuals with OCA2 have a visual acuity greater than 6/60, compared with 40 per cent of individuals with OCA1. Significant refractive error is common, with 14 per cent having more than 10D of ametropia.[79] Strabismus is also frequently seen in albinism. Nystagmus presents in the first 3 months of life, but tends to reduce with age.[80] Some individuals with albinism do not have nystagmus.

Electrodiagnostic tests are an important tool with which to verify the diagnosis of albinism. The ERG demonstrates a supranormal response, but more importantly the visual evoked potential (VEP) shows characteristic crossed asymmetry because of the increased decussation of nerve fibres at the optic chiasm. VEP crossed asymmetry is not unique to albinism and has to be viewed in the context of the subject's other findings.[81]

References

1 Duane A (1905). Congenital deficiency of abduction associated with impairment of adduction, retraction movements, contraction of the palpebral fissure and oblique movements of the eye. *Arch Ophthalmol.* **34**, 133–159.
2 Huber A (1974). Electrophysiology of the retraction syndrome. *Br J Ophthalmol.* **58**, 293–300.
3 Miller NR, Kiel SM, Green WR, *et al.* (1982). Unilateral Duane's retraction syndrome (type 1). *Arch Ophthalmol.* **100**, 1468–1472.
4 DeRespinis PA, Caputo AR, Wagner RS and Suqin G (1993). Duane's retraction syndrome. *Surv Ophthalmol.* **38**, 257–288.
5 Velez G (1970). Duane's retraction syndrome associated with Goldenhar's syndrome. *Am J Ophthalmol.* **70**, 945–946.
6 Gupte G, Mahajan P, Shreenivas VK, *et al.* (1992). Wildervanck syndrome (cervico-oculo-acoustic syndrome). *J Postgrad Med.* **38**, 180–182.
7 Ro A, Gummeson B, Orton RB and Cadera W (1989). Duane's retraction syndrome: Southwestern Ontario experiences. *Can J Ophthalmol.* **24**, 200–203.
8 Kubota N, Takahashi H, Hayashi T, Sakaue T and Maruo T (2001). Outcome of surgery in 124 cases of Duane's retraction syndrome (DRS) treated by intraoperatively graduated recession of the medial rectus for esotropic DRS, and of the lateral rectus for exotropic DRS. *Binocul Vis Strabismus Q.* **16**, 15–22.
9 Kumar D (1990). Syndrome of the month. Moebius syndrome. *J Med Genet.* **27**, 122–126.
10 Larrandaburu M (1999). The occurrence of Poland and Poland–Moebius syndromes in the same family: Further evidence of their genetic component. *Clin Dysmorphol.* **8**, 93–99.
11 Baraitser M (1977). Genetics of Moebius syndrome. *J Med Genet.* **14**, 415–417.
12 Bouwes-Bavinck JN and Weaver DD (1986). Subclavian artery disruption sequence: Hypothesis of a vascular etiology for Poland, Klippel–Feil, and Möbius' anomalies. *J Med Genet.* **23**, 903–918.
13 Ghabrial R, Versace P, Kourt G, Lipson A and Martin F (1998). Möbius syndrome: Features and etiology. *J Pediatr Ophthalmol Strabismus* **35**, 304–311.
14 Borck G, Wirth J, Hardt T, *et al.* (2001). Molecular cytogenetic characterisation of a complex 46,XY,t(7;8;11;13) chromosome rearrangement in a patient with Moebius syndrome. *J Med Genet.* **38**, 117–120.
15 Cronemberger MF, de Castro Moreira JB, Brunoni D, *et al.* (2001). Ocular and clinical manifestations of Möbius syndrome. *J Pediatr Ophthalmol Strabismus* **38**, 156–162.
16 Laughlin R (1956). Congenital fibrosis of the extraocular muscles. A report of six cases. *Am J Ophthalmol.* **41**, 432–438.
17 Engle E, Marondel I, Houtman WA, *et al.* (1995). Congenital fibrosis of the extraocular muscles (autosomal dominant congenital external ophthalmoplegia): Genetic homogeneity, linkage refinement, physical mapping on chromosome 12. *Am J Hum Genet.* **57**, 1086–1094.
18 Engle EC, Goumnerov BC, McKeown CA, *et al.* (1997). Ocular motor nerve and muscle abnormalities in congenital fibrosis of the extraocular muscles. *Ann Neurol.* **41**, 314–325.
19 Sener EC, Lee BA, Targut B, Akarsu AN and Engle EC (2000). A clinically variant fibrosis syndrome in a Turkish family maps to the CFEOM1 locus on chromosome 12. *Arch Ophthalmol.* **118**, 1090–1097.
20 Wang SM, Zwaan J, Mullaney PB, *et al.* (1998). Congenital fibrosis of the extraocular muscle type 2, an inherited exotropic strabismus fixus, maps to distal 11q13. *Am J Hum Genet.* **63**, 517–525.
21 Nakano M, Yamada K, Fain J, *et al.* (2001). Homozygous mutations in ARIX (PHOX2A) result in congenital fibrosis of the extraocular muscles type 2. *Nat Genet.* **29**, 315–320.
22 Doherty EJ, Macy ME, Wang SM, Dykeman CP, Melanson MT and Engle EC (1999). CFEOM3, A new extra-ocular congenital fibrosis syndrome that maps to 16q24.2-q24.3. *Invest Ophthalmol Vis Sci.* **40**, 1687–1694.
23 Bell JA, Fielder AR and Viney S (1990). Congenital double elevator palsy in identical twins. *J Clin Neuro-ophthalmol.* **10**, 32–34.
24 Ziffer AJ, Rosenbaum AL, Demer JL and Yee RD (1992). Congenital double elevator palsy: Vertical saccadic velocity utilising the scleral search coil technique. *J Pediatr Ophthalmol Strabismus* **29**, 142–149.

25 Candera W, Bloom JN, Karlik S and Viirre E (1997). A magnetic resonance imaging study of double elevator palsy. *Can J Ophthalmol.* **32**, 250–253.
26 Munoz M and Page LK (1994). Acquired double elevator palsy in a child with pineocytoma. *Am J Ophthalmol.* **18**, 810–811.
27 Namba T, Browns SB and Grob D (1970). Neonatal myasthenia gravis: Report of two cases and review of the literature. *Pediatrics* **45**, 488–504.
28 Brueton LA, Huson SM, Cox PM, *et al.* (2000). Asymptomatic maternal myasthenia as a cause of the Pena–Shokeir phenotype. *Am J Med Genet.* **92**, 1–6.
29 Brook JD, McCurrah ME, Harley HG, *et al.* (1992). Molecular basis of myotonic dystrophy: Expansion of a trinucleotide (CTG) repeat at the 3′ end of a transcript encoding a protein kinase family member. *Cell* **68**, 799–808.
30 Andrews PI and Wilson J (1992). Relative disease severity in siblings with myotonic dystrophy. *J Child Neurol.* **7**, 161–167.
31 Petty RKH, Harding AE and Morgan-Hughes JA (1986). The clinical features of mitochondrial myopathy. *Brain* **109**, 915–938.
32 Bosche J, Hammerstein W, Neuen-Jacob E and Schober R (1989). Variation in retinal changes and muscle pathology in mitochondropathies. *Graefe's Arch Klin Exp Ophthalmol.* **227**, 578–583.
33 Ringel SP, Wilson WB and Barden MT (1979). Extra-ocular muscle biopsy in chronic progressive external ophthalmoplegia. *Ann Neurol.* **6**, 326–339.
34 Ashery-Padan R and Gruss P (2001). Pax6 lights-up the way for eye development. *Curr Opin Cell Biol.* **13**, 706–714.
35 Walther C and Gruss P (1991). Pax-6, a murine paired box gene, is expressed in the developing CNS. *Development* **113**, 1435–1449.
36 Cvekl A, Sax C, Bresnick EH and Piatigorsky J (1994). A complex array of positive and negative elements regulates the chicken αA-crystallin gene: Involvement of Pax-6, USF, CREB and/or CREM, and AP-1 proteins. *Mol Cell Biol.* **14**, 7363–7376.
37 Kamachi Y, Uchikawa M, Tanouchi A, *et al.* (2001). Pax6 and SOX2 form a co-DNA-binding partner complex that regulates initiation of lens development. *Genes Dev.* **15**, 1272–1286.
38 Plaza S, Prince F, Jaeger J, *et al.* (2001). Molecular basis for the inhibition of *Drosophila* eye development by Antennapedia. *EMBO J.* **20**, 802–811.
39 Vetter ML and Brown NL (2001). The role of basic helix–loop–helix genes in vertebrate retinogenesis. *Cell Dev Biol.* **12**, 491–498.
40 Jean D, Ewan K and Gruss P (1998). Molecular regulators involved in vertebrate eye development. *Mech Dev.* **76**, 3–18.
41 Shields MB (1983). Axenfeld–Rieger syndrome: A theory of mechanisms and distinctions from the iridocorneal endothelial syndrome. *Trans Am Ophthalmol Soc.* **81**, 736–784.
42 Fitz N and Kaback M (1978). The Axenfeld syndrome and the Rieger syndrome. *J Med Genet.* **15**, 30–34.
43 Semina EV, Reiter R, Leysens NJ, *et al.* (1996). Cloning and characterisation of a novel bicoid-related homeobox transcription factor gene, RGS, involved in Rieger syndrome. *Nat Genet.* **14**, 392–399.
44 Doward W, Parveen R, Lloyd IC, *et al.* (1999). A mutation in the RIEG1 gene associated with Peter's anomaly. *J Med Genet.* **36**, 152–155.
45 Nishimura DY, Swiderski RE, Alward WL, *et al.* (1998). The forkhead transcription factor gene FKHL7 is responsible for glaucoma phenotypes which map to 6p25. *Nat Genet.* **19**, 140–147.
46 Phillips JC, del Bono EA, Haines JL, *et al.* (1996). A second locus for Riegers syndrome maps to chromosome 13q14. *Am J Hum Genet.* **59**, 613–619.
47 Nischal KK, Naor J, Jay V, MacKeen LD and Rootman DS (2001). Clinicopathological correlation of congenital corneal opacification using ultrasound biomicroscopy. *Br J Ophthalmol.* **86**, 62–69.
48 Ozeki H, Shirai S, Nozaki M, *et al.* (2000). Ocular and systemic features of Peter's anomaly. *Graefe's Arch Clin Exp Ophthalmol.* **238**, 833–839.
49 Traboulsi EI and Maumenee IH (1992). Peter's anomaly and associated congenital malformations. *Arch Ophthalmol.* **110**, 1739–1742.
50 Kivlin JD, Fineman RM, Crandall AS and Olsen RJ (1986). Peter's anomaly as a consequence of genetic and non-genetic syndromes. *Arch Ophthalmol.* **104**, 61–64.
51 Hanson IM, Fletcher JM, Jordan T, *et al.* (1994). Mutations at the PAX6 locus are found in heterogeneous anterior segment malformations including Peter's anomaly. *Nat Genet.* **6**, 169–173.
52 Semina EV, Brownell I, Mintz-Hittner H, *et al.* (2001). Mutations in the human forkhead transcription factor FOXE3 associated with anterior segment ocular dysgenesis and cataracts. *Hum Mol Genet.* **10**, 231–236.
53 Yang LL, Lambert SR, Lynn M and Stilting RD (1999). Long-term results of corneal graft survival in infants and children with Peter's anomaly. *Ophthalmology* **106**, 833–848.
54 Elliott JH, Feman SS, O'Day DM and Garber M (1985). Hereditary sclerocornea. *Arch Ophthalmol.* **103**, 676–679.
55 Mietens C and Weber H (1966). A syndrome characterized by corneal opacity, nystagmus, flexion contracture of the elbows, growth failure, and mental retardation. *J Pediatr.* **69**, 624–629.
56 Lin C, Lueder GT and Kass MA (1995). Ocular abnormalities in a patient with Rothmund–Thomson syndrome. *J Pediatr Ophthalmol Strabismus* **32**, 132–134.
57 Stoilov I, Akarsu AN and Sarfazi M (1997). Identification of three different truncating mutations in cytochrome P4501B1 (CYP1B1) as the principle cause of primary congenital glaucoma (buphthalmos) in families linked to the GLC3A locus on chromosome 2p21. *Hum Mol Genet.* **6**, 641–647.
58 Russell-Eggitt IM, Rice NS, Jay B and Wyse RK (1992). Relapse following goniotomy for congenital glaucoma due to trabecular dysgenesis. *Eye* **6**, 197–200.
59 Ton CCT, Hirvonen H, Miwa H, *et al.* (1991). Positional cloning and characterization of a paired box- and homeobox-containing gene from the aniridia region. *Cell* **67**, 1059–1074.
60 Abitol M, Gerard M, Delezoide A, *et al.* (1995). PAX6 gene expression during human embryonic development at the cellular level. *Am J Hum Genet.* **57**, A132,742.
61 Margo CE (1983). Congenital aniridia: A histopathological study of the anterior segment in children. *J Pediatr Ophthalmol Strabismus* **20**, 192–198.
62 Walton DS (1979). Aniridia with glaucoma. In: *Glaucoma*, p. 351–354. Eds Chandler PA and Grant WM (Philadelphia: Lea & Feibiger).
63 Clericuzio CL (1993). Clinical phenotypes and Wilms tumor. *Med Pediatr Oncol.* **21**, 182–187.
64 Crolla JA, Cawdery JE, Oley CA, *et al.* (1997). A FISH approach to defining the extent and possible clinical significance of deletions at the WAGR locus. *J Med Genet.* **34**, 207–212.
65 Weiss AH, Kousseff BG, Ross EA and Longbottom J (1989). Simple microphthalmos. *Arch Ophthalmol.* **107**, 1625–1630.
66 Warburg M (1991). An update on microphthalmos and coloboma: A brief survey of genetic disorders with microphthalmos and coloboma. *Ophthalmic Pediatr Genet.* **12**, 57–63.
67 Warburg M (1992). Update of sporadic microphthalmos and coloboma: Non-inherited anomalies. *Ophthalmic Pediatr Genet.* **13**, 111–122.
68 Biswas S and Lloyd IC (1999). Oculocutaneous albinism. *Arch Dis Child.* **80**, 565–569.
69 Boissy RE and Nordlund JJ (1997). Molecular basis of congenital pigmentary disorders in humans: A review. *Pigment Cell Res.* **10**, 12–24.
70 Summers CG and King RA (1994). Ophthalmic features of minimal pigment oculocutaneous albinism. *Ophthalmology* **101**, 906–914.
71 Giebel LB, Tripathi RK, King RA and Spritz RA (1991). A temperature-sensitive tyrosinase in human albinism: A human homologue to the Siamese cat and the Himalayan mouse. *J Clin Invest.* **87**, 1119–1122.
72 Lee S-T, Nicholls RD, Schnur RE, *et al.* (1994). Diverse mutations of the P gene among African–Americans with type II (tyrosinase-positive) oculocutaneous albinism (OCA2). *Hum Mol Genet.* **3**, 2047–2051.
73 Lee S-T, Nicholls RD, Bundey S, *et al.* (1994). Mutations of the P gene in oculocutaneous albinism, ocular albinism, and Prader–Willi syndrome plus albinism. *New Engl J Med.* **330**, 529–534.
74 Boissy RE, King RA, Nordlund JJ, *et al.* (1996). Mutation in and lack of expression of tyrosinase-related protein-1 (TRP-1) in melanocytes from an individual with brown oculocutaneous albinism: A new subtype of albinism classified as 'OCA3'. *Am J Hum Genet.* **58**, 1145–1156.
75 Charles SJ, Moore AT and Yates JRW (1992). Genetic mapping of X linked ocular albinism: Linkage analysis in British families. *J Med Genet.* **29**, 552–554.

76 Charles SJ, Moore AT, Grant JW and Yates JRW (1992). Genetic counselling in X-linked ocular albinism: Clinical features of the carrier state. *Eye* **6**, 75–79.
77 Boissy RE and Nordlund JJ (1997). Molecular basis of congenital pigmentary disorders in humans: A review. *Pigment Cell Res.* **10**, 12–24.
78 Kriss A, Russell-Eggitt I, Harris CM, Lloyd IC and Taylor D (1992). Aspects of albinism. *Ophthalmol Paediatr Genet.* **13**, 89–100.
79 Kinnear PE, Jay B and Witkop JR (1985). Albinism. *Surv Ophthalmol.* **30**, 75–101.
80 Collewijn H, Apkarian P and Spekreijse H (1985). The ocular motor behaviour of human albinos. *Brain* **108**, 1–28.
81 Kriss A, Russell-Eggitt I and Taylor D (1990). Childhood albinism. Visual electrophysiological features. *Ophthalmic Paediatr Genet.* **11**, 185–192.

11
Spectacle Dispensing for Children

Andrew Keirl

Initial considerations

A review of several texts concerned with the subjects of paediatric optometry and general dispensing surprisingly showed little understanding of what is meant by 'paediatric dispensing', as the words do not appear to form an officially defined term.

It is, however, generally accepted by most practitioners that a different approach needs to be taken when dealing with children. So what makes paediatric dispensing different? Clearly, the facial structures of younger children, in particular, differ considerably from those of an adult, but any answer to this question must include reference to what some authors refer to as the duality of the patient.[1]

This term has come about because, in such cases, we usually deal with two patients, the parent and the child, often with conflicting interests. Communication difficulties and an understanding of the psychology involved in dealing with both the parents and the child present challenges in paediatric dispensing (see Chapter 15 for further discussion of this point) that may not be encountered in general adult optometric and/or dispensing practice.

In recent years some frame manufacturers, suppliers and optical groups have paid little attention to differences in facial measurements between adults and children. This decision, presumably taken from a commercial standpoint, has sometimes produced difficulties in frame selection for younger patients, which has resulted in frames that fit inadequately.

With regard to spectacle lenses, adult prescriptions are usually given to correct a refractive error. While this is also the case in paediatric optometry, lenses can be supplied for reasons other than refractive error, such as for occlusion therapy and the treatment of accommodative strabismus.

The practitioner with an interest in paediatric dispensing should attempt to answer the following questions:

- What features should manufacturers incorporate into the design of children's spectacle frames? Children are not merely small adults, as their facial features are quite different from those of a mature person.
- Should manufacturers be doing more to incorporate these differences into the design of children's frames? In the opinion of the author, scaled-down adult spectacle frames or children's frames manufactured using components from adult frames should not be accepted by practitioners.
- What are the visual demands that need to be addressed in paediatric dispensing? The visual demands placed on children today are vast. Children are encouraged to and, perhaps more importantly, want to use technology from a very early age. Indeed, children appear to be born with a mouse in their hands these days!
- Should safety be the paramount concern in paediatric dispensing? Children tend to be rougher with themselves and their spectacles than do adults. On the whole, adults understand their limitations and tend to treat themselves with some degree of care. Children, however, act as though they are invincible. Their spectacles and, more importantly, their eyes are not.
- When or where does paediatric dispensing stop and adult dispensing start? Until the early 1980s children were rarely given much thought when it came to dispensing spectacles or designing frames, so opticians had little to offer. Children today are more demanding and brand conscious. We rarely see children wearing ordinary trainers or an unmarked baseball cap. Now we have designer frames (to match the designer trainers) and lightweight lenses.

The primary considerations in paediatric dispensing are, therefore, comfort and fit, function, eye protection and fashion.

Spectacles and frame selections

Frames selected for children should not be based solely on aesthetics. A frame selected must:

- Ensure an anatomically correct fit;
- Place the lenses correctly in front of the eyes;
- Be comfortable, stable and not damage the forming features;
- Not inhibit the natural development of the nasal structure.

Plastic frames can achieve the primary goal of anatomical correctness if the frame is shaped and sized correctly and the bridge is of the correct structure. If the bridge of the frame does not conform to that of the child, it seeks out the area of the nose on which it does conform. In other words, it slips! Since 90 per cent of the frame's weight rests upon the bridge, no single fitting feature of a child's frame is more important. The main feature in a good bridge fit is the amount of the frame's bridge surface that rests flush upon the nose. The general rule is the larger the area of contact, the more support and the less pressure.[2]

Unfortunately, frames worn today by children are often miniature or 'scaled-down' adult spectacle frames. As a result of this situation, a poor relationship often exists between the dimensions of the child's face and the spectacle frame, with the result that a frame may neither be acceptable nor comfortable to wear. Adult patients who are unhappy with their spectacles may simply go elsewhere. A poorly fitted frame or, more importantly, a frame that is not worn because it is so uncomfortable may cause a child permanent visual and/or developmental harm.

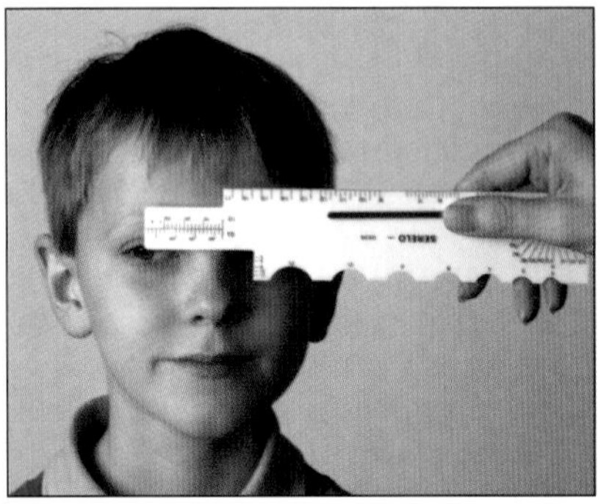

Figure 11.1
Crest height facial measurement

The main features of spectacle frames for children[3] compared with those for adults are that the:

- Crest height is lower;
- Frontal angle is larger;
- Splay angle is larger;
- Frontal width is smaller;
- Angle of side is smaller.

In addition, and as a consequence of the child's smaller cranial features, the:

- Boxed lens size is smaller;
- Lens aperture must have a shape that differs from adult designs;
- Length to bend and length of drop are shorter;
- The vertex distance is often very short.

We often forget the world that we live and work in was built by (and for) adults. As a consequence, children often have to look upwards, which results in a direction of gaze through the gap between the upper rim of the frame and their eyebrows. This may be of little consequence for myopic children, but could have repercussions for esophoric hypermetropes, as an uncorrected accommodative esophoria may become decompensated and break down into an esotropia. Spectacles do not slide upwards!

Also, the mechanical problems caused by the lenses might compound the problem of slipping. Stock uncut lenses that are much larger than the minimum uncut diameter may increase the weight of the appliance, which may cause further dispensing problems, such as slipping frames and sore nasal areas.

The prerequisites of a child's frame do not significantly differ from those of an adult's frame,[4] and are:

- To hold the lenses in the required position;
- The frame must display stability, rigidity and strength;
- The frame must be comfortable to wear and give acceptable cosmesis;
- Best use must be made of the natural field of view.

Dermatological problems of a spectacle frame in contact with the skin of a child have been documented and need to be considered in paediatric dispensing.[5] It has been known since the early 1960s that children's skin can withstand a remarkable degree of physical insult without permanent damage, with speedy recovery and adaptation to pain. This relative insensitivity to badly fitting frames may lead to irritation and malformation of the developing ears and nose.

Anthropometry for spectacle frames

Before the early 1960s little interest was shown in the problems concerned with children's spectacles. The literature does, however, contain several primary research articles that discuss the relationship between facial measurements of children and the manufacture of spectacle frames for use in paediatric dispensing.[4,6–8]

Important facial measurements in paediatric dispensing are the bridge measurements, specifically the crest height, bridge projection, frontal angle and splay angle. These measurements are illustrated in *Figures 11.1–11.4* and defined in *Table 11.1*.

The corresponding frame measurements are illustrated in *Figures 11.5–11.9* and defined in *Table 11.2*.

The bridge projection can be positive, negative or 'zero'. Negative and zero bridge projections are often encountered when dispensing to younger age groups. Negative bridge projections are sometimes referred to as 'inset' bridges.

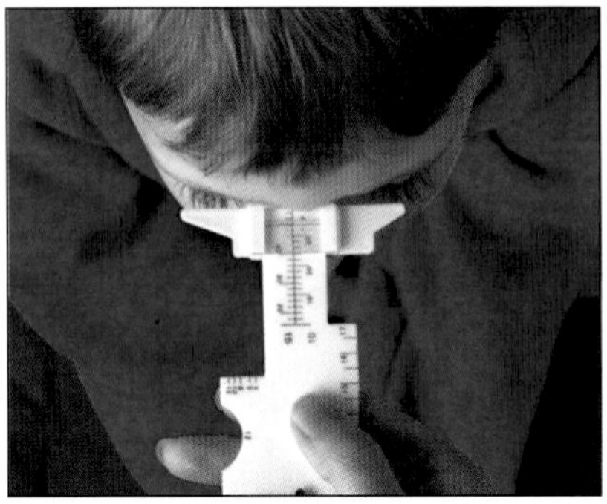

Figure 11.2
Bridge projection facial measurement

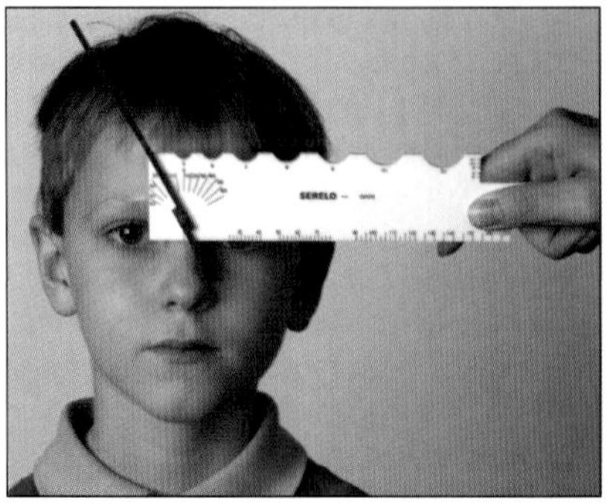

Figure 11.3
Frontal angle facial measurement

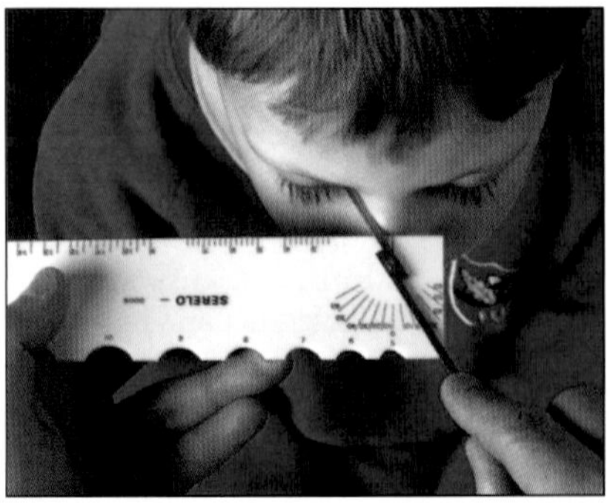

Figure 11.4
Splay angle facial measurement

Table 11.1 Facial measurement definitions

Term	*Definition*
Crest height	Distance, measured in the assumed spectacle plane, between the lower limbus and the nasal crest
Bridge projection	Horizontal distance between the assumed spectacle plane and the eyelashes in their most projecting position
Frontal angle	Angle between the vertical in the assumed spectacle plane and a parallel to the assumed bearing surface on the side of the nose
Splay angle	Angle between the assumed pad-bearing area on the nose and a normal to the assumed spectacle plane

Table 11.3 is a compilation of the results of various studies found in the available literature and shows the mean values for children's bridge measurements. The data show that at around 13 years of age the bridge dimensions are more or less equivalent to adult dimensions.

The results and conclusion of the various studies show that:

- Children's faces do not grow at a steady rate;

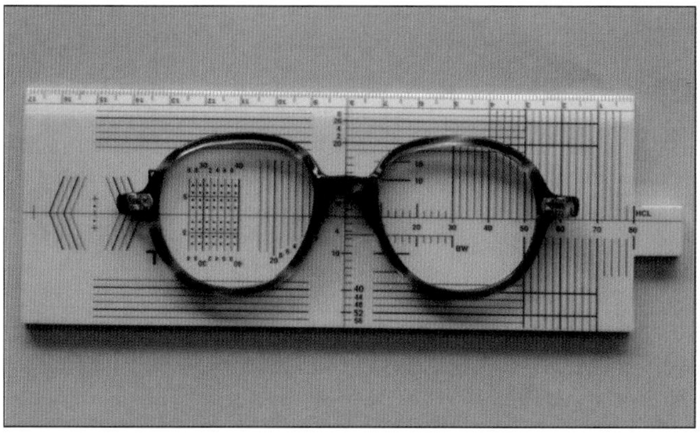

Figure 11.5
Crest height frame measurement

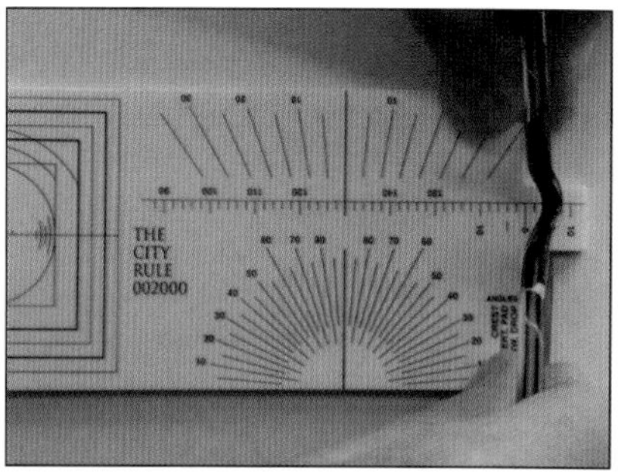

Figure 11.6
Positive bridge projection frame measurement

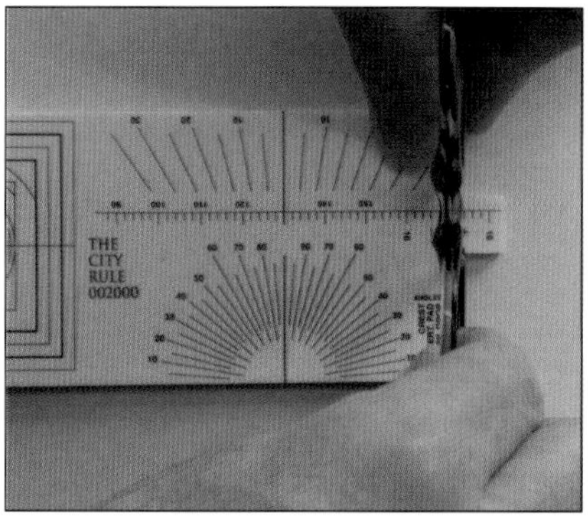

Figure 11.7
Negative bridge projection frame measurement

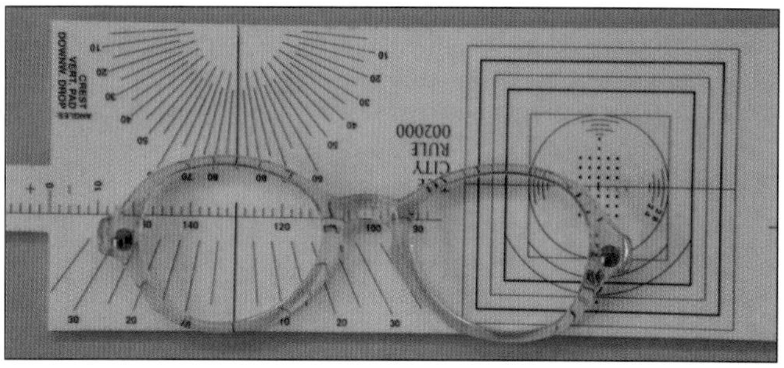

Figure 11.8
Frontal angle frame measurement

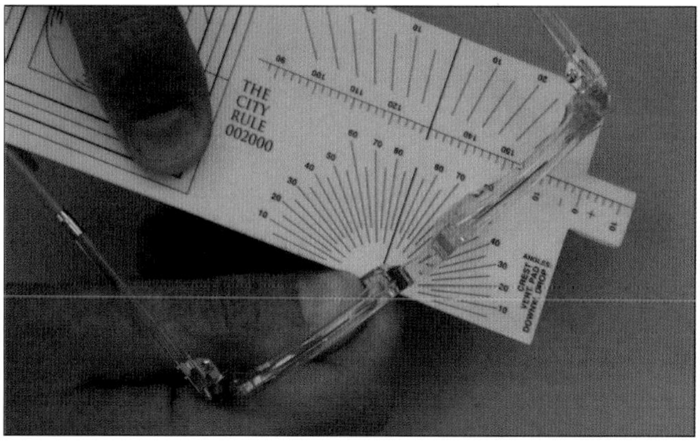

Figure 11.9
Splay angle of pad

Table 11.2 Frame measurement definitions

Term	*Definition*
Crest height	Vertical distance from the horizontal centre line of the front to the mid-point of the lower edge of the bridge
Bridge projection	Minimum horizontal distance from the back plane of the front to the centre of the back of the bridge
Frontal angle of pad	Angle between the vertical and the line of intersection of the pad plane with the back plane of the front
Splay angle of pad	Angle between the pad plane and a normal to the back plane of the front

- Facial structures differ in proportion to those of adults;
- The nose alters considerably during development;
- Only two dimensions remain practically unchanged – the angle of crest and apical radius.

At 5–7 years of age children seldom show a bridge on the nose. There is a smooth flat area that grades from the forehead to nose bulb. Many children older than 6 years of age show true noses and the beginning of a nasal bridge. At over 9 years of age there are formed noses, but the projections are small and from 11 years of age the nose is well formed. Most children's facial measurements equal those of adults by 13 years of age. The exceptions to this are the head width and the front to bend, which both increase by approximately 10mm after 13 years of age. Adult bridges have heights of 5–7mm and splay and/or frontal angles of 20–25°.

The facial measurements of Afro-Caribbean children have also been studied,[4] and a summary of available data is given in *Table 11.4*. These differences are significant and indicate that the demographics of a practice may influence the designs of frames selected.

In 1993 a study into the facial characteristics in children with Down's syndrome was carried out by Woodhouse *et al.*[9] This important and interesting study measured the facial characteristics in children with Down's syndrome and compared them with two previous studies.[4,8] The results of the study showed that between 7 and 14 years of age, the facial characteristics of children with Down's syndrome do not change with age and rarely coincide with those of other children, either of a similar age or younger. The authors stated that children with Down's syndrome cannot be fitted satisfactorily with conventional children's frames and suggest that a specially designed range of frames be made available.

Significant refractive error is very common among children with Down's syndrome so the requirement for spectacles for this group is high. It has been reported that 77 per cent of children with Down's syndrome suffer from a refractive error.[10]

The nature of the ametropia can be myopia or hypermetropia and there is often a significant astigmatic error. Another study has shown that accommodative problems may require correction in up to 80 per cent of school-age children with Down's syndrome.[11] Other ocular problems associated with Down's syndrome include cataract, nystagmus, strabismus and keratoconus.

Table 11.3 Mean children's bridge measurements

Age (years)	3.0–4.5	4.5–6.0	6.5–8.5	10.0–11.5	13.5
Crest height (mm)	−0.8	−0.5	+0.5	+2.4	+4.5
Projection (mm)	+0.2	+1.0	+1.4	+1.6	+3.0
Frontal angle (°)	34	34	32	31	35
Splay angle (°)	35	34	32	29	29

Subjects measured in the Woodhouse *et al.*[9] study were divided into three groups based on age. *Table 11.5* gives the results for crest height, bridge projection, frontal angle and splay angle. Crest height in normal children shows a general increase with age, starting with a negative crest and becoming progressively more positive with age. The Down's syndrome group showed a slight, but insignificant, increase with age. Bridge projection in normal children also increases with age, starting at around zero and increasing to about 4–5mm by 14 years of age. Bridge projection in Down's syndrome appears to decrease with age. Children with Down's syndrome have frontal angles that are smaller than normal and splay angles that are larger than normal. Other points of interest from the Woodhouse *et al.*[9] study are summarised in *Table 11.6*.

The Woodhouse *et al.*[9] study clearly shows that the Down's syndrome child presents a special case in paediatric dispensing, as there was not a single child in whom all facial measurements fell within the normal range. The other problem highlighted by the study was that the facial measurements of Down's syndrome children are not consistently smaller or larger than the normal for age. If the measurements were consistently larger or smaller, one could simply fit a frame designed for an older or younger child. On occasions, the only option for a Down's syndrome child is to the supply a hand-made frame.

Plastic frame selection

So, bearing in mind the above regarding the facial measurements of children, what can we now say about the selection of plastics spectacle frames in paediatric dispensing?

Table 11.4 Facial measurements of Afro-Caribbean children

Measurement	*Approximate difference in Afro-Caribbeans*
Crest height (mm)	−2
Projection (mm)	−1
Frontal angle (°)	+7
Splay angle (°)	+9

Table 11.5 Means of crest height, bridge projection, frontal angle and splay angle for the three age groups in the Down's syndrome study[9]

Age (years)	Crest height (mm)	Bridge projection (mm)	Frontal angle (°)	Splay angle (°)
7.0–8.9	−3.0	−1.0	26.25	33.8
9.0–11.9	−1.3	−2.4	26.4	35.0
12.0–14.0	−1.4	−2.8	26.3	33.8

Table 11.6 Summary of other facial measurements included in the Woodhouse study[9]

Interpupillary distance	Smaller than normal in older Down's syndrome children
Apical radius	Smaller than normal
Front to bend	Shorter than normal
Temple width	Larger than normal
Head width	Larger than normal in younger children, but smaller than normal in older children

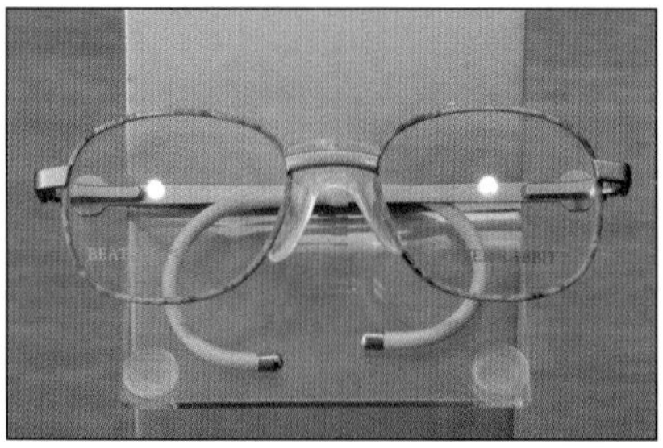

Figure 11.10
Sample child frame

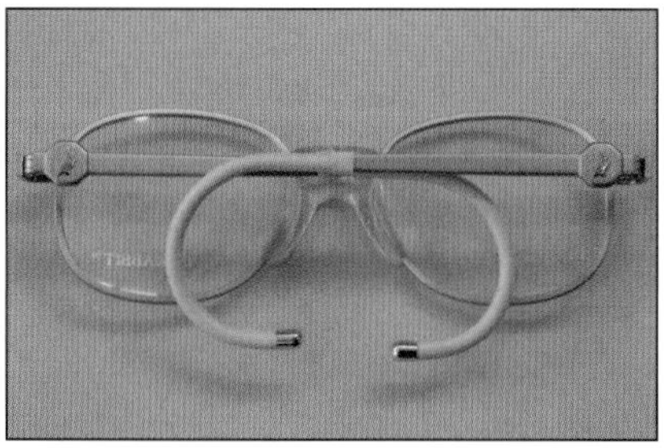

Figure 11.11
View of frame from behind

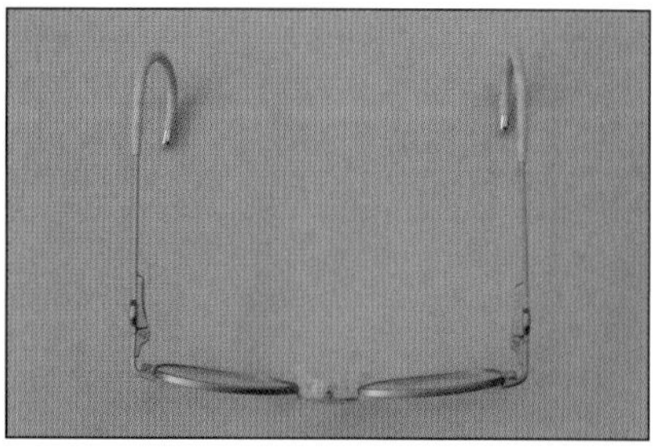

Figure 11.12
View of frame from above

The most important point is that the bridge of the frame must be compared with the child's bridge – these should have the same shape and be of equal width.

A regular bridge with a negative projection is often the most suitable design for the underdeveloped nasal structure common to the infant or toddler, while a keyhole bridge is useful for older children. The crest height controls the vertical position of the front and is measured from the horizontal centre line (HCL) to the bearing surface (nasal crest) of the nose. A larger crest height causes the frame to sit lower on the face. In younger children with underdeveloped noses, the bearing surface and the HCL are very close, which gives a crest height of around zero.

The function of the bridge projection is to control the horizontal position of the front. A negative bridge projection pushes the frame away from the face and compensates for the underdeveloped nasal bridge of the very young child. This prevents the eyelashes from rubbing against the back surface of the lenses.

The main feature of the frame in *Figure 11.10* is its insert bridge. Note also the low crest height and the curl sides. *Figures 11.11* and *11.12* show the frame from *Figure 11.10* viewed from behind and above. Note the negative bridge projection and the low crest height.

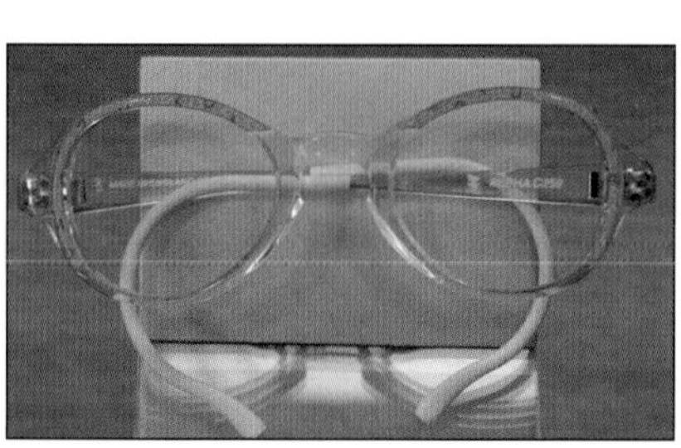

Figure 11.13
Frame with keyhold bridge

Keyhole bridges

For some children, keyhole bridges can have definite advantages, as the design distributes the weight along the sides of the nose and not on the crest. Prolonged pressure can break down the fatty tissue and, in extreme cases, causes deviation of the septum.

Figure 11.13 shows a front manufactured using a keyhole bridge. The purpose of this type of bridge is to provide clearance at the crest. Without the keyhole, the crest height of this frame would be around zero. Note also the large frontal angle.

Metal frames

Metal frames can solve many fitting problems when dispensing to children. However, safety considerations are of utmost concern when fitting children with metal frames. Recognition of an age-appropriate frame is critical in the dispensing of a metal frame to a child.[12]

Age-appropriate frames consist of components sufficiently stable for age-related activities and sized correctly to fit the anatomical features at a given stage of development. Paediatric frames that are scaled-down versions of adult styles or manufactured using adult components cannot be considered age appropriate.

Bridge design

Bridge design is probably the most important feature to consider when selecting an age-appropriate metal frame.

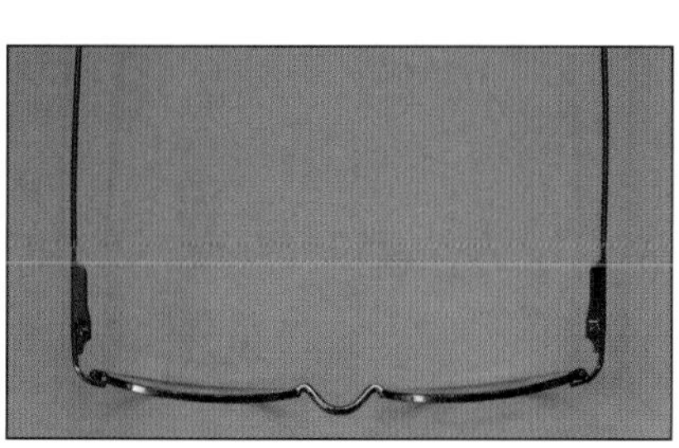

Figure 11.14
Frame with 'w' bridge

Bridges of metal frames are either adjustable or fixed. Metal frames with saddle or 'w' bridges (*Figure 11.14*) are inappropriate for paediatric dispensing as they cannot be adjusted and are designed to distribute the weight solely on the crest of the nose; they cannot be considered age appropriate.

Adjustable bridges

Metal frames with adjustable pad bridges or pads on the arms are useful in paediatric dispensing. However, to give the correct vertical positioning and/or centration, pad arms should be soldered along the nasal rim at a height to present the pad-arm box assembly at approximately the same height as the sides. If the box assembly is too high, the frame sits low on the child's face (*Figure 11.15*). This may have a knock-on effect as far as centration and decentration is concerned, which produce lenses with unnecessarily thick edges.

Another important item to consider in the design of metal frames with adjustable pads is the shape of the bridge bar, as the shank of the bridge bar can be a significant

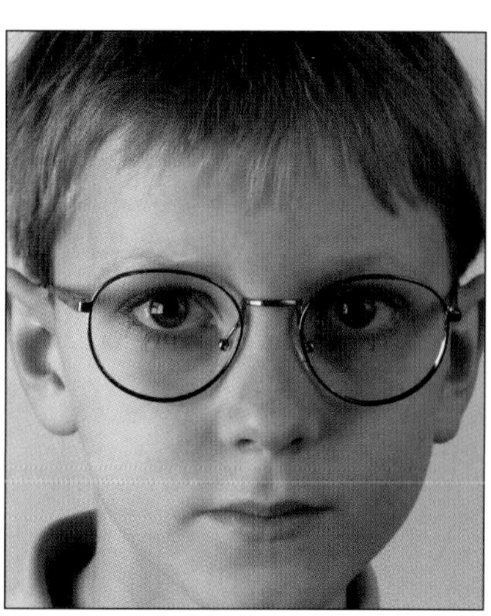

Figure 11.15
Box assembly sits too high, frame sits low

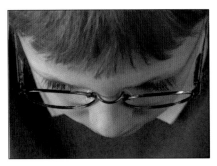

Figure 11.16
Shanks of bridge bar too close to face

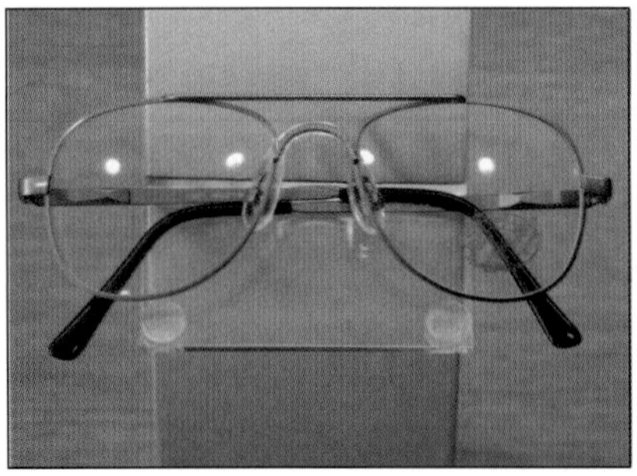

Figure 11.17
Frame with strap bridge

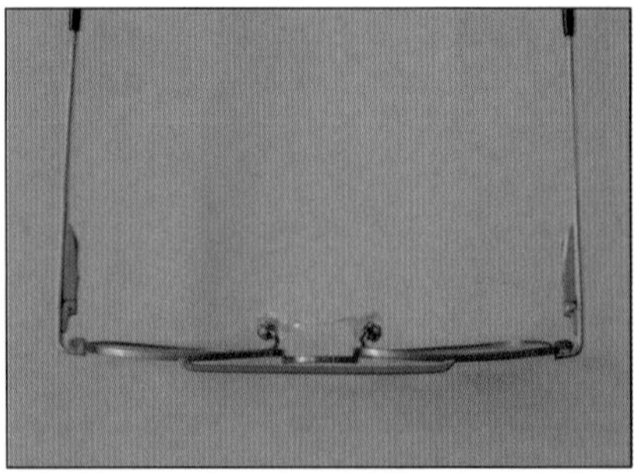

Figure 11.18
Strap bridge seen from above

safety concern. A metal frame may not be considered age appropriate if the shanks of the bridge bar extend inward too far to be considered safe as, under impact, this area of the frame could injure the wearer (*Figure 11.16*).

Yet another important feature to consider in the design of metal frames with adjustable pads is the type and size of the pad itself. Adjustable pads and ribbon pads assist in correctly distributing the weight of the spectacles, which should be distributed over as great an area as possible. This is best achieved by the use of larger nose pads, although strap bridges can also be used to distribute the weight of the glasses over a wider area. However, while a toddler's size might indicate the use of small round pads, strong plus lenses may be too heavy to be supported comfortably by this pad type.

In general, select the pad size that distributes the weight of the spectacles over as much surface as the facial structure will allow. The selection of pad size is totally subjective. When dispensing metal frames with adjustable pad bridges, practitioners should be prepared to change the pads from those supplied with the frame to produce the best possible fit by providing adequate support.[13]

Strap bridges

Another option for use with a pads-on-arms metal frame is the strap bridge. As strap bridges absorb more impact and retain adjustment better than adjustable pads, they can be used for very young children.

A strap bridge must be selected so that it conforms to the bridge bar that connects the right and left rims. Practitioners should be aware that a small nose might not be able to support the bulk of a strap pad. *Figures 11.17* and *11.18* show a strap bridge that conforms to the shape of the bridge bar of the frame.

Clearly, the major labour of love in paediatric dispensing is frame adjustment! One of the most frequently needed adjustments arises because the pad arms that hold the strap bridge spread too far apart. If this occurs, the crest of the child's nose carries the entire weight, which is uncomfortable and, if not corrected, the fatty tissue breaks down to leave a permanent ridge.

Side styles

Three types of side are used in paediatric dispensing. For very young children loop-end sides can be used.

Curl sides are very useful for toddlers and older children, and for school-age children curl or drop-end sides are appropriate. The drop-end sides supplied on children's frames are generally too long to produce a satisfactory adjustment. If curl sides are to be used they should have a silicone covering to provide comfort and durability. The curl should rest along the back of the ear and extend around the ear root, stopping just short of the ear lobe.[14]

Speciality frames

The main problem in the dispensing of a frame to very small children is one of rigidity. When dispensing to babies, frames need to fit the facial structures perfectly. Frames also need to be accepted without negative reactions from either the patients or their children.

An example of a speciality frame, which can be used for tiny babies and also older children, is the Comoframe (WT Rees; *Figure 11.19*). The characteristics of this frame that make it particularly suitable for use with very young children are that it is made using a soft and pliable material, has no hinges or metal parts and uses elastic to hold the frame in place on the face.

As far as tiny babies are concerned, when they start to walk their face is protected, the frame adapts to the facial contours and it is indestructible.

For older children the use of frames of this type reduces the risk of facial and ocular trauma, permits any kind of sports activity and is unlikely to inhibit any kind of play, however rough.

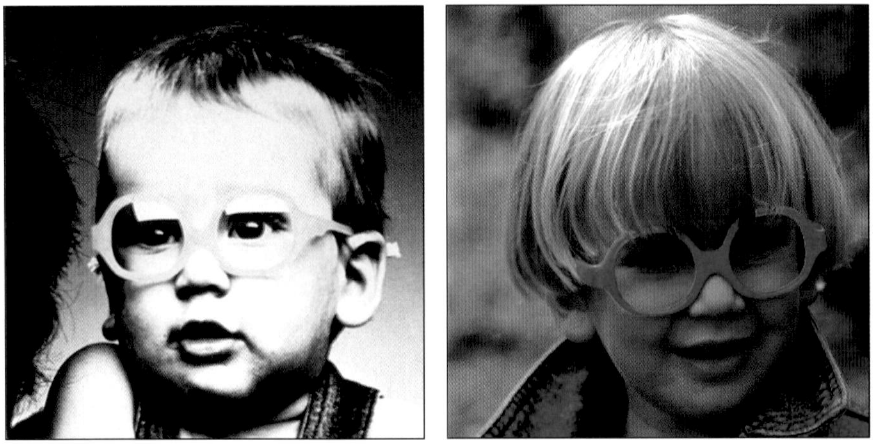

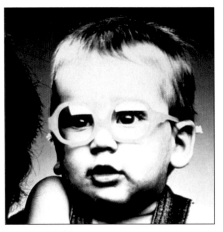

Figure 11.19
Comoframe wearers

The use of holes and elastic helps to keep the frame in place and therefore keeps the lenses well centred. This prevents the child from looking above the lenses and, if required, guarantees occlusion.

From a practical point of view, the use of elastic keeps little ones from pulling off their spectacles. As far as the optometrist is concerned, the use of this frame allows the early correction of refractive errors, permits strabismus treatment from a very early stage, facilitates the spectacle correction of infantile aphakia and permits the early treatment of anisometropic amblyopia.

With reference to the duality of the patient, from the parent's point of view use of this frame reduces the fear of facial and ocular trauma, removes resistance to traditional frames and resolves the problem of broken and/or distorted frames.

A very useful range of children's frames is available from Menrad. These include several metal frames with small eye sizes, adjustable pad bridges and side lengths of 120mm. In addition, Menrad produces frames specifically designed for younger children. *Figure 11.20* shows Menrad model 15310, a well-designed frame that is suitable for the older child and features sensibly positioned pad arms to ensure that the frame does not sit low on the child's face. The importance of position of the frame on the face is also reflected in the design of Menrad model 15314 (*Figure 11.21*). Here, the pad arms are actually below the HCL and, in addition, the joints are positioned very close to the HCL. The design of this frame makes it very age appropriate. *Figures 11.22* and *11.23* show Menrad models 155935 and 155545, which are designed for the younger child and feature negative bridges, curl sides and side lengths from 115 to 130mm.

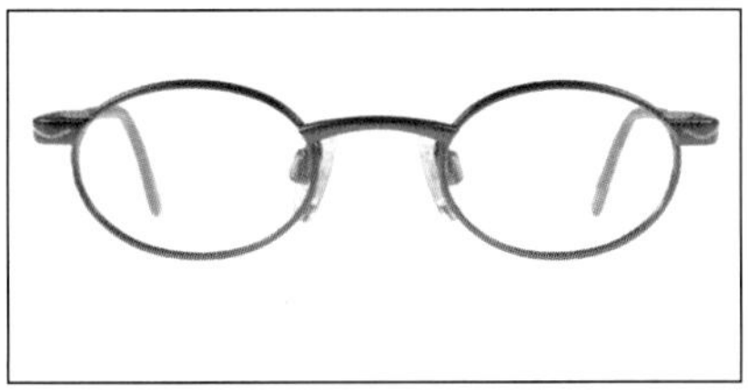

Figure 11.20
Menrad 15310 frame

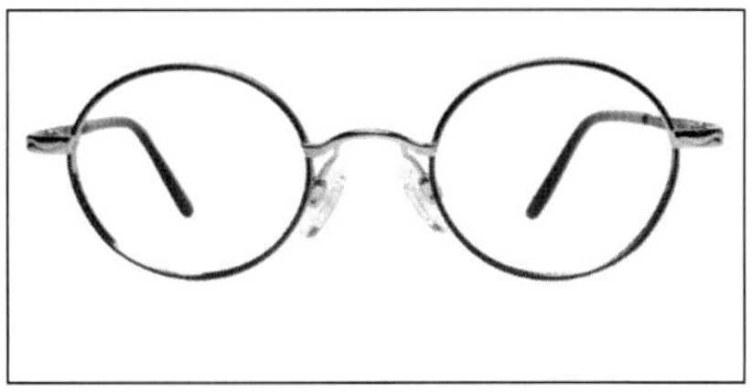

Figure 11.21
Menrad 15314 frame

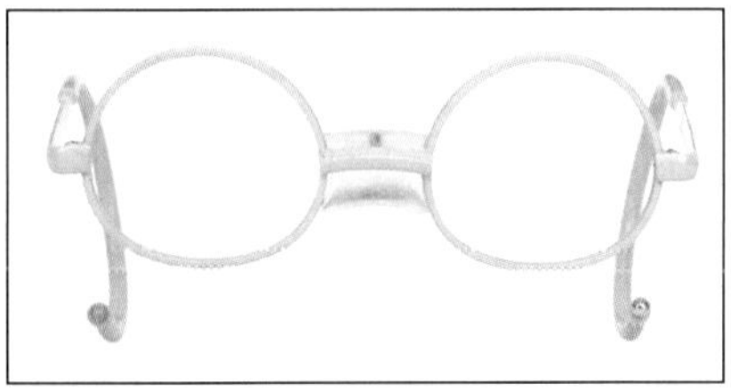

Figure 11.22
Menrad 155935 frame

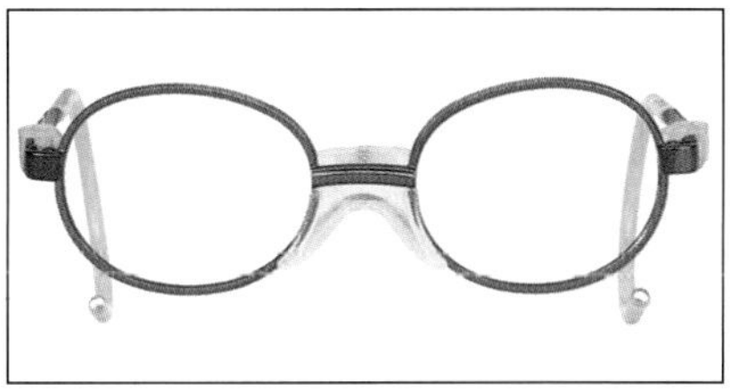

Figure 11.23
Menrad 155545 frame

Spectacle lenses

Prescription analysis

Compared with prescription analysis in general adult dispensing, prescription analysis in general paediatric dispensing requires additional considerations based on the following criteria:

- The child's age and stage of visual development;
- Common conditions encountered within the child's age group;
- The prescription being presented;
- Information obtained from parents.

Adult and children's prescriptions may look identical, but their purposes may be quite different. In general adult dispensing the usual objective of a spectacle prescription is to correct a refractive error. Children's prescriptions are not always intended to accomplish this same objective, for example, in amblyopia therapy or in strabismic anisometropia.

Lens material

Polycarbonate is the lens material of choice in paediatric dispensing. The recent growth of the polycarbonate lens market results from the high impact resistance of this material. In the USA, it has become the default material for children. The refractive index of polycarbonate is 1.586, V-value 30 and density 1.2.

The advantages of polycarbonate are:

- Very high impact resistance (greatest impact resistance of all ophthalmic materials, which, if it does fracture, crazes and does not break into particles);
- No age-related warping, chipping or discoloration;
- Polycarbonate has a relatively high refractive index (1.586);
- One of the lightest lens materials available (density 1.2);
- Absorbs UV radiation below 380nm;
- Resistance to distortion by heat and has electrical resistance properties.

The disadvantages of polycarbonate are:

- Compared with CR39 or glass, the surface quality of polycarbonate is poor;
- The V-value of polycarbonate is low and may cause visual problems when viewing off-axis;
- The surface of polycarbonate is soft and has been found to scratch easily;
- Surface coatings reduce the impact resistance of polycarbonate;
- Solvents such as acetone reduce impact resistance.

Polycarbonate has a wide product availability, which includes single-vision lenses, single-vision aspheric lenses, bifocal lenses, polarising lenses, progressive power lenses and photochromic lenses.[15]

The major drawback of polycarbonate is its low V-value. However, since the arrival on the market of Trivex, a plastics material manufactured by PPG and used by Hoya as 'Phoenix' and Younger as 'Trilogy', practitioners now have an alternative to polycarbonate. Trivex has the following properties:

- It passes FDA at 1mm centre thickness;
- It meets ANSI Z87.1 standards;
- Withstands a pulling force of 80kg;
- Withstands pressure of 10kg.

In addition, Trivex:

- Displays a good resistance to scratching;
- Absorbs UV to 395nm;
- Displays resistance to high temperatures;
- Displays resistance against solvents;
- Requires no special edging equipment;
- Can be manufactured with a centre thickness of 1.3mm for minus lenses.

Polycarbonate is extremely difficult to process compared with other plastics lens materials. A lens with high impact resistance and straightforward processing ability will be very welcome. In terms of impact resistance, Trivex is comparable to polycarbonate, but its main advantage lies in its V-value (46 compared with 30 for polycarbonate).

Impact resistance of lens materials
Impact resistances of glass lens materials are:

- Toughened glass 18m/s;
- Conventional glass 12m/s;

Impact resistances of plastics lens materials are:

- CR39 18m/s;
- Polymethyl methacrylate (PMMA) 34m/s;
- Polycarbonate (coated) 152m/s;
- Polycarbonate (uncoated) 244m/s.

Data for both glass and plastics were obtained using 3mm samples.[16] The above information illustrates why polycarbonate or Trivex should be the materials of choice in paediatric dispensing.

Even when uncoated, polycarbonate outperforms other materials in terms of impact resistance. It is generally agreed, however, that in paediatric dispensing, the superior impact resistance of polycarbonate outweighs any possible disadvantages associated with its low V-value.

In paediatric dispensing, safety is the critical issue. It can be argued that nothing else deserves higher priority.

The practitioner has a duty of care to warn parents and children of the dangers of not providing adequate eye protection and must discuss with the child's parents the materials available to assist the parent in selecting the appropriate lens. In this age of litigation, it is sensible that the practitioner documents on the patient's permanent record that the patient and parent were informed about lens material choice and indicated the material selected.

Interestingly, in the USA some practitioners ask parents and/or patients to countersign the permanent record if polycarbonate was not selected.

Positive powered spectacle lenses
Far too many children are being dispensed with thicker lenses than necessary, because large diameter stock lenses are being edged into small frames, which results in finished lenses with unnecessarily large edge and centre substances.

Rather than using stock lenses, minimum substance surfacing should now be standard practice for hypermetropic prescriptions. Minimum substance surfacing results in a lighter, less bulbous and more attractive lens, which means that the likelihood the child will wear the spectacles is greater. The cosmetic benefits of correct surfacing are illustrated in *Figure 11.24*, in which the right and left prescriptions are the same. The right lens has been surfaced and the left is a stock lens.

Aspheric lenses also provide an improvement in the cosmetic appearance of a spectacle lens, particularly in hypermetropic cases. Aspheric lenses are available for both plus and minus prescriptions. In paediatric dispensing, they are advantageous in the correction of hypermetropic prescriptions, as the use of an aspheric lens greatly improves the cosmetic appearance and therefore the potential wearability of the lenses.

The advantages of aspheric lenses compared to a lens manufactured using traditional spherical surfaces for the normal power range are well known, but are given here for completeness:

- Flatter by 2–3D;
- Slightly thinner;
- Good oblique vision;
- Less spectacle magnification.

Special lenses
While most paediatric prescriptions can be satisfied using single-vision lenses, there are a few special lenses for use in paediatric dispensing.

One such is the Excelit AS produced by Rodenstock, designed for use in the treatment of accommodative esotropia. The Excelit AS is a CR39 40 × 25mm curved top segment on the convex surface of the lens. The segment is outset by 4mm to discourage convergence for near. As with all bifocals for use in accommodative esotropia, the segment should be positioned so that it bisects the pupil and the distance portion should be centred to correspond with the monocular centration distances.

An E-type bifocal is an alternative to the Excelit AS in this case. In addition to the use of specialist lenses, the practitioner can, with a little imagination, adapt lenses designed for adult dispensing. An example here is the use of an E-style bifocal for the management of convergence weakness exophoria, whereby an emmetropic patient could have the lenses glazed upside down! A −2.50D lens with a +2.50D add would then give plano in the upper part of the lens and −2.50D in the lower part.

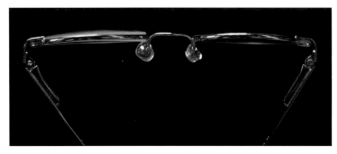

Figure 11.24 *Minimum substance surfacing on the right lens of this isotropic correction*

Optical centration
Horizontal centration
There are several schools of thought as to how this is best performed in paediatric dispensing. For younger children, a 'manual' PD measurement using a millimetre ruler is generally recommended, while a pupillometer may be used with older children.

It is suggested that practitioners try to use a 'child-friendly' ruler and keep distractions to a minimum to prevent head and eye movements. As a result of facial asymmetry in children, monocular PDs should be taken for maximum precision.

Again, opinions differ on the best measurement procedure for very young children. Using a penlight to locate the corneal visual points of distance-fixated eyes or measuring between the corneal–scleral margins are two common methods. An alternative approach is to measure the distance between the nasal and temporal canthi.

Neither a child's eye movements nor problems like strabismus or amblyopia affect the measurement obtained using this technique. In the case of strabismus, each eye must be occluded in turn. A suggested method is as follows:

- Cover patient's left eye, so if the right eye was deviating it now takes up fixation;
- Patient to fixate dispenser's left eye, who measures right mono PD;
- Cover patient's right eye, so the patient's left eye now fixates;
- Patient to fixate dispenser's right eye, who measures left mono PD.

This method can be performed by using a standard millimetre ruler or by using a pupillometer. In both cases, each eye is occluded in turn.

Vertical centration
Achieving the correct pantoscopic angle helps to ensure the best possible vision and helps to provide a comfortable fit. It has been recommended[17] that the pantoscopic angle (the angle between the visual axis of the eye when in the primary position and the optical axis of the lens) for a child's frame be 0° (the average pantoscopic tilt for an adult fitting is between 8 and 10°).

As a consequence of this, the optical centre should coincide with the pupil centre. In view of the underdeveloped nasal bone in most children, the lower rim of the frame is likely to rest against the cheek if the pantoscopic tilt is larger than zero. However, some pantoscopic angle is useful to prevent the child's long eyelashes coming into contact with the lenses.

In all cases, the pantoscopic angle and the vertical centration of the lenses should correspond.

Paediatric frame adjustment

The basics of frame adjustment can be summarised by simply stating the functions of the bridge and the sides:

- The bridge is responsible for holding the spectacles up;
- The temples and/or sides are responsible for holding them on.

The suggested procedure for paediatric frame adjustment involves seven steps.[18] In reality, this system is essentially the same as procedures used in the adjustment of an adult frame:

- Pre-adjustment – the frame is first trued or set up;
- Removing temple pressure – all pressure is removed from the temples;
- Verifying equal vertex distance – the right and left angles of letback should not create unequal vertex distances;
- Pantoscopic angle – should be close to zero to correspond to the facial plane;
- Alignment of the bridge – the bridge of the frame should now be adjusted to fit the child's bridge;
- Temple adjustment – the temples are adjusted to match the contours of the child's head;
- Snugging – equal tension is returned to the temples from the top of the ears throughout the area behind the child's ears.

I am sure that, as a result of bitter experience, readers of this chapter will agree that the two most abused components of a child's spectacle frame are the pad arms and the sides.

What other adjustment skills does the practitioner involved in paediatric dispensing need? In addition to routine adjustment, the two essential skills are:

- The conversion of a drop-end side to a curl side using cable adapters;
- The shortening of a metal side.

These skills can often be used to solve common fitting problems in paediatric dispensing. Kits and advice are available from companies such as Hilco to help practitioners perform these essential tasks.

Monitoring the fit of a frame

Whenever a spectacle-wearing child comes into the practice for whatever reason it is important to have a good general look at the overall fit of the frame. This is something that the optometrist, in particular, is well placed to do.

Be alert to any signs of an improperly fitting bridge as, since the child's nose is still developing, changes can occur that would render a previously well-fitting frame unsatisfactory. Remember that the burden of fit is always on the bridge. In particular, observation skills are necessary when a strap bridge has been fitted, as one of the most frequently needed adjustments arises because the pad arms are spread too far apart, which results in the entire weight of the spectacles resting on the crest of the nose.

If left untreated, this causes the fatty tissue to break down and leaves a permanent ridge. The parent should be warned to look out for this.

In addition to the fit of the bridge, the side length should be checked at regular intervals, possibly every 2–3 months. If necessary, the length-to-bend can be altered. Once the drop is no longer in contact with the mastoid process, it must be replaced. Curl sides should be restructured approximately every 3 months. A well-adjusted side places the maximum amount of temple surface on the greatest temporal area. The drop should rest comfortably over the back of the ear and into the side of the head. Ideally, the temple should not touch the side of the head before reaching the ear.

Special-purpose eyewear

Special-purpose eyewear is a growing market, particularly in the areas of sports appliances and eye protection. Products currently available are:

- Sun protection eyewear;
- Sports protection eyewear;
- Swimming goggles;
- Scuba masks;
- Ski goggles.

Figure 11.25 shows an example of paediatric sports eyewear.

Summary

More children are wearing spectacles than ever before. We are testing children earlier, more screening programmes are in place and the link between poor vision and learning difficulties has been recognised. As a result, children are less likely to have to struggle through school, unable to read comfortably or see the board.

Paediatric dispensing can be fun and often very rewarding. Definite challenges are presented in paediatric dispensing and it is commonly accepted that children can be difficult to fit with prescription spectacles. As eloquently summed up by Katheryn Dabbs Schramm, children come in different sizes, shapes and colours from different economic backgrounds and have different tastes – they have a limited attention span, frequently squirm and can be quite vocal when displeased!

The complexity and intimidation of paediatric dispensing is even greater when the practitioner and/or dispenser is required to fit a child less than 2 years of age. For older children, fashion, trends and peer pressure are important social factors for the child of the 21st century.

As registered professionals, we have a responsibility to the children we serve and also to their parents. We must constantly strive to improve both the products that we dispense and the methods that we use to dispense them.

If you are not satisfied with products being supplied, do something about it! If we fit an adult incorrectly, he or she may be uncomfortable and not return to the practice.

If we fit children incorrectly, we can do them permanent harm. However, if we fit children correctly, the practice-building opportunities from paediatric dispensing are enormous.

Acknowledgement
The author would like to thank Menrad, Michelle and Thomas Owen, WT Rees, Norville Optical Group and Rodenstock for their help in compiling this chapter.

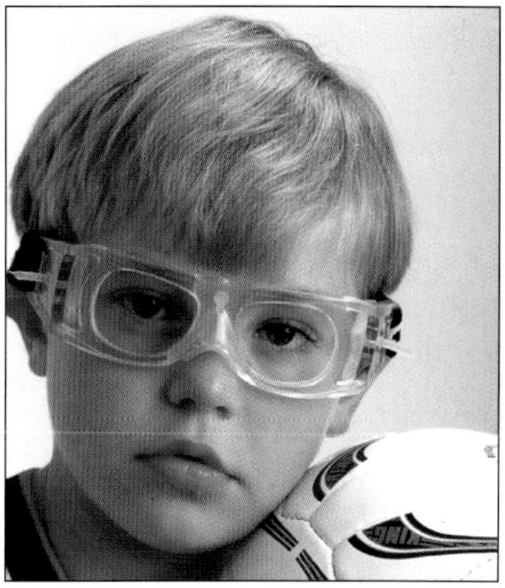

Figure 11.25
Paediatric sports eyewear

References

1 Wilson D (1999). *Practical Optical Dispensing*, p. 265 (New South Wales: Australia Open Training and Education Network).
2 Schramm KD (2000). *Dispensing Paediatric Eyewear*, p. 51–56 (Boston: Butterworth–Heinemann).
3 Obstfeld H (1997). *Spectacle Frames and their Dispensing*, p. 188–189. (London: WB Saunders).
4 Kaye J and Obstfeld H (1989). Anthropometry for children's spectacle frames. *Ophthalmic Physiol Opt*. **9**, 293–298.
5 EHirsch MJ and Wick RE (1964). *Vision in Children*, p. 272. (London: Hammond, Hammond and Co).
6 Marks R (1961). Some factors for consideration in the fitting and selection of children's eyewear. *Am J Optom Arch Am Acad Optom*. **38**, 185–193.
7 Zhuk GV (1974). Investigation of the parameters of spectacle frames for school children. *Biomed Eng*. **7**, 223–225.
8 Earlam R and White K (1990). Developing a frame for children. *Optician* **200**, 16–18.
9 Woodhouse JM, Hodge SJ and Earlam RA (1994). Facial characteristics in children with Down's syndrome and spectacle fitting. *Ophthalmic Physiol Opt*. **14**, 25–31.
10 Pueschel SM (1987). Health concerns in persons with Down's syndrome. In *New Perspectives in Down's Syndrome*. Eds Pueschel S, Tingley C, Rynders J, Crocker A and Coutcher D. (Baltimore: Brookes).
11 Woodhouse JM, Meades JS, Leat SJ and Saunders KJ (1993). Reduced accommodation in children with Down's syndrome *Invest Ophthalmol Vis Sci*. **34**, 2382–2387.
12 Schramm KD (2000). *Dispensing Paediatric Eyewear*, p. 66–72 (Boston: Butterworth–Heinemann).
13 Schramm KD (2000). *Dispensing Paediatric Eyewear*, p. 71–72 (Boston: Butterworth–Heinemann).
14 Schramm KD (2000). *Dispensing Paediatric Eyewear*, p. 173–176 (Boston: Butterworth–Heinemann).
15 Polycarbonate Lens Council, 1655 North Fort Myer Drive Suite 200, Arlington, VA 22209, USA.
16 North R (2000). *Work and the Eye*, Second Edition, p. 79 (Oxford: Butterworth-Heinemann).
17 Størseth G, Lundemo T and Lundemo B (1985). Barn og briller 0-7 ar. *Optikeren Oslo* **4**, 15–16.
18 Schramm KD (2000). *Dispensing Paediatric Eyewear*, p. 161–178 (Boston: Butterworth–Heinemann).

Further reading

Obstfeld H (1997). *Spectacle Frames and their Dispensing* (London: WB Saunders).
Schramm KD (2000). *Dispensing Paediatric Eyewear* (Boston: Butterworth–Heinemann).

12
Paediatric Contact Lenses

Lynne Speedwell

Prescribing contact lenses for use by children is a specialised area of optometry that is sometimes overlooked. There are a host of situations in which contact lenses may be the most appropriate correction, some for therapeutic and protective purposes, some for cosmesis and, increasingly, as a safe option to correct simple ametropia. As many diseases that benefit from contact lens intervention are congenital, techniques for fitting children with lenses have had to be developed. These have had to address both the physical challenges of fitting lenses to small and ever-growing eyes, and also the psychological barriers to a small child having contact lenses. Both are considered in this chapter.

General considerations

Motivation

As with adult patients, the practitioner is likely to be the one to introduce the idea of contact lenses. Remember that the child is the patient: treat each on his or her own merits and avoid generalisations.

In most instances, if the child is keen to wear lenses, he or she should be able to insert, or at least remove, the lenses themselves.

Many children initially appear keen to try lenses, but on closer questioning some of them do not actually know what contact lenses are or that they have to be inserted into the eye. The practitioner therefore needs to discuss with the children what they want out of their lenses and why they want to wear them (and to try and stop the parents answering for the children).

At this point, the practitioner can usually elicit whether it is the child or the parent who is most keen. At a remarkably young age, peer pressure or even bullying can make a child want to be rid of their glasses; changing to a cosmetically more acceptable frame may be preferable to being fitted with contact lenses.

However, psychological reasons for the child wanting contact lenses may influence the practitioner to fit lenses to a child who might not otherwise be an ideal candidate.

There are occasions when the parents bring pressure to bear on both the child and the practitioner either to fit lenses initially or to maintain the child in lenses when the practitioner advises otherwise. From a fitting point of view, this rarely works. A child may be coerced into trying lenses, but the actual day-to-day wear becomes less regular as the novelty wears off.

Time restraints on a school morning and the reluctance of the child to have the parent insert the lenses can result in the number of days' wear becoming fewer. By the time such children return for follow up, they have often reverted to spectacles.

All potential contact lens patients, including children, need a full eye examination, including slit lamp, prior to commencing lens wear. During the eye examination it is easy to tell how co-operative a child is likely to be. For example, if fluorescein instillation proves difficult, it is unlikely that the child will allow contact lens insertion.

Conversely, most children who allow eversion of the upper eyelids are not difficult when a contact lens is inserted. Bear in mind that if lenses are fitted to a child who cannot be examined adequately, it may prove impossible to carry out a thorough aftercare examination.

As with all dealings with children, several short appointments are usually better than one lengthy one. Even children who are keen may need several visits before they feel confident enough to have lenses inserted. Be patient and try to encourage them as much as possible, even if they don't achieve lens wear. They usually try their best if you are positive with them. Don't tell children that they look better in contact lenses, as they may not be able to manage lenses initially. Such an approach can further affect their confidence, and upset them even more if they experience difficulty.

The first visit

The build-up to the first visit can be such a worrying time for children that they perform badly. Give them a chance to redeem themselves. They are usually upset if they could not let you put a lens in the first time. Be patient, and at the second or third visit they are often completely different.

Advise the parents to instil artificial tears for a few weeks and also encourage the children to touch their conjunctiva with a clean finger. By the subsequent appointment they are usually more relaxed and keen to show off their achievements.

There is no particular age at which lenses should be first attempted. Some 5-year-olds are excellent candidates for lens wear and some 15-year-olds are definitely not. The decision about whether to fit lenses is similar to that in adults, in that it is made on an individual basis.

As with adults, some children who start off well become lazy and abandon lenses after a short time, while many who find lenses difficult at the beginning do very well, given time and perseverance. Only if the best contact lens type or modality is out of reach financially for the parent should fitting be postponed for a child who is otherwise suitable.

No single type of lens suits all children. They can do remarkably well with rigid gas-permeable (RGP) lenses if these are deemed to be the best lens of choice. Before commencing lens wear, explain to both the parent and the child the different types of lenses available and the advantages and disadvantages of each.

Always give reasons for your decisions. Provide as much information as possible, preferably in written form so that they can go home and discuss what they have been told. If the reason not to fit is because of reluctance on the part of the child, leave the way open to trying again at a later date.

Lens hygiene

Stress the need for lens hygiene. Children are often enthusiastic at this stage and are prepared to clean their own lenses. Parental supervision is advisable initially, but after a time children should be able to care for their own lenses.

Communication

Allow both child and parent time to ask questions. When dealing with children, remember that because they may be young doesn't mean they don't understand (see Chapter 15 for a further discussion of this). Some children are very astute and their level of comprehension astounding.

Give choices so that the child can feel more in control. For example, 'Which eye do you want me to put the first lens in?'

It can help with co-operation, especially if RGP lenses are to be fitted, to instil local anaesthetic drops first. Ask the patient whether he or she prefers to have drops or not.

Never tell lies! Children will remember and not trust you again. If something is likely to hurt, warn them in advance. If you say nothing, you might manage to insert the first lens or drop more easily, but it is unlikely that you will manage the second.

Give lots of encouragement and try to talk about other topics (hobbies, birthdays, holidays) while the lenses are settling. If anaesthetic drops are instilled and the lenses left to settle for more than 15 minutes, the drops wear off by the time the patient returns. If at that stage the eyes are comfortable, the practitioner can explain that this is how the lenses feel when they are worn regularly. (These ideas also apply when fitting adults with lenses, although the topics of conversation may differ.)

Lens choice

Sometimes it is advisable to start with a different type of lens than the one you would choose for an adult. A child with myopic astigmatism may do better initially with spherical soft lenses, even though the vision may not be as good, rather than toric soft or RGP lenses.

This is both to build confidence and to keep expenses down. Once they have mastered the handling and shown that they are keen to wear lenses, the lens type can be changed to give better acuity.

Cleaning solutions depend on practitioner preference, although with young infants heat sterilisation of soft lenses can avoid any risk of a reaction to the cleaning solutions. If the parents have a steam steriliser for a baby's bottles, they can also use it to sterilise the lenses in fresh saline in a heat-resistant case.

When the child is older, the method can be changed to hydrogen peroxide or multipurpose solutions, although it is still advisable to continue to use a rub and rinse step.

Indications for paediatric contact lenses

Refractive error and squint

Children with high refractive errors benefit visually from contact lenses at any age, although they may not be mature enough to cope with them. High myopes especially do well with lenses, as the image is magnified, but with hypermetropes the image size is reduced.

Fully accommodative squints do just as well with contact lenses as with spectacles, but beware the child who will not wear spectacles: they may also be poor at following instructions for their contact lenses.

Contact lenses provide less aniseikonia and potentially better stereopsis than spectacles[1] and should therefore, where possible, be attempted. Unilateral myopes do better than unilateral hypermetropes,[2] but they all require extensive patching of the good eye to improve any concomitant amblyopia. Even with treatment, the amblyopia is frequently too dense to respond much, in which case the benefits of contact lens wear are also not apparent.

Fitting young myopes with RGP lenses may retard any increase in refractive error. Conventionally fitted rigid lenses have been used to attempt to slow the progression of myopia.[3–5] The reason for this is controversial (see Chapter 5), but as long as lenses are well fitted and hygiene maintained, it is up to the individual practitioner to decide whether or not to try.

Orthokeratology can be carried out on young myopes and can be successful, but only if the children themselves are compliant and so usually it is not attempted with children younger the teens (although in Asia children are fitted from a very young age).

Congenital and pathological disorders

Most children with congenital or pathological conditions are fitted with contact lenses through the hospital eye service. However, emergencies may be seen in practice and older children and adults with such conditions, who have no active pathology, may be discharged or their care shared with private practice.

Where possible, it is easier to examine young children using hand-held instruments. Soft lens insertion is upwards under the upper eyelid and removal is by scooping the lens out using the eyelids – similar to rigid lens removal. All lenses should be removed and cleaned daily, as the risks of hypoxia, especially with thick lenses, is high.[6] Parents, once they understand the risks, are keen to remove the lenses daily and the large majority are adept at lens management once they have been shown what to do. If parents are unable to handle the lenses, it is safer to prescribe spectacles. The conditions described below are the main ones that may benefit from contact lens wear; types of lenses are also suggested.

Aphakia

Aphakia is the most common indication for contact lenses in children and they are first fitted in infancy.

It is important when refracting to be aware of the back vertex distance (BVD) as, for example, a +20.00DS spectacle lens at 16mm BVD requires a +29.41DS contact lens.

As infants tend to be interested only in their immediate environment, they are overcorrected by 2–3D for close-up focus. Therefore, the power of the first lens required is typically +32.00DS. By school age (or younger, depending on the child), the correction is changed to a distance contact lens with bifocal spectacles for close work. Astigmatism is usually not corrected in the very young as it commonly alters and reduces over the first 2 years.[7]

Bifocal contact lenses are not practical in young aphakes. Some bifocals are thick and move too much on blink; they need good subjective feedback, which children are not able to provide, and acuity can be compromised. However, they may be considered for older children.

Where there is a choice, an ultraviolet inhibitor should be incorporated into aphakic lenses to try to reduce long-term damage to the macula. Unfortunately, not all types of lens provide this option.

Intraocular lenses (IOLs) are used now for some babies and many older children, although their safety is still a matter of debate. Post-operatively, a combination of corrective devices may be necessary in the infant eye as the prescription of the IOL used is lower than that needed for an older child, to allow for eye growth.[8,9] A contact lens and/or spectacle lens is fitted in addition.

For children who do not have IOLs, the two main options are either spectacles or contact lenses and both have advantages and disadvantages. Remember that, although the visual field is better with contact lenses or IOLs, spectacle lenses magnify the image that an aphake sees, thus improving the visual acuity, because of the BVD effect.

Aphakes with poor acuity derive much visual benefit from this effect, which can enable them to cope without extra magnification. Many such aphakes are keen to use spectacles for school or work and to wear contact lenses for social events or sports. If they have an IOL inserted they would lose this advantage. Patients who are considering secondary implants should think carefully before going ahead with the operation. They should try wearing their contact lenses full time first before doing so.

Soft lenses need to be high water content to maximise oxygen permeability, although they should still be removed at night. Silicone hydrogel lenses are not currently available in the necessary parameters. If keratometry (K) readings are taken, the radius is fitted on K. If Ks are not possible, the first lens tried should be 7.0mm to 7.2mm radius, which is approximately the known average K for a neonate.[10]

Some microphthalmic eyes need lenses as steep as 6.4mm. The total diameter (TD), as with adults, is approximately 2mm larger than the corneal diameter. This can be as small as 10.5mm for microphthalmic eyes, although some of these do better with lenses of larger diameter.

Table 12.1 Available parameters for Bausch & Lomb Silsoft lenses

Total diameter (mm)	*Back optic zone radii (mm)*	*Power (D)*
11.3mm	7.50, 7.70, 7.90	+23.00, +26.00, +29.00, +32.00
12.5mm	7.50, 7.70, 7.90, 8.10, 8.30	+7.50 to +20.00 (0.50 steps)

Reducing the front optic diameter (FOD) reduces the centre thickness, increases oxygen permeability and can prevent the lens from disappearing into the upper fornix if children with tight lids cry or squeeze their eyes. A lens with a 12.0mm TD is normally manufactured with a FOD of 8.5mm, which can be reduced to 6.0mm.

Silicone rubber lenses may be used for infants and children,[11] especially if soft lenses are rubbed out or fall out because of poor blinking or dryness, or if they won't centre well – they are, however, expensive, and parameters are limited.

Down's syndrome patients are frequently born with cataracts. They also suffer from dry eyes[12] and they rub their eyes. Silicone rubber lenses can be especially useful for such patients. Where lens handling is difficult and where occasional overnight wear is necessary, silicone rubber lenses carry the lowest risk of problems as their oxygen permeability is so high.[13,14]

The only silicone rubber lenses currently available are Silsoft lenses from Bausch & Lomb. These are only available in limited parameters (*Table 12.1*).

K readings should be taken before fitting any silicone rubber lenses and the lenses fitted on the flattest K for toric corneas and the flattest K + 0.1mm for spherical corneas. The lenses should be slightly flat initially, as they usually tighten and a steep lens is very difficult to remove.[15] Assess the lenses immediately after insertion, using fluorescein and an ultraviolet lamp, and remove the lenses at once if they show central pooling. Check again 10 minutes later before allowing them to settle for at least 45 minutes, when final assessment and over refraction can be carried out. The ideal fitting lens shows some central touch with slight-to-moderate edge clearance (*Figure 12.1*).

Lenses are cleaned using a surfactant cleaner for both soft lenses and RGP lenses, and then soaked overnight in a soaking solution for RGP lenses.

Most infants do well with RGP lenses,[16] although if the child squeezes his or her eyes shut corneal abrasions can be caused during lens insertion. In such cases, a different type of lens should always be used. Older children vary in their response to rigid lenses.

If possible, carry out keratometry, although if K readings are not available, the first lens can be fitted empirically for the known average K, namely 7.1mm for a neonate. Instil a local anaesthetic before inserting the first trial lens.

The diameter of the lens should be approximately 1.0–1.5mm smaller than the horizontal visible iris diameter (HVID). This relatively large diameter, together with an aspheric design, reduces the risk of the lens being rubbed out. Reducing the edge clearance further reduces lens loss. The fit is checked with an ultraviolet lamp or the blue filter on a slit lamp, and any necessary parameter changes can be ordered. The lenses are cleaned with the practitioner's system of choice.

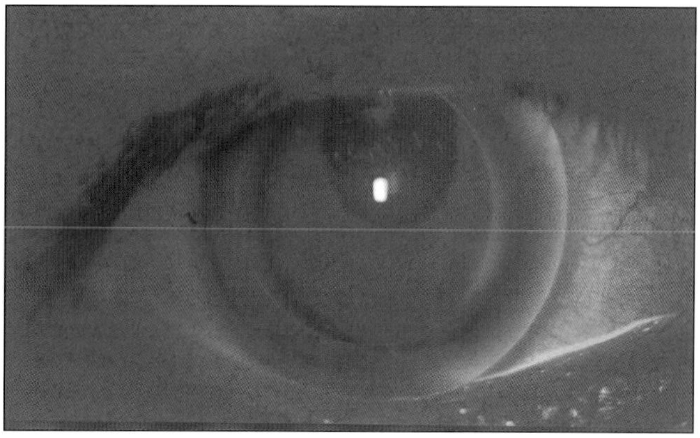

Figure 12.1
A silicone rubber lens that fits well centrally, but has more edge clearance than necessary. This lens causes no problem with wear

RGP scleral lenses can also be fitted using Pullum's controlled clearance RGP scleral lenses[17] or impression lenses. These are useful in cases with an irregular corneal surface caused by injury or surgery, and they can be modified as the prescription changes.[18] Fitting may be better managed with a sedated infant.

Unilateral aphakes are treated in much the same way as bilaterals, except that they usually need a lens in one eye only and patching is necessary for up to half the waking hours for the first 7 years of life.[19]

Dislocated lenses
Dislocated lenses (*Figure 12.2*) usually have a high degree of lenticular myopia and astigmatism, unless the lens has dislocated sufficiently for the patient to see with the aphakic portion of the pupil. If lenses are removed surgically, it is rare that both eyes are operated on at the same time, and at present it is not possible to insert an IOL safely, especially in children. One eye is rendered aphakic, while the other eye is highly myopic, which is difficult to correct with anything other than contact lenses, although if the child is extremely upset by the idea of lenses, spectacles can be prescribed as an interim measure.

In patients with Marfan's syndrome, both the corneal diameter and the radius of curvature are often increased. HVID can be more than 13.50mm and it is not uncommon to have keratometry readings flatter than 9.50mm. Lenses tend to drop on the cornea, especially RGP lenses, so soft lenses may be a better choice, as they are more likely to centre.[20]

Congenital glaucoma (buphthalmos)
Eyes with congenital glaucoma, regardless of whether they have undergone surgery, tend to be more sensitive than normal and cannot always tolerate RGP lenses. The size of the cornea may be 15mm or more, and pannus may exist, especially in eyes that have undergone surgery. Large soft lenses are required and care is needed to ensure that there is adequate oxygen to prevent neovascularisation.

Nystagmus
Wearing contact lenses, especially rigid lenses, can reduce the symptoms of nystagmus,[21,22] and possibly reduce the amplitude. It is unlikely this can improve the acuity in the long term, but nystagmus is not a contraindication to contact lens wear at any age.

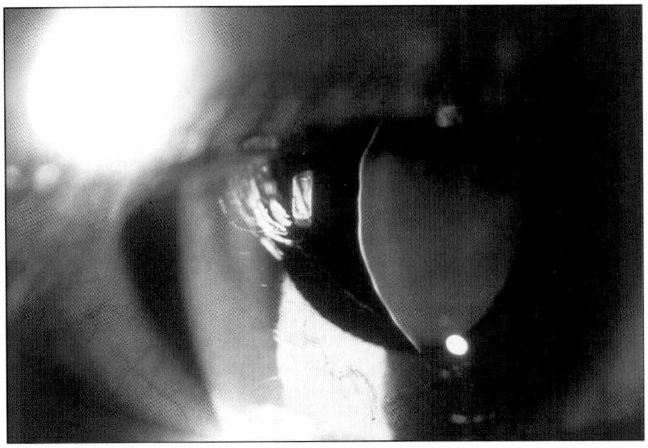

Figure 12.2
A dislocated lens. There is a large aphakic section of pupil, which is easy to refract through. The aphakic acuity can be demonstrated to a patient who is uncertain whether surgery will benefit them or not

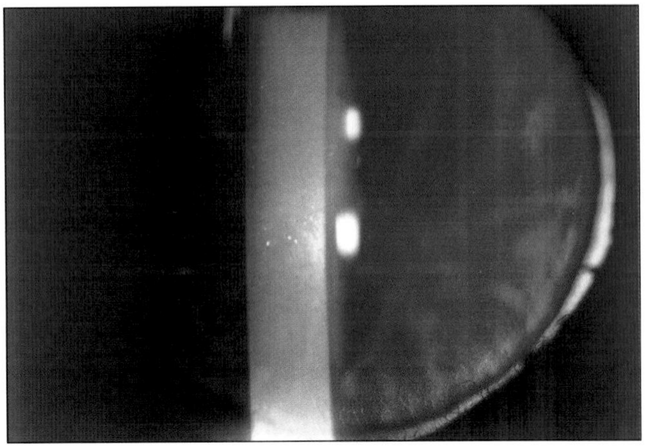

Figure 12.3
Early lens opacities in an eye with aniridia

Nanophthalmos
Eyes with nanophthalmos are small, highly hypermetropic (often more than 20D) and have small steep corneas and thick sclera.[23] Lenses are fitted as for aphakic infants, but no allowance is made for loss of accommodation.

Corneal grafts
Corneal grafts are carried out on infants with sclerocornea or Peter's anomaly. The graft tissue is larger than the removed button of diseased cornea, which results in a steep cornea and high myopia. A small RGP lens with adequate edge lift is needed and is similar to a keratoconus fit. As the graft settles down, it can become steeper and more myopic so frequent follow up is required.

Tinted or cosmetic lenses
Congenital aniridia
Tinted lenses do not improve acuity in congenital aniridia. However, older children do appear more comfortable with tinted soft lenses, especially so where lens opacities develop (*Figure 12.3*). Care must be taken as aniridics have a corneal stem cell deficiency[24] and pannus is a common problem (*Figure 12.4*). In adulthood, the cornea may become opacified so RGP lenses give a better acuity and may delay the need for a stem cell graft.

Albinism
Infants with oculocutaneous albinism anecdotally appear to be more sensitive to having contact lenses inserted. Those who do manage to wear lenses seem to derive little benefit from them, and reducing the amount of light that enters the eyes does not improve visual acuity.[25] In addition, the lenses need to be darkly tinted on pale blue or pink eyes, which makes them cosmetically unacceptable (unless hand-painted lenses are used, which is prohibitively expensive). Wearing dark glasses and a hat or shading the pram is usually more beneficial.

Tinted lenses, RGP or soft, do benefit some older children. When fitting soft lenses, the cylindrical correction common in albinos does not always produce much improvement in acuity, so spherical lenses are adequate. In those patients who do appreciate their astigmatic correction, RGP lenses work well.

Iris coloboma
Cosmetic iris lenses do not help young children with iris coloboma, as the vision is not usually affected. They may help older children if the cosmesis is unacceptable especially if the coloboma is unilateral. The lens can then be fitted as a tinted segment, which makes colour matching easier.

Achromatopsia (rod monochromatism or stationary cone dystrophy)

Photophobia is a problem with achromatopsia[26] and a tint is needed constantly. Tinted pupil lenses (*Figure 12.5*), which leave the iris colour unaffected, reduce reliance on spectacles. Some patients do not find this type of lens adequate as light still enters the pupil obliquely, so it is better to fit a tinted iris lens, especially in brown-eyed individuals and those who are not concerned if their eye colour is altered. Dark glasses are still required in addition for outdoors.

The optimum colour of the tint varies between individuals, as some achromats can be very specific about the colour. Many find a medium brown tint is most beneficial, but colours such as red or grey suit others. Some older children (and adults) may have a pair of sunglasses with their 'perfect' colour. In such cases, a sample spectacle lens can be sent to the contact lens laboratory to match.

Microphthalmos

Microphthalmos can occur with or without cataracts. In patients who are microphthalmic and aphakic, the power can be more than 40D. Where only one eye is microphthalmic to fit a cosmetic soft lens with an iris size that matches the fellow eye improves cosmesis. A prescription can be incorporated into the lens for a sighted eye; for a severely amblyopic eye, a plano cosmetic lens is prescribed.

Scars and opacities

For cases in which the eye is unsightly, parents can be upset by other people's comments. Fitting the infant for the parent's sake can help enormously.

Aftercare

Aftercare in children is not very different from that in adults, with a few extra precautions. Care must be taken to avoid hypoxia, especially with soft lenses in aphakic eyes. These lenses are very thick and, unfortunately, are not available in either of the silicone hydrogel materials. Microphthalmic corneas show the worst neovascularisation and the blood vessels have the shortest distance to grow before they reach the pupillary margin. If these new vessels leak lipid it can compromise the vision, and in a young eye can result in amblyopia.

As the aphakic eye grows, the radius and diameter of the lenses increase and the power decreases. An infant who requires soft lenses of 7.00/12.00/+32.00 is likely to need 7.80/13.50/+22.00 by 2 years of age. However, in microphthalmic eyes the growth is less, so a lens that fits in infancy may fit an older child or adult, although the power usually reduces.

Many conditions, have a high risk of glaucoma, in particular aphakia,[27,28] nanophthalmos,[29] aniridia[30,31] and dislocated lenses,[32] so intraocular pressure should be checked at every aftercare visit. Some conditions, such as aphakia[33] and Stickler's syndrome, among others, are at risk of retinal detachment.[34]

Children's eyes are just as likely as adult's to develop giant papillary conjunctivitis (GPC). Disposable lenses are also not available in high prescriptions, so protein removal tablets should be used and, if necessary, the lenses changed to RGP. Poor hygiene can lead to infections in all lens wearers and it is important to stress the risks to both parent and child.

Corneal scars in infancy, however they are caused, can result in amblyopia and will affect the vision for life, especially if the scar is central. Corneal scars also lead to neovascularisation, which can in turn lead to lipid leakage and reduced vision.

Children's tears are usually adequate, but the blink rate may be low, especially in infants, which leads to dryness: tear supplements can help. Older children can develop blepharitis or meibomitis, which requires lid hygiene. Tinted or high prescription lenses are not usually replaced frequently, so deposit formation can occur.

Summary

There is no minimum age below which contact lenses can be fitted, and there are few ocular conditions in infancy and childhood for which lenses must be worn. Many conditions are corrected optimally with contact lenses and lenses may also provide the most acceptable cosmetic appearance as well as the best chance for binocular vision.

However, it is important to weigh up the advantages to be gained against the possible distress caused to a young child who is pushed into lens wear. Conversely, young myopes can become happier and more confident if they no longer need to wear spectacles.[35] Many aphakes change to glasses for a few years until they decide that they would like to revert to lenses.

Children forced into lens wear at a young age may be put off for a long time if they decide for themselves that they want lenses, fitting becomes so much easier.

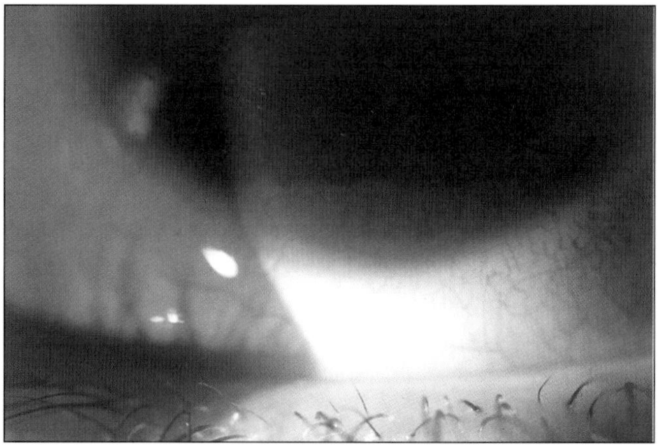

Figure 12.4 *Early pannus in the same eye as that shown in Figure 12.3 (child 6 years of age)*

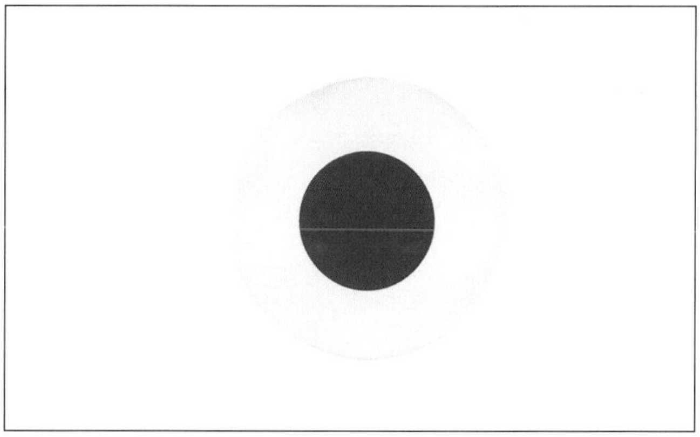

Figure 12.5 *Tinted pupil lens used for patient with achromatopsia*

References

1 Winn B, Ackerley RG, Brown CA, Murray FK, Prais J and St John MF (1988). Reduced aniseikonia in axial anisometropia with contact lens correction. *Ophthalmic Physiol Opt.* **8**, 341–344.
2 Morris J (1979). Contact lenses in infancy and childhood. *Contact Lens J.* **8**, 15–18.
3 Stone J (1976). The possible influence of contact lenses on myopia. *Br J Physiol Opt.* **31**, 89–114.
4 Grosvenor T, Perrigrin D, Perrigrin J and Quintero B (1989). The use of silicone-acrylate contact lenses for the control of myopia: Results after 2 years of wear. *Am J Physiol Opt.* **66**, 41–47.
5 Grosvenor T and Scott R (1993). Three year changes in refraction and its components in youth-onset and early adult-onset myopia. *Optom Vis Sci.* **70**, 677–683.
6 Amaya L, Speedwell L and Taylor D (1990). Contact lenses for infant aphakia. *Br J Ophthalmol.* **74**, 150–154.
7 Atkinson J, Braddick D and French J (1980). Infant astigmatism: Its disappearance with age. *Vis Res.* **20**, 891–893.
8 Enyedi LB, Peterseim MW, Freedman SF and Buckley EG (1998). Refractive changes after pediatric intraocular lens implantation. *Am J Ophthalmol.* **126**, 772–781.
9 McClatchey SK, Dahan E, Maselli E, *et al.* (2000). A comparison of the rate of refractive growth in pediatric aphakic and pseudophakic eyes. *Ophthalmology* **107**, 118–122.
10 Asbell P, Chiang B, Somers M and Morgan K (1990). Keratometry in children. *CLAO J.* **16**, 99–102.
11 Aasuri MK, Venkata N, Preetam P and Rao NT (1999). Management of pediatric aphakia with Silsoft contact lenses. *CLAO J.* **25**, 209–212.
12 Filippello M, Cascone G, Zagami A and Scimone G (1997). Impression cytology in Down's syndrome. *Br J Ophthalmol.* **81**, 683–685.
13 Koch JM, Refojo MF and Leong FL (1991). Corneal edema after overnight lid closure of rabbits wearing silicone rubber contact lenses. *Cornea* **10**, 123–126.
14 Tighe, B (1997). Contact lens materials In: *Contact Lenses*, Fourth Edition. Eds Phillips AJ and Speedwell L, p. 50–92 (Oxford: Butterworth–Heinemann).
15 Refojo MF and Leong FL (1981). Water pervaporation through silicone rubber contact lenses: A possible cause of complications. *Contact Intraocul Lens Med J.* **7**, 226–233.
16 Amos C, Lambert S and Ward M (1992). Rigid gas permeable correction of aphakia following congenital cataract removal during infancy. *J Pediatr Ophthalmol Strabismus* **26**, 290–295.
17 Pullum K (1997). The role of scleral lenses in modern contact lens practice. In: *Contact Lenses*, Fourth Edition. Eds Phillips AJ and Speedwell L, 566–609 (Oxford: Butterworth–Heinemann).
18 Ezekiel D (1995). A gas-permeable paediatric aphakic scleral contact lens. *Optician* **35**, 25–27.
19 Lloyd IC, Dowler JG, Kriss A, *et al.* (1995). Modulation of amblyopia therapy following early surgery for unilateral congenital cataracts. *Br J Ophthalmol.* **79**, 802–806.
20 Speedwell L and Russell-Eggitt I (1994). The long and the short and the tall. *J Br Contact Lens Assoc.* **17**, 135–139.
21 Abadi RV (1979). Visual performance with contact lenses and congenital idiopathic nystagmus. *Br J Physiol Opt.* **33**, 32–37.
22 Safran AB and Gambazzi Y (1992). Congenital nystagmus: Rebound phenomenon following removal of contact lenses. *Br J Ophthalmol.* **76**, 497–498.
23 Stewart DH, Streeten BW, Frockhurst RJ, *et al.* (1991). Abnormal scleral collagen in nanophthalmos: An ultra-structural study. *Arch Ophthalmol.* **109**, 1017–1019.
24 Nishida K, Kinoshita S, Ohashi Y, Kuwayama Y and Yamamoto S (1995). Ocular surface abnormalities in aniridia. *Am J Ophthalmol.* **120**, 368–375.
25 Ruben, M. Albinism and contact lenses Contact Lens Journal 1967; **1**(2).
26 Moore A (1997). Inherited retinal disorders. In: *Paediatric Ophthalmology*, Second Edition. Ed. Taylor D, 557–599 (Oxford: Blackwell Science).
27 Simon JW, Mehta N, Simmons ST, Catalano RA and Lininger LL (1991). Glaucoma after pediatric lensectomy/vitrectomy. *Ophthalmology* **98**, 670–674.
28 Johnson CP and Keech RV (1996). Prevalence of glaucoma after surgery for PHPV and infantile cataracts. *J Pediatr Ophthalmol Strabismus* **33**, 14–17.
29 Calhoun FP Jr (1976). The management of glaucoma in nanophthalmos. *Trans Am Ophthalmol Soc.* **73**, 97–122.
30 Mackman G, Brightbill FS and Optiz JM (1979). Corneal changes in aniridia. *Am J Ophthalmol.* **87**, 497–502.
31 Khaw PT (2002). Aniridia. *J Glaucoma* **11**, 164–168.
32 Nelson LB and Maumenee IH (1982). Ectopia lentis. *Surv Ophthalmol.* **27**, 143–160.
33 Chrousos GA, Parks MM and O'Neill JF (1984). Incidence of chronic glaucoma, retinal detachment and secondary membrane surgery in pediatric aphakic patients. *Ophthalmology* **91**, 1238–1241.
34 Scott JD (1980). Congenital myopia and retinal detachment. *Trans Ophthalmol Soc UK* **100**, 69–71.
35 Barnard N (1991). The psychological effect of contact lenses on a seven year old child. *Contact Lens J.* **18**, 282.

13
Low-Vision Assessment and Management

Robert Harper

Introduction

There are estimated to be some 1.4 million children (aged 14 years and under) with blindness worldwide, as defined by an acuity in the better eye of less than 3/60 or a visual field of less than 10°.[1]

The major causes of worldwide blindness vary by region, a factor recognised in the region-specific strategies adopted by the World Health Organisation (WHO) in its Vision 2020 priorities. In developing countries, the leading causes of childhood blindness include xerophthalmia, measles and, at a later stage, onchocerciasis and trachoma. In the developed countries, congenital and inherited conditions represent the most common causes of low vision in children, including cataract, nystagmus, optic atrophy, retinopathy of prematurity, albinism and aniridia.

Cortical visual impairment (or cerebral visual impairment, CVI) probably deserves special mention, since this condition is increasingly being recognised as the most common cause of visual impairment (VI) in children in the developed world. CVI refers to pathology in the retrogeniculate visual pathways, with an absence of pathology in the anterior visual pathway and visual loss greater than would be expected on the basis of an ophthalmic examination.

In the UK, information on blindness and partial sight is derived from the registration statistics compiled by local authority social services departments. In March 2000, some 306,000 people were registered blind or partially sighted, of whom 8130 (2.7 per cent) were 0–17 years of age.[2]

Overall registration statistics are widely considered to underestimate the true scale of the population with VI. In children, it has been suggested that there is large-scale underidentification of children with VI by local education authorities (LEAs), and that the true figure for children with VI in Britain might be as high as 25,000.[3] While this revised figure for children still comprises only a small proportion of all VI, when measured in terms of 'years with low vision' children form a much more significant section of the population with low vision.

The initial developmental and educational issues, and the subsequent social and economic impact of low vision throughout a lifetime, make the assessment and management of children with VI of fundamental importance. The optometrist has a key role to play as part of the multidisciplinary team involved in the provision of paediatric low-vision care. In this chapter the assessment and management of children with low vision by optometrists is described. Reference is made to the role played by other disciplines, with emphasis on the need for good communication with all concerned in the child's welfare.

Education support services for children with visual impairment

The current emphasis on inclusion is resulting in mainstream schools taking responsibility for the education of a large proportion of children with special educational needs (SENs), including those who have VI. A child has SEN if he or she has a learning difficulty that calls for special provision to be made for him or her.

A learning difficulty, in this context, is regarded as 'significantly greater difficulty in learning than the majority of children of the same age' or 'a disability that either prevents or hinders the child from making use of educational facilities'. Arrangements to identify and provide for children with SEN are set out in the Education Act 1996, supported by the Code of Practice on the identification and assessment of SEN, to which LEAs and schools must have special regard.

The Code of Practice sets out five recommended stages for addressing children's SEN. Stages 1–3 are school based, with stages 2 and 3 now being called School Action and School Action plus. The vast majority of these children will have their needs met in mainstream schools. Stage 4 involves the LEA considering the need for, and arranging for, a multidisciplinary assessment of needs. Stage 5 involves the LEA making a statement of SEN and the monitoring of this statement.

In England, approximately 258,000 of the 8.4 million pupils on school rolls have a statement of SEN (referred to as a 'recognition of need' in Scotland), which is about 3.1 per cent of children. A much higher proportion of children have SEN without a statement (approximately 20 per cent). In 2000, about 60 per cent of children with a statement of SEN were placed in mainstream schools and figures over the 5 year period 1995–2000 suggest a fall in the number of pupils with a statement being educated in special schools.

The author is not aware of national statistics on the proportion of children with SEN that is attributable to VI. While it is reasonable to assume that the majority of children with VI are being educated in mainstream schools, it is estimated that some 40 per cent of children with a VI may also have an additional disability or learning difficulty.[4] Children with SEN educated in mainstream schools remain the responsibility of the host institution, but for inclusion to be successful the appropriate specialist services must be available to provide practical help and advice. In practice, this support is usually arranged by a qualified teacher of the visually impaired (QTVI).

The amount of support may vary according to local circumstances and the level of impairment, but it may include input from learning support assistants (usually qualified nursery nurses) and adaptive equipment (see below) to enable the child to follow the curriculum. Some mainstream schools have a special resource unit within the school that provides additional facilities. While local circumstances may result in variations in educational provision, a few 'special' schools cater specifically for children with more severe VI (although such pupils can be integrated into mainstream schools), or those with a learning or physical impairment in addition to VI. These schools may have smaller class sizes and a wider range of specialist equipment and often have facilities for children with other disabilities.

The publication of a recent document on quality standards in education support for children and young people with VI[4] aims to provide markers for LEAs when they review their service provision. Although no specific mention is made of the role of optometrists, one of the general principles within these quality standards relates to the need for LEAs to work collaboratively with other agencies, including the health sector. Equally, it is important for optometrists to bring to the attention of the LEA any particular educational concerns that they may have about a child with VI.

Low-vision assessment

Referrals

Referral for a low-vision assessment is initiated, in most cases, by an ophthalmologist, a paediatrician, an optometrist, an orthoptist or a QTVI. Assessment is often considered at school age, although pre-school assessment can be very valuable, and it has been suggested that any child with a cognitive age equivalent of 3 years or older might use and benefit from a simple magnifier.[5]

Since many cases of childhood VI are congenital, and since VI can affect all areas of general development, it has been argued that children with VI who receive services at school age or later may be receiving services too late.[6]

Preliminary discussion

The nature of the initial discussion varies with the age of the child (i.e., pre-school, primary or secondary), but it is likely to include a discussion on what problems are perceived by the child and/or parents or guardians and their understanding of the VI.

While recognising that advice, general strategies and low-vision devices may have implications beyond the classroom, the educational issues are paramount. Thus, the optometrist needs to establish the following:

- Type of school attended;
- Whether or not there is a statement of SEN;
- Level of input from a QTVI or learning assistant;
- Use of spectacles and/or devices;
- Use of enlarged print;
- Access to adaptive equipment;
- Position in the classroom;
- Amount of board work and sharing of texts.

Since children may not express their difficulties, it is important to question proactively both the child and parents (or guardians) about potential difficulties, such as reading the board, attention span for reading, headaches or asthenopia, and so on. A more comprehensive discussion of the appropriate questioning of a child with VI is given in Chapter 15.

Assessment of visual functions

In common with low-vision assessment in adults, careful assessment of visual functions is necessary to inform the appropriate management strategies. The assessment of visual acuity in infancy and early childhood is covered in Chapter 3.

For the typical ages of children assessed in a low-vision clinic (usually 4 years and older), letter-matching tests (e.g., Sheridan Gardiner or Sonksen–Silver tests) or letter-naming tests (e.g., a Snellen chart or, preferably, a logMAR chart) are likely to be appropriate. Picture tests or other alternatives may be necessary, for example, with a child who has multiple disability. The advantages of logMAR charts are now well documented and paediatric versions of this chart design that feature symbols can be used, if appropriate. Arguably, the assessment of near vision and near acuity is more valuable, and charts with words or sentences that use a log scale and M or N notation are the most preferable.

The McClure Reading Test (*Figure 13.1*) has reading material of varying difficulty

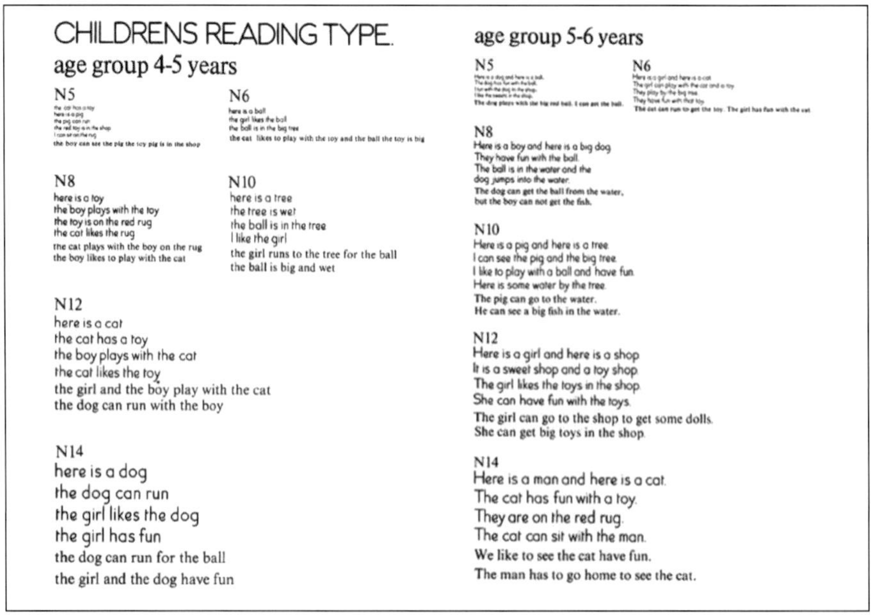

Figure 13.1
Samples from the McClure Reading Test showing print for different age groups

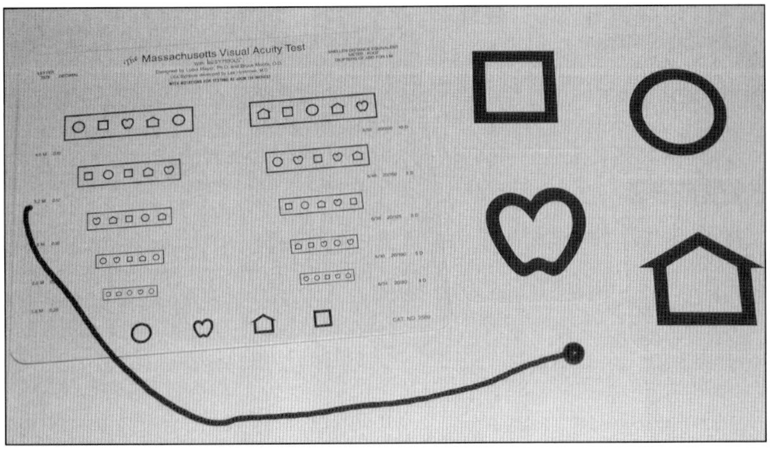

Figure 13.2
The Massachusetts visual acuity test. The cord attached to the test card is 40cm (acuity range 4M to 0.2M). The test is supplied with a response key and training cards. Threshold near acuity is a correct response for 3/5 symbols

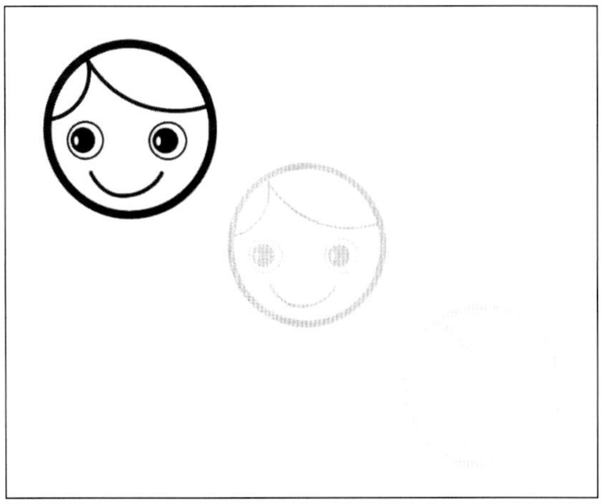

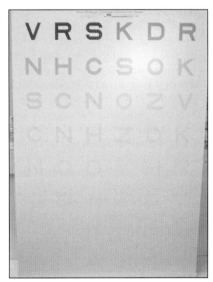

Figure 13.3
Hiding Heidi contrast sensitivity test. The set has four cards (printed on both sides) with varying contrast levels from 1.25 per cent up to full contrast (only three of the different contrast levels are illustrated here)

appropriate for different ages. This design feature is useful, since in many cases it assists in determining whether poor performance is caused by the VI itself versus the child's reading ability. For some children a test that uses symbols, such as the Massachusetts near chart (*Figure 13.2*), may be necessary.

More comprehensive methods to assess reading ability (and not just acuity), such as the Neale Analysis of Reading Ability (which considers speed, accuracy and comprehension), are desirable arguably, but are not routinely feasible in a clinical setting.

Refraction is a key part of the assessment process. Provision of a spectacle correction is more likely than not in a child with VI, because of the association of the ophthalmic diagnostic groupings that cause childhood VI with either refractive error and/or the requirement for a tint (see below). Assessment of refraction is, therefore, essential and if a cycloplegic examination is deemed necessary, a follow-up appointment can be arranged to reassess function with a spectacle correction and to proceed with device evaluation.

Assessment of accommodative function is also essential, not least because the use of this facility in children with VI can often obviate the need for other magnification strategies, since relative distance magnification can be provided by holding the material or object close (see Management, below). Similarly, assessment of binocular status can also be of value in a low-vision assessment, a function that is perhaps given less attention than required in people with low vision.[7]

As is the case with adult VI, the measurement of acuity alone may not provide an adequate description of visual function, and so the measurement of visual fields, contrast sensitivity (CS) and colour vision can be useful. CS is related to the performance of many real-world tasks and activities, and sometimes shows a better correlation with performance than measures of visual acuity do.

While studies to examine the relationship between visual functions and task performance have tended to use adult subjects, the results are considered applicable to a paediatric population and can be used to help predict performance or understand problems with 'real-world' functioning. For example, it is possible to estimate the maximum reading rate likely to be achieved with magnification and decide whether or not supplementary vision-substitution strategies might be necessary (see Management, below).

For younger children or where comprehension for a letter-based test is problematic, the 'Mr Happy' or 'Hiding Heidi' CS tests may be suitable. The Hiding Heidi low-contrast face stimulus (*Figure 13.3*) has four cards (printed on both sides) with contrast levels of 1.25 per cent, 2.5 per cent, 5 per cent, 10 per cent, 25 per cent and maximum. A blank card is included to cover the stimulus before presenting it. The tester slides both cards out to reveal 'Heidi' and the response can be verbalising, pointing or preferential looking. While there are few instructions for the mode of use of this test, a good protocol is described by Leat *et al.*[8] For older children, the Pelli–Robson low-contrast letter chart (*Figure 13.4*) is arguably the most useful measure of CS, and the mode of administration is more intuitive to optometrists used to letter-based tests.

Visual field assessment is not easily achieved in young children, but has implications for registration status, predicting the functional impact of VI and the parent's and/or professionals' understanding of the VI. The Goldmann can provide reliable results in some children from about 6 years of age, but is not widely available. Leat *et al.*[8] propose confrontation testing using internally illuminated stimuli or white Styrofoam balls as stimuli, to provide an approximate alternative that might be valuable for those of all ages with multiple impairments and/or minimal visual responses.

Figure 13.4
Pelli–Robson low-contrast letter chart. Threshold is determined as the last triplet for which at least two of the three letters are recognised correctly, although miscalling the letter 'C' an 'O', or vice-versa, is permitted as this improves test reliability

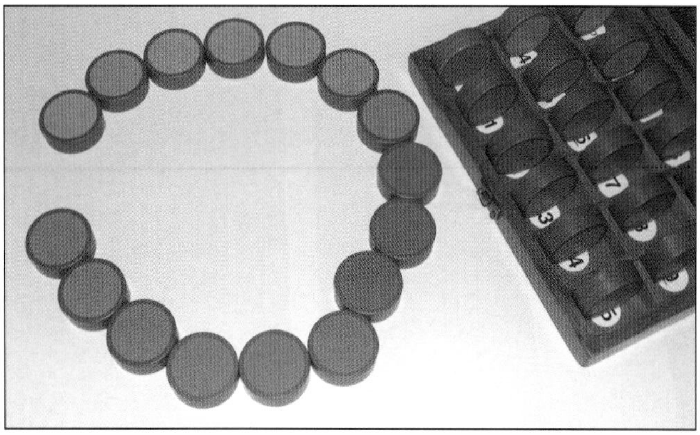

Figure 13.5
PV16 quantitative colour vision test, a large panel derivative of the D15

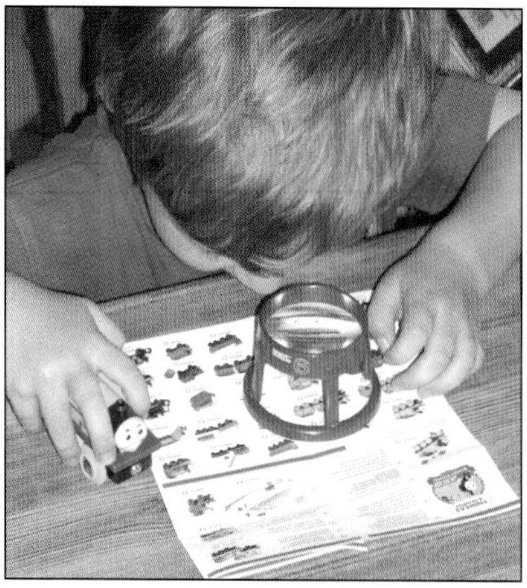

Figure 13.6
Pre-school child using a 6× Coil ('lobster-pot') stand magnifier with high emergent vergence

Finally, colour-vision assessment (e.g., using the PV16 test, *Figure 13.5*) may be useful to be able to offer advise on confusions that might give rise to difficulty with particular teaching materials.

Management

Pre-school years

In the pre-school years, key information for parents or guardians includes the diagnosis, prognosis, level of visual functioning, optimal use of residual vision and availability of support services. Visual function terminology should be translated into meaningful information. The Snellen fraction can be 'translated'; for example, at 6/24 the child is able to see the same detail as a child with normal sight if the detail is made 4× as large or if the child moves 4× nearer. However, it might be preferable to use more functional examples, such as the child can recognise familiar faces or specified objects at a particular distance.

Reports can be offered to the parents, the nursery professional and the paediatrician and should include advice about lighting control, the use of spectacles, the use of tints or filters and the use of low-vision aids. While a device may not be necessary for reading at this age, children of about 3 years of age may make more general use of a stand magnifier for inspecting small objects, such as stamps, coins, leaves and even insects! Stand magnifiers with high emergent vergence and about 5–6× magnification are probably the most suitable devices (*Figure 13.6*). Distance binoculars (typically 8× magnification) should be tried, since these are often easier for a young child to handle than are monoculars (*Figure 13.7*).

Both pre-school and younger school-age children can become quite animated with the extent of detail and distance that they can see with binoculars, and the broad smile in the clinic is a rewarding reaction for the practitioner to be able to observe.

Primary school years

Optometric management in school-age children with VI should be considered as part of the broader educational support, with the aim to ensure that children with VI have equal opportunity, learning experiences alongside their peers and opportunities that maximise their independence.

Children face changing visual demands (especially print size and demands on near vision), particularly during the early stages of their schooling, and regular follow-up is important to ensure that the appropriate management is being offered. Assisting a child's access to the curriculum is clearly a key goal and the use of low-vision devices for reading assumes an increasing importance as visual tasks become more demanding. While the threshold near acuity often appears satisfactory at a closer working distance in young children, either unaided or with their conventional spectacle correction, the sustained use of high levels of accommodation may hamper fluent reading for prolonged periods.

Practitioners need to be mindful of both the association between low vision and reduced accommodation[8] and of the visual requirements for extended reading versus spot (i.e., short-term) reading at a close working distance. In relation to the latter issue, optometrists need to consider the acuity reserve (i.e., the ratio of the print size required to be read to the threshold near acuity) and the contrast reserve (i.e., the ratio of the contrast for the print required to be read to the contrast threshold).

Recommendations for the acuity reserve and the contrast reserve have been derived from research work on adult subjects,[9] but are likely to have similar implications in children with low vision. For fluent reading, an acuity reserve of >2:1 is considered necessary. For example, a child who needs to read a print size of N16 (2.0M) is likely to need a threshold near acuity of at least N8 (1.0M) to provide sufficient acuity reserve to be comfortable in prolonged reading. Similarly, a contrast reserve of >10:1 is probably desirable. For example, if the child is reading a book with a print of 80 per cent contrast, the child's contrast threshold on the Pelli–Robson chart needs to be <7.8 per cent (i.e., correct recognition of low-contrast letters to at least half-way down the chart in *Figure 13.4*). Consideration needs to be given to methods of contrast enhancement (i.e., local task lighting, glare reduction or electronic systems, including CCTV).

The visual requirements for reading can often, therefore, create the need for magnification. While a number of options to provide this magnification can be considered, high reading additions, stand magnifiers, bar magnifiers or 'brightfield' magnifiers (*Figure 13.8*) are likely to be the main near-vision devices employed. *Table 13.1* summarises the process used to determine a suitable reading addition (after Leat[6]).

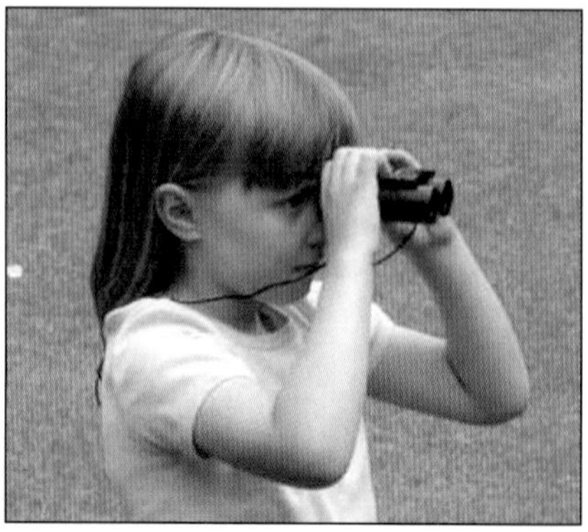

Figure 13.7
Child using 8× distance binoculars

Table 13.1 Steps to assessing a reading addition in a child (after Leat)[6]

Identify the print size the child needs to read, using samples of the print being used. Use this information to determine the matching N or M notation
Measure the child's near acuity at his or her habitual near distance
Calculate the expected accommodation for age: Amplitude = $15 - (0.25 \times \text{age})$
Calculate the estimated add. We assume that children, as adults, can exert half of their amplitude for sustained tasks:
Estimated add = working distance in D – 1/2 amplitude
Re-measure near acuity with estimated add, and note threshold, fluency of reading (or sounding out symbols or letters), any changes in working distance and, with older children, subjective preference
If the child is reading the target print size easily (ideally with at least a 2× reserve of acuity without a reduction of working distance), consider prescribing this add
If the child is not reading the target print easily, try increasing the add further (which means decreasing the working distance)
The reading add may be prescribed as a bifocal (generally an executive or large D segment bifocal to give the maximum field of view), a multifocal, a single vision or a microscopic lens

While a multifocal can be considered, remember that the initial add is often 3D or more and in subsequent years, when the addition needs to increase, it may move out of the range of a multifocal design (+3.50 Add). Furthermore, the field of view is not as good as that of a bifocal, although the improved cosmesis of these lenses may outweigh these limitations for some children, especially since 'not wanting to appear to be different' is likely to be an important consideration. If bifocals are prescribed, the segment should be placed high, usually at the lower pupil margin.

Stand magnifiers have the advantage of a wide available magnification range, whereas bar and brightfield magnifiers provide restricted magnification (approximately 1.5–2×), although the latter limitation can be offset to some extent when these optical devices are used at a very close working distance (i.e., with relative distance magnification). Bar or brightfield magnifiers appear to be popular with QTVIs, possibly because these are considered more 'acceptable' in the classroom, with the availability of different lengths and line guides being additional features (*Figure 13.8*). These devices also allow the habitual close working distance to be retained. Similarly, if using a stand magnifier, moderate-to-high magnification (i.e., above 5×) is desirable to encourage the closer working distance.

All of these devices are readily portable and reasonably robust, factors that are important when considering devices for young children. Even where relative size magnification (i.e., simple enlargement of the print, either at source or by photocopying) is commonly employed, there will be occasions where access to small print may be necessary. Thus, an introduction to the use of magnification devices is to be encouraged and considered complementary to the use of large print.

Telescopes can be considered for board work, although given the availability of other options for board work their use outside the classroom may be of more significance (e.g., on school trips and days out or holidays with family). As mentioned above, binoculars may be easier for the younger child to handle, although older children may find a compact monocular more practical to carry about.

Early use of a telescope is arguably helpful to encourage their subsequent use as an aid to independent travel when the child is older. While bioptic telescopic designs offer the potential for spectacle mounting a telescope to copy board work, these devices are not prescribed commonly in the UK, and some people might consider their use in the classroom to be unacceptable. Probably of more practical relevance in this regard is the recommendation for the child to be allowed to move much closer to the board or for photocopies of board work (large print if necessary) to be made available. A conventional full-field hand-held telescope may still prove useful, however, for demonstrations or for watching educational videos in the classroom.

Children at primary school may often undertake supplementary activities that create additional visual requirements, such as a child with VI needing to see to read music (*Figure 13.9*). Depending on

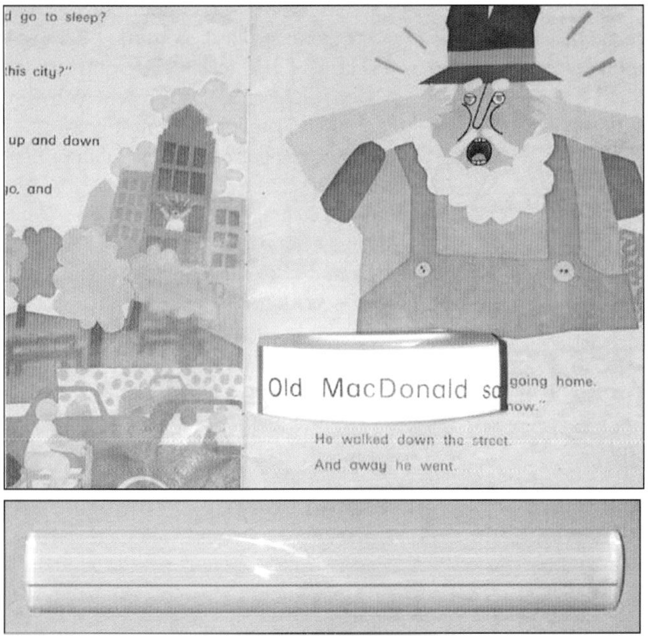

Figure 13.8
(a) Brightfield 'dome' magnifier and (b) a ruled bar magnifier

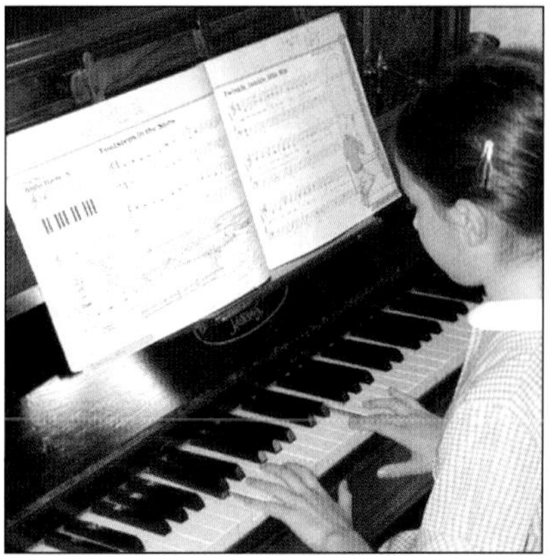

Figure 13.9
Reading music presents a challenge to children with VI

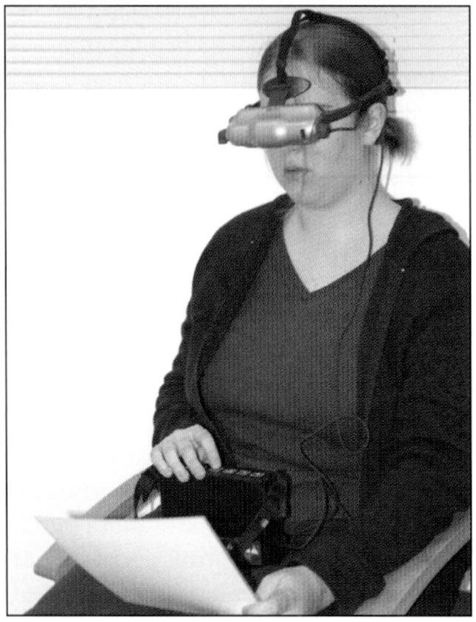

Figure 13.10
NuVision head-mounted electronic magnifier uses a purpose-designed Keeler optical system, and offers 5× magnification at optical infinity to 10× at 13cm

the child's visual function, simple enlarged photocopies of the relevant music may provide a satisfactory solution. While low-powered near or intermediate telescopes may be considered for this purpose (about 2–3× magnification), higher magnification is unlikely to offer a sufficient field of view. Leat *et al.*[8] consider the use of head-mounted video-magnification devices (such as the Keeler NuVision device, *Figure 13.10*) for this purpose when higher magnification is required.

Secondary school years

While many of the issues discussed above for younger children also apply to older children, other considerations important to children in their secondary school years may influence the management.

Firstly, children in the secondary school years are often much more conscious of their appearance in their peer group. Not wishing to be seen to be different may make use of optical devices difficult, if not impossible in the classroom, at least for some children. Concerns might also be expressed about bullying and isolation. Electronic devices, including CCTV and adapted PCs, might be perceived by the child to be better solutions than optical devices, as electronic aids may cause less, if any, peer ridicule and so may be more successful in the classroom, with optical devices reserved for independent access to small print at home.

Secondly, considerably more demands are likely to be placed upon children in terms of the magnitude and scope of near work (rather than the print size itself, which is likely to have reached standard print sizes in the final few years of primary school).

Adaptations and equipment

Enlargement of print (relative size magnification) is a widely used strategy to support children with VI at school, although the use of low-vision devices should be considered complementary. Indeed, as children progress throughout their school years, it would seem essential that they be able to access regular print size independently, at least for a proportion of the time. Exercise books can be made available with bold lines, and the use of local task lighting and black felt-tip pens can enhance contrast for writing. A reading stand or angled desk can improve comfort and performance when reading, by positioning the print at a more accessible angle with a close magnifier to object distance (*Figure 13.11*).

Given the widespread use of computers in everyday life, an adapted PC is also an important tool for a child with VI. An enlarged screen (20inch or more) can provide a degree of magnification, with further enhancement being available for a range of applications with text-enlarging software. Speech synthesis can also be considered, if appropriate. CCTV technology can be funded through the LEA, and many children with VI make use of such equipment both at school and at home. The possible benefits of head-mounted video-magnification systems are currently under evaluation, including the NuVision system, Jordy II, Maxport and Flipperport (for a review, see Chabra and Culham[10]). While such devices are unlikely to replace the need for optical devices, they may in some circumstances offer a more acceptable 'high tech' solution for some school activities, although their role here is not yet fully established.

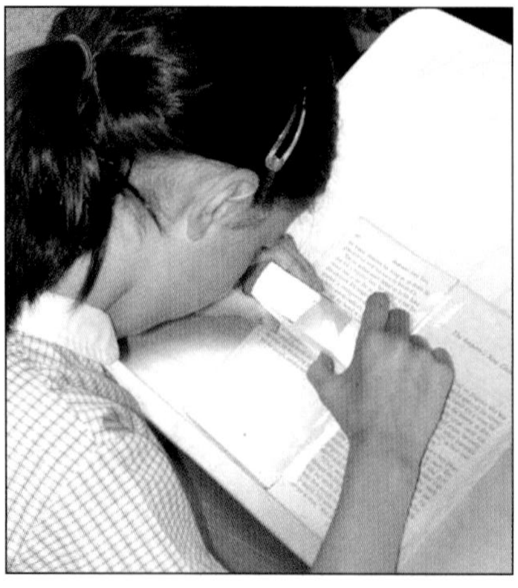

Figure 13.11
Use of an angled desk or reading stand can improve comfort and posture for a child with VI, as it enables her to 'get in close'

Other considerations

Some of the ophthalmic pathologies that cause VI in children are likely to result in photophobia and a tint can be considered for a child of any age. While discomfort from glare can be removed by reducing the light level with a tint, a reduction in disability glare and improvement in visual performance is considered more controversial.[11]

A neutral tint is arguably preferred where colour vision is not specifically affected by the disorder (albeit performance may be affected by the low vision itself), and a brown or grey tint of approximately 15 per cent light transmission factor (LTF) should be tried, for example, in children with albinism or aniridia. Children with other pathologies, for example a cone dystrophy, may benefit from the use of lenses with more selective wavelength attenuation, including the Corning CPF photochromic lenses or the fixed tint PLS 530-550 lenses (yellow, amber or red in colour), although a standard dark brown tint may suffice.

However, no prescribing rules from the research that has been conducted to date are commonly accepted, and the final choice may have to be based on observation of the behaviour or subjective preference of an older child. Consider the possible requirement for different tints for different circumstances (e.g., indoor versus outdoor), the possible use of Transitions photochromic lenses or a graduated tint and other methods of lighting control (e.g., a baseball cap). It is important to remember that the control of illumination is the key issue, since a child with VI who requires a tint may still need local task lighting to enhance contrast.

Many children with VI present with nystagmus and the use of a null point (i.e., where the oscillation has less influence on visual function) can be encouraged. While optical (i.e., prismatic correction) or surgical intervention may be indicated,[11] simple advice may also be useful. For example, reading may be more comfortable with the book held laterally, rather than straight ahead, or a child may see the board better when viewing from a desk on the right-hand side of the classroom rather than one on the left.

Recommendations and written reports

The QTVI should receive a report on the child's assessment, a document that can be copied to both the parents and the community paediatric team responsible for the child's development. As mentioned above, the communication must be meaningful (i.e., use appropriate terminology).

Consent for the release of information should be sought, most usually from the parents or guardians in the case of a younger child, although children under 16 years of age may have the capacity to consent under the 'Gillick' test (whereby the child has an understanding of 'nature, purpose and hazards'). The content is likely to include the child's visual capabilities (resolution, contrast, colour, visual field, etc.) and the implications of these with respect to strategies for reading print and access to board work. Other details might include the use of spectacles (including the possible requirement for protective eyewear), the use of devices (with implications for reading speed and extra time allowances for exams), adaptive equipment, recommendations for lighting and glare control and, if not provided previously, information on the eye condition and support groups.

This chapter describes the optometrist's contribution to the management of children with VI, but, as is recognised elsewhere in healthcare, it is essential that our contribution be integrated with that of other professionals through good communication, and thereby enhance the prospects for the wider social and educational development of children with VI.

Acknowledgements

The author thanks Chris Dickinson, Cindy Tromans and Gill Rudduck for helpful comments on this article, and Louise Culham, Julie Sznapka and Ophthalmic Imaging, MREH, for selected illustrations.

References

1 Thylefors B, Negrel AD, Pararajasegaram R, *et al.* (1995). Global data on blindness. *Bull World Health Org.* **73**, 115–121.
2 Department of Health. www.doh.gov.uk/public/blindandpartiallysighted.htm.
3 Walker E, Tobin M and McKennell A (1992). *Blind and Partially Sighted Children in Britain: The RNIB Survey*. RNIB (London: HMSO).
4 Department for Education and Skills (2002). *Quality Standards in Education Support Services for Children and Young People with Visual Impairment*. (London: DFES Publications).
5 Gould E and Sonksen PM (1991). A low vision aid clinic for pre-school children. *J Vis Impairment* **9**, 44–46.
6 Leat SJ (2002). Paediatric low vision management. *CE Optom.* **5**, 22–25.
7 Rundstrom MM and Eperjesi F (1995). Is there a need for binocular vision evaluation in low vision. *Ophthalmic Physiol Opt.* **15**, 525–528.
8 Leat SJ, Shute RH and Westall C (1999). *Assessing Children's Vision*. (Oxford: Butterworth–Heinemann).
9 Whittaker SG and Lovie-Kitchin JE (1993). Visual requirements for reading. *Optom Vis Sci.* **70**, 54–65.
10 Chabra A and Culham C (2002). Technically advanced low vision aids: A comparison of four new devices. *CE Optom.* **5**, 17–21.
11 Dickinson CM (1998). *Low Vision Principles and Practice*. (Oxford: Butterworth–Heinemann).

14
Vision Screening

Jane Henderson

Introduction

Screening has been defined as 'a public health service in which members of a defined population, who do not necessarily perceive they are at risk of or are already affected by a disease or its complication, are asked a question or offered a test, to identify those individuals who are more likely to be helped than harmed by further tests or treatment to reduce the risk of a disease or its complications'.[1] Vision screening and assessment occurs in the UK from birth to puberty in diverse forms with wide variations in methods and programmes across the country. This chapter provides an overview of different practices from birth to puberty, with a review of and reference to national guidelines and recommendations.

National Screening Committee

In 1996 the National Screening Committee (NSC) was inaugurated with the remit to review the huge variation in screening practice,[2] conditions sought, adequacy and appropriateness of tests provided and, perhaps most importantly, evidence base.[3] In 1998 antenatal and child health subgroups were constituted to gather and interpret information that pertained to their speciality.

In June 2000 the Child Health Screening Sub-Group chaired by Dr David Elliman, a consultant community paediatrician, and comprising representatives from the Royal College of Ophthalmologists, the College of Optometrists and the British Orthoptic Society, defined two grades of vision defect and associated degree of disability.[4]

Conditions that cause a serious and permanent impairment of vision leading to substantial disability

One child in every 1000–2000 has a major disorder that affects the eyes. There is a higher incidence of serious visual impairment, one in 500 live births, but a significant number of these have associated neurological abnormalities. It is recognised that early diagnosis and appropriate treatment of retinoblastoma, cataract and glaucoma are beneficial to the long-term visual outcome for the infant concerned. It is relatively easy to screen for congenital cataract and guidance in line with the medical evidence presently available (see below), given the age at screen is acknowledged.[5] Undetected retinoblastoma has serious repercussions, but presentation of this and of childhood glaucoma, which also has the potential to cause severe vision defect, varies tremendously, and no single screening test or specific optimum age at screen can be established.

Conditions that cause little disability

Common eye defects occur in a significant percentage of children. The actual percentage obviously varies significantly according to what definition of 'common eye defects' a researcher adheres to. Refractive error, squint and supervening amblyopia account for the large majority of such defects. Disability attributable to these conditions is immensely difficult to quantify and, as such, treatment benefit is equivocal.

Treatment itself (glasses and/or occlusion of the 'good eye') can be distressing for both the child and parent, and as Snowdon and Stewart-Brown identified in 1997 in a major systematic review of research on the effectiveness of pre-school vision screening (PVS),[6] 'an invitation to PVS carries with it the implicit assumption that screening is going to benefit the child. In the absence of sound evidence that the target conditions sought in the programmes are disabling and that the interventions available to correct them do more good than harm, the ethical basis for such interventions is very insecure'.

Controversy and debate over the treatment of amblyopia still prevails. The first national, multicentre randomised controlled trial of the treatment of unilateral, 'straight-eyed' reduced vision is near completion.

It may be of value to consider the advantages and disadvantages of intervention and correction when reflecting on the perceived benefits of present screening programmes:

- What does the programme set out to achieve?
- For what purpose?
- What are the potential health benefits to be gained?
- On what evidence is this supported?

Current screening procedures

Neonatal

Retinopathy of prematurity

Improved neonatal care has resulted in a significant increase in the survival rate for pre-term babies with birth weight less than 1000g, which has increased from 5 per cent to 65 per cent over the past 40 years. Likewise, the survival rate of babies with birth weight 1000–1500g has risen from 35 per cent to 90 per cent. The aims of retinopathy of prematurity (ROP) screening are to detect severe, stage three ROP (see Chapter 9), which may then be treated in its early stages, and to identify those babies about to be discharged from the hospital in whom the ROP has the potential to develop into a more severe form. Low birth weight babies of less than 1500g or pre-term babies of less than 31 weeks gestational age are automatically screened for ROP by an ophthalmologist in the hospital.

Screening guidelines for ROP were initially drawn up in 1990 by a working party of the Royal College of Ophthalmologists and the British Association of Perinatal Medicine after a report that severe ROP could be treated effectively. These guidelines were reviewed in 1997 and are accepted and followed nationally.

Congenital cataract

Current practice follows guidance based on the reports of two national joint working parties, the Royal College of Ophthalmologists and the Royal College of Paediatrics and Child Health, which have recommended that all babies should be screened for 'red reflex' before the age of 8 weeks. This screen is usually performed prior to discharge from hospital by a paediatrician, although on a national scale variations in training and clinical practice have been identified.[7]

There may be a deficit in service for those children born in the home environment, for whom the eyes are not examined as early as desired by an appropriately trained health professional. General practitioners (GPs) are encouraged to repeat the screen for red reflex at the 6–8 week check. The NSC recently recommended that the examination should be repeated before the baby's seventh week, in conjunction with an assessment of visual behaviour and to detect squint. If the red reflex is absent, babies are referred directly to a paediatric ophthalmologist within the hospital eye service (HES) for urgent assessment.

Infancy to age 4–5 years

Sure Start programmes

Sure Start is the government initiative to support children, parents and communities through the integration of early education, child care and health and family support services.[8] These programmes are being introduced in areas of social deprivation in the first instance, with the intention to provide benefits for children from lower socio-economic groups.

Although health education is one of the key issues to be covered, Sure Start programmes are still in their early stages, and inclusion of 'vision awareness' for parents may not yet have been addressed. The Sure Start centres, however, provide an opportunity to capture those infants who may not otherwise have attended a more formal pre-school vision assessment.[9]

Secondary or request screening

At present, different services are offered in different regions for parents or carers who raise concerns. For babies and young infants the first point of contact is generally a health visitor or a GP, who then refers according to personal preference or knowledge of specific local services. The referral route may be to an optometrist, the HES or to a community orthoptist who holds clinics at local premises.

Pre-school vision screening

In one survey, 94 per cent of responding health districts in England and Wales were undertaking PVS.[10] The format and age at which the assessment was carried out was found to vary greatly, and this is still the case nearly 20 years later. Using Newcastle upon Tyne as an example, in a relatively small geographical area the range of primary vision and muscle balance screening extends from no screening in one area to a service offered to infants as young as 3 years and 6 months in another area, but not until the age of 5 years in yet another.

Tests employed are age-related and therefore assessment methods vary in complexity, sensitivity, specificity and repeatability. Vision tests employed vary from single optotypes, such as Kay Pictures and single Sheridan Gardiner, recorded using Snellen-based notation, to crowded LogMAR, the latter being the linear test designed by McGraw and Winn[11] in which visual acuity is documented using a decimal notation.

Not only do tests (and their inherent accuracy and robustness) vary, but referral criteria are also diverse. The majority of programmes 'fail' children with a visual acuity of 6/9 or worse. However, in some areas children need to achieve 6/5 with single Sheridan Gardiner (i.e. 'fail' at 6/6).

Different programmes also employ different referral routes: some areas refer direct to the HES, while others (such as the Northumberland model) in the first instance refer 'straight-eyed' amblyopes with single optotype visual acuity of 6/9 to 6/18 to local optometrists who have signed up to follow a defined protocol.

The Birmingham model, however, refers those children who fail to meet the standard 0.100 (6/6 Snellen equivalent) using a crowded LogMAR test to a specific clinic at which each child is reassessed by an orthoptist in addition to refraction by an optometrist. Both models, as do the majority of vision and/or squint screening programmes, fast-track more complex cases directly into the HES. Both models, as with many PVS programmes nationwide, are currently under review and evaluation.

School entry

Most districts undertake some form of vision assessment at school entry. School nurses, school health advisers, audio/vision screeners, vision technicians or orthoptists perform this screen. The advantage of this method is that it meets one of the screening criteria of 100 per cent coverage.[12] This system may render the service more cost-effective per capita because of the more extensive coverage.

Age 8 years to teens

Visual acuity testing

There is again diversity in screening programmes, with a wide variation of age at testing, methods used and testing conditions.[13] In some areas there is only one screening contact at either 8 or 11 years of age. In others, vision assessment is undertaken twice, at 9 and 13 years of age.

The role of vision screening after school entry remains unclear as there is a paucity of evidence to support the benefits of screening in this age group. For example, what degree of disability is caused at this age by uncorrected refractive error?

Parents of school-age children may attend an optometrist for an eye test if teachers raise concerns or if academic achievement is below expectations.

Colour vision assessment
Total colour blindness is extremely rare. Congenital deficiencies in colour vision essentially affect the recognition and interpretation of reds and greens in approximately 8 per cent of boys and only 0.5 per cent of girls.

Evidence to demonstrate an association between a colour vision deficit and its effect on education and learning difficulties is poor,[14] yet colour vision assessment is still undertaken in an *ad hoc* manner throughout schools nationwide. Obviously, it may have a bearing on the choice of future career and so is a relevant finding before later school years, when course options are made.

Children with special needs – Down's syndrome
Different areas again have different policies for the vision assessment of children with special needs. Some have strict protocols to follow: for example, the first vision assessment by the age of 2 years with annual review until 6 years of age, and then subsequent biannual reviews until the age of 16 years. In certain areas, vision is monitored in the community jointly by orthoptists and optometrists, with the involvement of ophthalmologists only in those cases with identified cataract or squint.

Vision defects in individuals with Down's syndrome are common. A recent study produced evidence that 46 per cent of the target group (68 cases, between 5 and 19 years of age) demonstrated substantial visual deficits as a result of high refractive errors, anisometropia and amblyopia caused by squint.[15]

Personal child health record
Personal child health record (PCHRs, often referred to as the 'red book' or 'yellow book', dependent upon the colour of the booklet's sleeve) are designed and developed at a local level, and so reflect local health promotion and programmes of health surveillance and care. Occasionally, coterminous counties amalgamate programmes to provide a region-wide PCHR. Each PCHR is retained by an individual from birth through to the teens. Contacts with health professionals are recorded at each stage of development. The record thus provides a comprehensive yet concise overview of the child's health and health care needs.

David Elliman and Helen Bedford of the NSC are attempting to develop a working national PCHR.

The Ideal Model

The Hall Report – Health for all children
The basis of the Hall Report[16] is that there will be a universal or core health programme available to all, plus additional. services targeted to those who need them. The content of the universal programme should be justified, where possible, by evidence of effectiveness.

Any change to current screening programmes must be made using the Hall Report as a reference tool in conjunction with timely evidence-based practice.

Specific areas of ophthalmic screening
The NSC has identified five specific areas of ophthalmic screening, which are detailed in the Hall report:

- Retinopathy of prematurity in pre-term and/or low birth weight infants;
- Congenital cataract and ocular anomalies in neonates and infants;
- Amblyopia and reduced vision in pre-school children;
- Refractive errors in school children;
- Congenital colour vision impairment in secondary school children.

Neonatal
Low birth weight infants
Approximately 6600 infants of birth weight <1500g are born in the UK every year, with a survival rate of 80 per cent. About 450 infants (8–10 per cent) develop severe, stage three ROP. The risk of severe ROP in larger or more mature babies is extremely low, and Royal College of Ophthalmologist guidelines state ROP screening in this group of infants to be unjustified.[17]

Screening of the defined age/weight group is extremely important as treatment by cryotherapy or laser is ineffective once the vitreous has become involved or cicatrisation has commenced. Once stage three has been identified, it is recommended that treatment be commenced within 2–3 days. The College Guidelines clearly and explicitly cover the whole ROP screening process.

Babies with a birth weight of under 1500g tend to have a higher incidence of vision and ocular problems, such as ROP, squint and myopia.[18,19] However, remember that such babies account for only 1 per cent of live births. Croft *et al.*, in 1998, identified the majority of severe vision loss cases in the low birth weight group to be associated with cerebral palsy rather than the result of ROP.[20] There is little evidence, however, to identify without selection bias the percentage of low birth weight children that contribute to the overall population of those with severe vision loss.

In 2002, Saunders *et al.* identified that pre-term infants without ROP had high rates of refractive error.[21] Cycloplegic refraction was undertaken at birth, term, 6, 12 and 48 months corrected age in a cohort of 59 pre-term infants and 40 full-term subjects. Although a degree of emmetropisation over time was demonstrated, it was felt that refractive development in pre-term infants was more erratic than that for full-term subjects and thus refractive error in pre-term infants warranted monitoring.

Congenital cataract
Congenital cataract occurs in one in 10,000 births (excluding births with multiple abnormalities). Infants born at 2500g or less demonstrate a three- to four-fold incidence of developing infantile cataract.[22] At present no national guidelines are available, but recommendations drawn from working parties of the Royal College of Ophthalmologists and the Royal College of Paediatrics and Child Health are published.

In many areas local protocols exist, yet documentary evidence recorded in a comprehensive national cross-sectional study of 235 children with congenital cataract identified that 29 per cent of cases remained undetected until after their first birthday.[23] This finding is disappointing given the importance placed on early detection and treatment of congenital cataract. More robust strategies are required to achieve effective and earlier diagnosis.

The NSC recommends examination for the red reflex perinatally and before a baby's seventh week of life. Evidence, albeit limited, supports the belief that early treatment initiated at 1–6 weeks postpartum increases the potential for near-normal visual development.[24] Paediatricians are the first health professionals to assess babies at discharge from hospitals. GPs provide the second contact within 8 weeks.

Although funduscopy *per se* is not essential, assessment of the presence or absence of the red reflex is a quick and relatively easy test for the detection and prevention of a major vision defect. Appropriate training and skill development in conjunction with enhanced awareness of recommendations by clinicians needs to be addressed. In theory, prompt referral to an ophthalmologist expedites early treatment and reduces disruption to the development of normal vision.

Genetic screening
Documenting family history, both at the antenatal and neonatal stages of care, is

perceived by the Child Health Screening Sub Committee of the NSC to be of import and relevance. This issue may be raised and details recorded by a paediatrician or health visitor.

Infancy to 4–5 years

Sure Start

The UK Government invested over £1 billion for the period 1999–2004. All programmes are expected to include a number of core services:

- Outreach and home visiting;
- Support for families and parents;
- Support for good-quality play, learning and child-care experiences for children;
- Primary and community health care, including advice about both family health and child health and development;
- Support for children and parents with special needs, including help to gain access to specialised services.

National targets provide a framework of consistency to the Sure Start programmes, yet more specific objectives and targets that address local needs should be included.

If primary vision screening of infants is abandoned by health visitors, it is implied that the Sure Start scheme increases parental awareness of the potential vision defects that may affect their child. Thus, the onus is placed on the parents to seek advice if they have any concern regarding their child's visual health. This is especially so in cases where there is a positive family history of squint, amblyopia and/or refractive error. It is essential, therefore, for eye care specialists, such as orthoptists and optometrists, to work alongside the Sure Start team to identify clear referral pathways to facilitate access to the appropriate eye care professional.

Parental concern

In the most recent publication of *Health for All Children*, Hall and Elliman propose that children should not be screened routinely by health professionals, but that the identification of squint and vision defects should be reliant on parental observation or concern.[16] GPs and health visitors are being urged to take an active role in health promotion by raising parental awareness, and enquiring about the family history of eye problems, such as spectacle wear or squint. It is generally assumed parents are aware that their child is entitled to free NHS eye examinations up to 16 years of age (19 if in full-time education) by community optometrists.[25] In this capacity, optometrists may be the first eye care professional to examine a child, and as such should be competent in vision assessment in pre-literate and illiterate individuals.

Vision screening in young children

The NSC has recommended that the only screening carried out before the age of 4 years should be that for ROP and media opacities.

Based on evidence currently available, it is proposed that primary vision screening of young infants by health visitors should be discontinued. PVS programmes need to be revisited, with the aim of achieving the perceived gold standard of examination using a linear vision test, for example a Crowded LogMAR, from the age of 4 years and preferably before the child's fifth birthday. The rationale behind the shift to an older age group is that a more robust, accurate, linear vision test may be undertaken. At this later age subjective responses are more reliable, yet the child is still young enough to respond to conventional treatment. Use of the Crowded LogMAR test, with the linear progression of letter size, is preferable to use of the less accurate Snellen chart.[26,27] During routine vision screening, assessment of near visual acuity adds little to the detection of significant vision defects and may therefore be omitted from routine testing. However, near vision should be assessed at secondary screening (i.e., in the situation where a child has been referred with a suspected visual problem).

As identified in the third edition of the Hall report,[28] PVS, if undertaken by doctors or health visitors, has a lower yield and less satisfactory sensitivity and specificity than a programme that involves orthoptists.

A model of direct referral to optometrists for children with an orthotropic vision deficit identified at the screening visit appears to work well, with orthoptists and optometrists working in conjunction towards an agreed protocol. The HES only becomes involved in cases where the visual acuity is poor (6/24 or worse), or when children fail to improve to a predetermined level of acuity after spectacle wear for a limited period of time. Any child with squint is referred directly to the HES for further assessment.

However, the exact nature of the ideal early-stage vision screening, in terms of who carries it out, where and with what, is still the subject of much debate.

Screening after school entry

Vision screening

Handicap or academic underachievement attributable to uncorrected refractive error has not been proved statistically, partly because of the difficulties in designing a study in which so many variables are involved. There is, however, much anecdotal evidence to support an argument that blurred vision adversely affects a child's educational development, and certainly many eye care professionals assume a link exists. Adolescents are likely to report their concerns if reduced visual acuity is perceived to be problematic, and so routine vision screening by either school nurses or audio/vision screeners may not be an effective use of resources.

Colour vision

Limited formal evidence is available concerning the benefits of colour vision screening in children of any age.

Two perceived benefits may be that:

- Children with a degree of colour blindness may be disadvantaged in the educational environment if colour-coded materials are used for teaching purposes.
- Certain careers require normal colour vision. Individuals with colour vision deficiencies may be precluded from particular professions and occupations. With this in mind, a case could be made to screen only boys at the beginning of secondary education. Affected individuals could then make informed and appropriate career choices. Hall advises that an optometrist or ophthalmologist should review such adolescents.

Personal child health record

It is intended that healthcare professionals use the PCHR as both a wide-reaching data collection tool and a reference document pertinent to a particular child's state of health. A national PCHR would provide commonality and potentially reflect equity of health education and healthcare provision nationwide. Data collected on such a wide scale would provide comprehensive evidence and hence permit audit on a scale not previously attainable.

What does the future hold?

Screening in the early neonatal period for ROP and cataract has been recognised as being effective, in that early detection permits early treatment of proved benefit to the individual. This screen relies upon the education, training and ability of the paediatricians, ophthalmologists and GPs concerned.

Low birth weight and premature babies have been identified as being at increased risk of having or developing ROP or congenital cataract. Again, screening promotes early identification, prompt treatment and increased health gain.

Health professionals, such as health visitors, orthoptists and optometrists, have a limited role in screening programmes to detect conditions that may cause severe vision deficit. It is the combined service provision, however, supplied by such individuals that maintains and promotes optimum levels of visual acuity in children.

An integrated approach appears to be the most effective for maintaining a high standard of visual health in the general population. The ethos behind the Sure Start programmes is to deliver health promotion and health care directly to the heart of the community. For this concept to be feasible and produce a viable service, communication barriers between health professionals need to be broken down, information disseminated and expertise shared. The introduction of systems for cross-professional co-operation and communication between health professionals, such as vision screeners, health visitors, paediatricians, orthoptists, optometrists and ophthalmologists, should support this process.

Education and training in conjunction with the demonstration of continuous professional development is paramount if high-quality health care is to be pursued. Simply relying on parents to take their children for eye examinations may not be sufficient and all eye care professionals, including optometrists, have a vital role in health education that emphasises the importance of regular eye examinations at all ages.

Ophthalmic screening and surveillance programmes need better evaluation and outcome monitoring to substantiate their effectiveness. Continuation of the present methods of screening, or the introduction of new standards, need a demonstrable evidence base before any changes are made.

References

1 National Screening Committee: http://www.nsc.nhs.uk/whatscreening/whatscreen_indhtm.

2 Smeeth L and Iliffe S (1998) Effectiveness of screening older people for impaired vision in the community setting: Systematic review of evidence from randomised controlled trials. *BMJ* **16**, 660–663.

3 National Screening Committee (1998). *Annual Report*. (NSC: Milton Keynes).

4 Child Health Sub-Group (http://www.nsc.nhs.uk/whatscreening/whatscreen_indhtm).

5 Taylor D (1998). Congenital cataract: The history, the nature and the practice. The Doyne lecture. *Eye*, **12**, 9–36.

6 Snowdon S and Stewart-Brown S (1997). *Pre-school Vision Screening: Results of a Systematic Review*. Centre for Reviews and Dissemination Report 9. (University of York: York).

7 Rahi J S and Lynn R (1998). A survey of paediatricians' practice and training in routine infant eye examination. *Arch Dis Child*. **78**, 364–366.

8 http://www.nsc.nhs.uk/whatscreening/whatscreen_indhtm.

9 Smith LK, Thompson JR, Woodruff G, *et al.* (1994). Social deprivation and age at presentation in amblyopia. *J Public Health Med*. **16**, 348–351.

10 Stewart-Brown SL, Haslum MN and Howlett B (1988). Pre-school vision screening: A service in need of rationalisation. *Arch Dis Child*. **63**, 356–359.

11 McGraw and Winn B (1995). Measurement of letter acuity in preschool children. *Ophthalmic Physiol Opt*. **15S**, 11–17.

12 Wilson JM and Jungner G (1968). *The Principles and Practice of Screening for Disease*. Public Health Papers 34. (Geneva: World Health Organisation).

13 Yang YF and Cole MD (1996). Visual acuity testing in schools: What needs to be done. *BMJ* **284**, 1856–1857.

14 Gordon NS (1998). Colour blindness. *Public Health* **112**, 81–84.

15 Tsiaras WG, Pueschel S, Keller C, Curran R and Geisswein S (1999). Amblyopia and visual acuity in children with Down's

syndrome. *Br J Ophthalmol.* **83**, 1112–1114.
16 Hall DM and Elliman D (2003). *Health for All Children*, Fourth Edition. Report of the 4th Joint Working Party on Child Health Surveillance. (Oxford: Oxford University Press).
17 The Royal College of Ophthalmologists and British Association of Perinatal Medicine (1995). *Retinopathy of Prematurity: Guidelines for Screening and Treatment*. Report of a Joint Working Party. (London: Royal College of Ophthalmologists).
18 Robinson R and O'Keefe M (1993). Follow up study on premature infants with and without ROP. *Br J Ophthalmol.* **77**, 91–94.
19 Powls A, Botting N, Cooke RWI, Stephenson G and Marlow N (1997). Visual impairment in very low birth weight children. *Arch Dis Child.* **76**, F82–F87.
20 Croft BJ, King R and Johnson A (1998). The contribution of low birth weight to severe vision loss in a geographically defined population. *Br J Ophthalmol.* **82**, 9–13.
21 Saunders KJ, McCulloch DL, Shepherd AJ and Wilkinson AG (2002). Emmetropisation following preterm birth. *Br J Ophthalmol.* **86**, 1035–1040.
22 SanGiovanni J, Chew EY, Reed GF, *et al.* (2002). Infantile cataract in the collaborative perinatal project: Prevalence and risk factors. *Arch Ophthalmol.* **120**, 1559–1565.
23 Rahi JS and Dezateux C for the British Congenital Cataract Interest Group (1999). National cross-sectional study of detection of congenital and infantile cataract in the UK: Role of screening and surveillance. *BMJ* **318**, 362–365.
24 Birch EE, Swanson WH, Stager DR, Woody M and Everett M (1993). Outcome after very early treatment of dense congenital unilateral cataract. *Invest Ophthalmol Vis Sci.* **34**, 3687–3699.
25 Royal College of Ophthalmologists, The College of Optometrists and the British Orthoptic Society (2002). *Guidelines for Children's Eye Care* (London: Royal College of Ophthalmologists).
26 Stewart C (2000). Comparison of Snellen and log-based acuity scores for school-aged children. *Br Orthoptic J.* **57**, 32–38.
27 McGraw PV, Winn B, Gray LS and Elliott DB (2000). Improving the reliability of visual acuity measures in young children. *Ophthalmic Physiol Opt.* **20**, 173–184.
28 Hall DM (1996). *Health for All Children*, Third Edition. Report of the Third Joint Working Party on Child Health Surveillance. (Oxford: Oxford University Press).

15
Paediatric Communication

William Harvey

It is important when communicating with children of various ages to consider how best to phrase sentences and to ensure the maximum understanding and co-operation on the part of the child.[1] As semantic development takes many years, the importance of good non-verbal skills when dealing with children cannot be emphasised too strongly.

The aim of this chapter is to argue 'what' should be asked of children in optometry practice in general and to expand further to describe 'how' such communication might best be carried out. More specific scenarios (such as the insertion of contact lenses discussed in Chapter 12), are described elsewhere in this book, with a more general outline provided here.

The 'problem' with children

Not every optometrist is happy to deal with children. When such an optometrist analyses the exact reasons for this, more often than not these are about problems in dealing with the behaviour of the patient than with any challenge to the technical or practical ability to carry out the examination.

Children often appear to behave in a greatly exaggerated manner, and openly express emotions that range from fear and anger to hilarity. It is this very expression that, whenever a problem for the child is solved, makes it all the more satisfying for the practitioner who has helped them. It therefore enhances a practitioner's satisfaction with his or her own role to include rather than exclude child patients, but to achieve this satisfaction effective communication skills are paramount.

An initial proposal

As well as changing physically, growing children are developing cognitively (in that their knowledge level increases) and are open to an ever-increasing number of experiences, preoccupations, problems and interests. Cognitive growth continues throughout life and this so-called 'lifespan development'[2] has a great influence on, among many other things, a patient's health beliefs.

It has been argued[3] that an individual's health beliefs, or the preconceived ideas that shape his or her perception and action during a clinical interaction, have an impact on the success of a clinician's communication with that individual. Success might be gauged in terms of how effectively information may flow between that individual and a clinician. It might therefore be proposed that for clinicians to be able to communicate with any patient of a particular age, they should have some awareness of the typical behavioural and personality traits of that age group.

It is fair to say, then, that to be effective in examining children, an optometrist needs to be flexible and change his or her own behaviour when dealing with a 2-year-old child. This interaction with a 2-year-old child will, in turn, be very different from the interaction with a 5-year-old and again with a 10-year-old. Chapter 1 gives a description of the expected ages at which visual and ocular processes and structures develop and reach full function, but readers may benefit from a reminder of the general pattern of behavioural development expected in children as they grow.

Milestones of development

Despite the great variety of environmental and genetic influences on a child's development, certain patterns emerge as common to the majority of individuals within a large social group. These have been studied and observed by many famous researchers into childhood development, such as Piaget,[4] and form the basis of most guides to development used by clinicians involved with monitoring the development of infants and ensuring that any particular infant is developing as might be expected. This is, for example, the basis of part of the Personal Child Health Record (PCHR or 'little red book') discussed in Chapter 14. *Table 15.1* gives a summary of the milestones or key events in the development of the child. It is based upon the Denver Developmental Screening Test,[5] which describes, albeit in more detail, the main events expected at any specified age in a child's development.[6] A thorough history and symptoms taking from a child, as outlined later, may well touch on several of these key events and so an awareness of the normal patterns of development are useful for any clinician who deals with children.

The Denver test is a useful guide and allows an optometrist who deals with very small children on a regular basis to have an idea as to the general level of expected function. The fuller version classifies the milestones into four distinct categories:

- Gross motor;
- Language;
- Fine motor;
- Personal/social.

While the first three put constraints upon the actual examination techniques an optometrist may use on a young child, the fourth category of personal/social development is the one that places the social and interactive skills of the practitioner most under the spotlight. It is, as already mentioned, a reason why some practitioners would rather avoid children. It is increasingly becoming realised, however, in all paediatric disciplines, that a mastery of recognising and responding appropriately to the personal and social development needs is as important as the objective clinical skills.

Slightly different developmental criteria have been proposed by Hyvärinen,[7] who considered four functional areas in which vision is important. These are:

- Communication (interpersonal, in a group or distance);
- Orientation and mobility;
- Everyday activity;
- Sustained near vision tasks, such as reading and writing.

It is safe to say that vision has a key role in these functions and that a thorough assessment of vision not only helps maintain development along established patterns, but also helps identify situations in which these patterns are not being followed.

Some psychologists have looked for patterns in the development of personality traits; one such classification is summarised in *Table 15.2*.[8] Each personality milestone is described in terms of conflicting emotions, which, it might be proposed, drive the behaviour of the child at the time.

Table 15.1 Behavioural events during normal development

Approximate age	*Developmental event*
2 months	Laughs, smiles spontaneously
3 months	Rolls over
3.5 months	Reaches for object
4 months	Cooing, gurgling noises
5.5 months	Sits without support, turns to voices
6 months	Stands holding on
	Plays peek-a-boo
	Good visual tracking and convergence
6–9 months	Babbles and imitates common sounds
8–9 months	Anxious in presence of unfamiliar individuals
	Distress at separation from mother figure (which may continue until around 20 months)
8–10 months	Creeps and crawls
9–10 months	Pulls self up to stand
9.5–10 months	Walks supported
10 months	Walks unsupported in short bursts
	Says 'mama' or 'papa'
11.5 months	Stands steadily
12 months	Walks
13 months	Says a few more words
17 months	Tackles stairs
20 months	Two-word sequences possible
2 years	Three-word sentences attempted
	First sign of handedness, which is fully established by 4.5–5 years
2.75 years	Repeats first and last names
7 years	Knows left and right on self
9 years	Knows left and right on others

Though unlikely to be the responsibility of the optometrist, any astute clinician might be the first to suspect communication difficulties that may require the intervention of a speech-language specialist. Danger signals might include:

- Lack of response by 6 months of age to the sound of others talking;
- Inability by 18 months to say any meaningful word or follow simple instruction;
- Inability by the age of 2 years to understand simple questions, use more than one word at a time or name easily identified objects in a picture;
- Inability at 3 years of age to use simple sentences or be understood by a stranger.

Several methods have been designed to assess children's ability to communicate. The Children's Communication Checklist

Table 15.2 A classification of personality traits with increasing age

Stage conflict	*Age (years)*	*Personality trait*
Trust/mistrust	0–1	Security, stability and trust required; new conditions create uncertainty and mistrust
Autonomy/shame	1–3	Striving to master physical environment, goals not yet attainable cause anxiety
Initiative/guilt	3–5	Having developed autonomy, makes efforts to join in and initiate activities with others
		Conflicts with others cause frustration
Industry/inferiority	5–11	Needs to meet demands of home and school
Identity/role confusion	11–18	Developing sense of identity, blending various roles into a cogent self-image

(CCC) designed by Bishop,[9] for example, has been used in research to assess children of 5–16 years of age and has proved sensitive to pragmatic difficulties, as it relies on completion by the parents. It is currently under review and an updated version, the CCC-R, is likely to be published shortly.

Visual versus semantic input

The majority of early learning is based on visual input. This is significant, not least when one considers the challenges to the development of a child with multiple impairment, such as the deaf–blind child, as discussed later.

A brief mention is made here of some interesting research on trying to establish the link between the development of perception and the development of language. It has been postulated that as language communication skills develop, a change occurs in how the perceptual processes analyse the visual image. This may play a role in influencing the way a child responds to visual stimuli in the very early years of development. The development of perception is the theme of many major psychology texts that interested readers may wish to read.[10,11]

The concept of 'photographic memory', or eidetic imagery (to give it its proper name), has long fascinated researchers and there are many accounts of infants able to recall complex and multistructured images presented to them, often after a long period of time. Recall usually is acknowledged not through verbal recollection, but by monitoring eye movements when a subject is presented with a blank surface subsequent to presentation of the complex image and after erasure of any after-image information.

The ability to recall in detail multifaceted visual stimuli deteriorates dramatically beyond a certain age and the very few adults able to perform such accurate visual recollection are often found to have significant social interactive difficulties, and more often than not are diagnosed as autistic. Many people recall the scene in the film *Rainman* when the autistic character is able to count rapidly the number of matches that have fallen to the floor.

More intensive neurological investigation has shown that as the brain centres that link language and social interaction (communication skills, as it were) develop rapidly during the first few years of life, the ability to perform eidetic imagery decreases dramatically. The hippocampus seems to be integral to this process. These centres may act differently in autism and the related Asperger's syndrome. It has thus been proposed that the processing of the image formed at the retina (the iconic memory) to that within the electrical network within the brain (long-term memory) becomes increasingly linked with semantic or language encoding as a child develops. It seems at this point that the ability to process memory purely in visual terms becomes lost.

If the reader tries to recall a familiar image now, most find it difficult to dissociate the image held within their head from the words used to describe it. The drive for social development in humans has increased the semantic role in perception. Though much further research needs to be done, our dealings with very small children need to be sensitive to the way the children may respond to word patterns and images presented to them.

Finally, it might, therefore, be the case that there is a physiological basis to the generally held view (though still disputed, see Chapter 14) that visual problems hinder social development and hence the need for accurate, and thorough eye care during the first few years of life.

Orientation and environment

It is well established that the flow of information between two people is very much influenced by the orientation of the interacting participants and the environment within which they interact. Although there are clinical situations in which a more authoritarian approach on behalf of the practitioner may be appropriate, such as in explaining a particularly complex and significant finding to an adult, generally speaking a very informal and friendly approach is best adopted when dealing with children. White coats and cold clinical environments are unlikely to improve the responses of a young child; a relaxed, colourful and friendly environment might.

The initial meeting with the child has a very important bearing on subsequent events; a useful way to establish a warm rapport from the start is for the practitioner to approach and greet the patient in the waiting area rather than to remain in the consulting room awaiting the child.

Sudden movements are to be avoided, including lights being suddenly turned on or off or the introduction of new pieces of equipment. Both may startle and detract from the overall control of the examination. Any necessary piece of equipment predicted to cause alarm, such as a refractor head or a slit lamp, may be introduced gently in a playful manner; the author often describes his refractor head as a space helmet (Skywalker's pod-racing attire has done optometrists throughout the world a great service).

The practitioner should also be aware of the often large size difference between themselves and the child patient. When there is a need to approach the patient, as with ophthalmoscopy, the child may see the practitioner as a giant. Although there is no easy way around this, the best approach, having first built up the confidence of the child, is to use gentle movements.

Gathering information

Children require accurate optometric assessment and consequently the information required should be based on the standard history and symptoms pattern,[12] which might be summarised as follows:

- Reason for attendance;
- Ocular and optical status;
- Symptoms (with appropriate probing questions as required);
- Ocular history (and that of family);
- Medical history (and that of family);
- Lifestyle, occupational (and educational) details.

At all ages, including for the very young, inclusion of the patient (i.e., the child) in all communications is important. The practitioner who addresses the parent or carer solely throughout the initial history and symptoms process runs a grave risk of alienating the child and reducing co-operation.

Conversely, when explaining the reason for particular questions or when, during the conclusion of the examination, the practitioner is giving advice to the parents with regards to their child, it must always be remembered that the child is usually the main point of focus in those parents' life. Throwaway comments or casual explanations of even seemingly (to the optometrist) innocuous conditions, for example astigmatism, may be the cause of serious concern to the parent. The practitioner must always be able to give clear instruction, be ready to give advice about the future implication of a visual finding and be suitably professional in communication to reassure the parent and avoid this potential conflict. Parents might need reassurance as to the need for certain questions being asked, for example those that concern the child's intellectual development, before accurate information is gleaned.

As has hopefully become obvious, the depth and nature of the questioning varies greatly according to both the patient's age and emotional status. However, certain child-specific questions might be included in these very basic categories.

Ocular and optical status

- Does the child report any difficulty seeing the blackboard or television?
- Does the child show any difficulty in reading?
- Is the child reluctant to carry out visually demanding tasks?
- Does the child have any unusual visual habits, such as holding books very close?
- Does the child have difficulty maintaining his or her place in a piece of text?
- Does the child rub his or her eyes very often, or blink excessively?
- Does the child 'squint' or screw up his or her eyes.

These and related questions may help to distinguish between an organic or a refractive visual problem, a behavioural or psychological problem, or one related to a particular disease process.

Educational details

When asking very detailed questions of a child and anyone with the child, great care must be taken to avoid stigmatising the child. Constant questioning of the child's intellectual ability may reduce the subsequent co-operation of the child throughout the rest of the examination. However, in certain situations, such as determining the presence of a specific reading difficulty independent of the child's intellectual status, or in trying to ascertain a distinct binocular status imbalance, further questions need to be pursued. In low vision practice, a clear understanding of any special educational provision is useful (see Chapter 13).

Developmental details

Questions that relate to the possibility of problems during the birth of a child are often relevant and need to be asked. Such questions may be expanded to look for the influence of developmental problems during the early years. For example, at what age did the child first walk, crawl, speak words and speak sentences? Is the child easily distracted, or overly active?

While the risks of such questions, not least in alienating the parents, should be obvious, careful questioning along these lines may well be worthwhile in establishing if a poor visual development performance has behavioural origins rather than an ocular or optical functional source.

It is useful to detail some more specific points that relate to the communication with children at various age groups, which reflect the expectations of children as they change during the early years.

Birth to 9 months

- Address the child as well as parent.
- Avoid sudden movements.

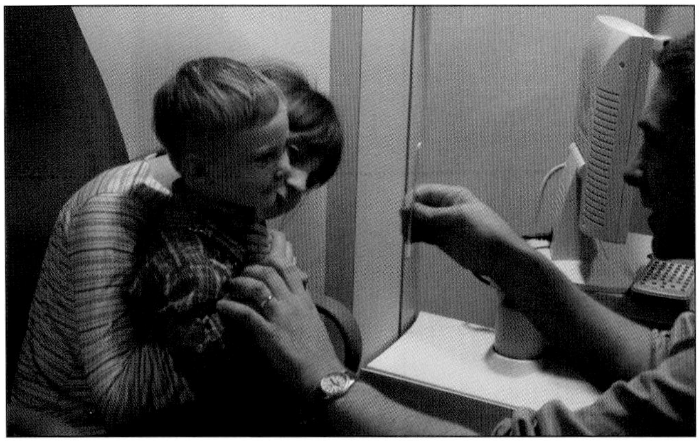

Figure 15.1 *This child responds very well while sitting on his sister's lap*

- Appropriate use of non-verbal cues, including touch, is effective at reassuring the very young. A warm and friendly tone of voice helps to convey a sense of security to the child.
- A generally friendly and informal environment is useful, but too many distractions at this early age, such as pictures and sounds, may be overly taxing to the child.
- At the end of this stage of development, loss of attention and distraction become more significant, so the use of reinforced visual targets (brightly coloured or with bells attached) may help maintain attention.
- Spending too long on any one task, including history taking, may fatigue the child and result in loss of attention. To maximise efficiency, the practitioner might consider asking some questions of the parent while carrying out the first visual examination procedures.
- Very young children still have an established diurnal pattern of wakefulness. The average newborn sleeps for 18–20 hours a day and by 1 month has developed a routine, which typically involves a period of wakefulness in the morning and a long afternoon sleep.[13] Morning appointments might, therefore, make it easier for the practitioner to maintain attention, and feeding times are best avoided as, even at this early stage, delayed feeding leads to fractiousness.

9 months to 3 years

- The need to prevent distraction becomes more important at this age and, again, sudden movements or events are to be avoided. Dimmer switches are a boon. It is also useful to avoid crowding an entire family in the consulting room.
- This age group has been described classically as developing 'stranger fear',[14] in which they have formed a particularly strong social bond with one person or a group of familiar people. Separation, even if just by a practitioner sitting in between, is enough to trigger a frightened and unco-operative response. The term 'stranger fear' is now falling out of favour,[15] as it appears that, though a child may well be wary of a stranger, fear is usually avoided by the child being aware that their parent figure is somewhere in the vicinity. The child responds very well if seated on the parent's (or sister's, as in *Figure 15.1*) lap, and it may be observed that parent involvement also helps allay any possible concerns on the part of the parent.
- Appointments should reflect the diurnal habits of the child still present at this stage.

Several appointments may be necessary, not just to complete all the necessary tests, but to enhance the child's familiarity with and hence confidence in the environment. This is particularly so when balancing the need for a cycloplegic assessment with the risk of deterring a child from having future eye assessments (*Figure 15.2*).

3 to 5 years

- The child now has established greater independence and language skills.
- A greater involvement in the history and symptoms process is now possible and advisable.
- Avoiding sudden movements may now be reinforced with a description of a procedure ('I'm going to shine a light at you now.').
- The increasing curiosity of this age group may be indulged by letting them push a button or touch an interesting looking piece of kit (obviously, safety and possible damage implications being considered) to aid rapport. The light to be shone in their eyes may first be shone on the back of their hand. This author has often found that a nervous child will

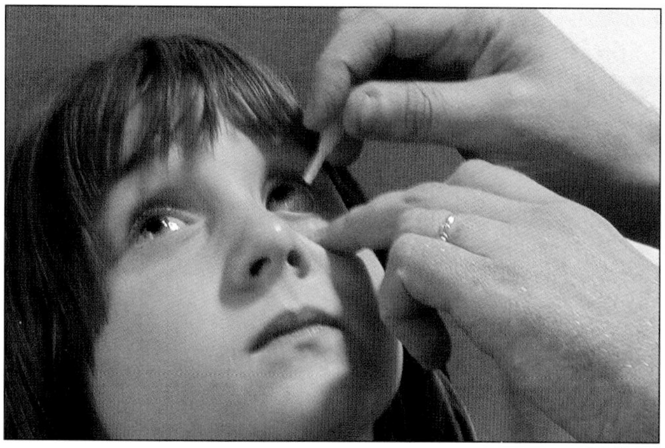

Figure 15.2
Care with the instillation of a cycloplegic can prevent unnecessary anxiety over future visits to the optometrist

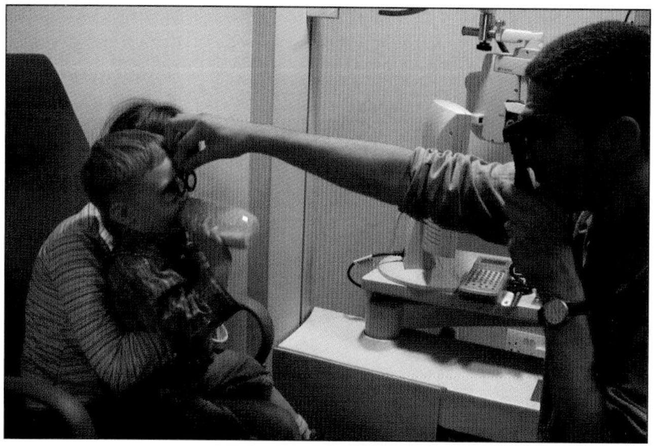

Figure 15.3
Some children respond better when a comfortable working distance is maintained

relax somewhat if involved in the choice of stop or colour of filter (a red-free filter usually still allows adequate fundus viewing) before ophthalmoscopy.

- In cases where a child clearly responds poorly to close proximity, much can be observed using indirect techniques. The often quoted advantage of a headset binocular indirect ophthalmoscope for examining children is sometimes offset by the brightness of the light and the strange appearance of the head-borne apparatus. Some of the newer spectacle-mounted systems are less imposing and, in extreme circumstance, a spot retinoscope and a +20D trial lens affords at least some view of the fundus (*Figure 15.3*).
- The developing language skills may not yet be sophisticated enough to respond appropriately to jokes or wordplay. Though obviously humour is an excellent way to diffuse any possible consulting room tension, the author has known of instances where children in this age group have been traumatised by comments such as 'Let's look in your eyes to see what you had for breakfast' or, as a chair is being raised 'Mind your head on the ceiling!'. Use humour with caution.
- Most of the clinical techniques (including field assessment and slit-lamp biomicroscopy) should be possible with children within this age category, often with only minor adjustment to technique.
- This author has found that hand-held autorefractors have improved significantly enough to allow a useful refractive assessment of even the most unco-operative child.[16]

5 to 11 years

- School-related questions become more significant with this group, and the practitioner must always be mindful of the need to avoid stigmatising the child's intellectual performance.
- Improved language ability should make it easier still to direct the majority of questions to the child. If there is still apprehension, it is useful to make sure that the majority of questions used are closed questions.
- Questions might digress to discuss a television programme or pop group (provided the practitioner is *au fait* with popular children's culture) as a useful way to gain confidence.
- Age is a poor indicator of intellect and it is often painful to watch others appear to act in a very child-friendly manner and actually sound very patronising. Most children in this age category actually respond very well to quite advanced ('adult') speech patterns.

11 to 18 years

- The very strong self-awareness of adolescence means that any leading questions or those that might imply a physical or behavioural anomaly are to be strongly avoided.
- The practitioner needs to be aware that answers to questions may be somewhat coloured by a particular need of the patient. Typically, this age group may want a spectacle correction to copy a classmate, or conversely dread the prospect of wearing a new correction and therefore altering their self-image, and so give misleading answers. Experienced practitioners should be able to spot inconsistencies of response without sounding as if they are trying to catch the patient out.
- The practitioner should be aware that the rules of patient confidentiality begin to have more bearing the older a child becomes and while, up until the age of 16 years the child is legally the responsibility of the parent or guardian who has full access to any information gained, sensitive subjects may be covered comprehensively in some instances if the child feels they can trust the practitioner to maintain a degree of secrecy. Obviously, discretion is needed here and parental involvement in the care of children under 16 years of age is usually the safest policy.

History and symptoms of the visually impaired child

All of the above points apply as much to the child with impaired vision as to the fully sighted child. However, as with all low-vision patients, if appropriate and adequate help is to be given, many extra details need to be addressed. The following list of suggested questions is by no means exhaustive, but covers important areas that need to be considered.[17]

Reason for attendance

- What problems does the child have?
- How is the child's performance at school or home affected?
- Do you understand the problem or diagnosis?
- How much vision do the parents think their child has? How do the parents understand the nature of the child's vision?

Expectations

- What expectations do the parents and child have of the future?
- What do they expect the optometrist's role to be? This point is particularly important and many practitioners who work in the field of low vision often give a summary of their role at the outset. Patients may have unrealistic expectations of miracle sight restoration and parents are often, understandably, guilty of this. The explanation need not be too negative and sentences such as 'My role is to discover exactly how much useful vision your child has and to help him or her to use it as best as possible' is suitably positive, but will gently quash any implications of 'improvement'.

Medical history

- Are there any other handicaps, ophthalmic or general, that are relevant?
- Is the child registered as blind or partially sighted?

Distance vision

- Details of targets need to be specific, such as the size of the television and if colour or black and white. How is the classroom laid out, what board is used, where is the teacher? A photograph of the school environment is useful.

Near vision

- Reading details need to be very specific, including discussion of duration of reading, environment and lighting details, size and nature of print and so on. Samples are very useful.

Mobility

- Does the child require a guide and, if so, what are the details?
- Is mobility dependent on vision or touch?
- Is the child able to orientate well, avoid collisions, maintain position?
- How does the lighting level affect the child's ability to move about?
- Does the child use tinted lenses, a visor or a hat?
- Can the child read signs, such as directional or warning notices?

Visual response

- Do the eyes appear abnormal?
- Is there a head tilt or turn that the child prefers to adopt?
- Can the child locate and track objects in his or her field?
- Can the child use vision sufficiently to play physical games with other children?

Details of the child's preferences at playtime may give important clues as to how confident they are at using their functional vision.

Current aids

- Full details of any aids in current use, preferably with a demonstration of how the child uses them, are important.

Educational considerations

- Does the child have an education statement?
- Does the child have access to specialist teaching, either equipment such as CCTVs or staff?

Home considerations

- Full details of the home environment, including any special equipment or adaptations, need to be ascertained.
- Can the child take care of him- or herself in the home?

Even though this is a generalised list to which further questions may be required for the needs of individual children, it is apparent that as soon as there is a special and specific need, a great deal of extra information is required. This may be over and beyond what most optometrists would recognise as a standard history and symptoms.

A word of caution

The danger of lists such as the above is that the assessment verges upon an interrogation. Much of the information may be gleaned from pre-assessment research. It has already been stated that visual input is essential for the normal development of behaviour. A clinician may thus have fewer clues as to the needs of a multiply impaired child who has established less well-defined methods of interpretation and feedback.

The same situation may have led to the child having been subjected to more questions from caregivers and providers than a normal child might expect. This may lead to overuse of questions and pronoun confusion by the children themselves as they grow older. For this reason, alternative communication systems and augmentative and reinforcing devices have been developed for particular use in dealing with the multiply impaired child.

Hearing-impaired children

When communicating with a child with a hearing impairment, the following general points should be considered:

- The practitioner should face the patient as much as possible. For times of significant communication, such as during history and symptoms, good lighting on both faces is important.
- The mouth should be as visible as possible. Some authorities point out that an untrimmed beard may inhibit the interpretation of speech!
- The practitioner should always attract attention before starting to speak.
- Any background noise may significantly reduce the ability of the patient to interpret the message from the practitioner. This is potentially a problem outside the consulting room, for example at reception or in a pre-examination area.
- As with most patients, the use of jargon or technical words (astigmatism, amblyopia and so on) adds to confusion.
- Specific instructions may be reinforced by being written down.
- Whole sentences are easier to interpret, though verbosity is best avoided.
- Complex messages, such as at the summing up of the practitioner's findings, should be given in short, concise bundles (categorisation).
- Speech should be slowed down to a steady, well-articulated pace of a sensible volume. If speech is too fast it becomes imperceptible; if it is too slow and the natural rhythm is lost, this makes interpretation harder.
- Though raising volume a little is helpful, shouting or speaking too loudly actually distorts clear speech and may even be painful (for either party).
- The practitioner should ascertain whether the patient has asymmetrical hearing loss and arrange to be seated nearer the side with reduced loss.
- The practitioner should not be shy or embarrassed to repeat important phrases.
- Speech can be reinforced very effectively by the appropriate body language without any need to resort to specialist sign languages.
- The practitioner must allow adequate time for the patient to respond. It is often forgotten that one has also to listen to a hearing-impaired patient.

Specialised languages

Thanks to the efforts of hearing-impaired people there has been an improved acceptance of sign languages to help communication. Many children with congenital hearing disability may use such a system fluently and patients with acquired disability (and, indeed, anyone interested in improving their communication skills) may learn such techniques at one of many specialised teaching centres throughout the country.

Such languages include:

- *British Sign Language (BSL).* BSL employs a range of gestures to represent words and meaning. It is closely allied to sign-supported English (SSE).
- *Makaton and Paget.* Both are popular symbolic languages learnt by many children. Instead of spelling out 'cup', for example, or having a gesture to represent it that needs to be learnt, Makaton illustrates it by the communicator mimicking the action of holding a cup. Again, these techniques are highly visual.
- *Hands-on signing.* These sign languages may be reinforced usefully for a patient with failing vision by allowing them to place their hands on the communicator to allow easier interpretation of the language.

Summary

The sometimes challenging behaviour of an unco-operative child in the consulting room should not deter the optometrist from attempting as thorough an investigation as possible. Good communication skills are essential to achieve this. In return, the practitioner is rewarded with one of the more satisfying aspects of their professional life; the chance to contribute to the well-being of future generations.

References

1 Franklin A and Harvey W (2000). Taking history and symptoms – Part 4. *Optician* **220**(5767), 16–21.
2 Shute R (1991). *Psychology in Vision Care*. (Oxford: Butterworth–Heinemann).
3 Harvey W (1998). Clinical communication – Part 4. *Optician* **215**(5658), 16–20.
4 Piaget J (1954). *The Construction of Reality in the Child*. (New York: Basic Books).
5 Frankenberg WK and Dodds JB (1969). *Denver Developmental Screening Test*. (Denver: University of Colorado Medical Centre).
6 Erickson EH (1963). *Childhood and Society*. (New York: Norton).
7 Hyvärinen L (1985). Classification of visual development and disability. *Bull Belgium Ophthalmol.* **215**, 1–16.
8 Ettinger ER. (1993). *Professional Communications in Eye Care*. (Oxford: Butterworth–Heinemann).
9 Bishop DVM (1998). Development of the Children's Communication Checklist (CCC): A method for assessing qualitative aspects of communication impairment in children. *J Child Psychol Psychiatry* **39**, 879–891.
10 Ferguson EJ (1977). The mind's eye: Non-verbal thought in technology. *Science* **197**, 827–836.
11 Gregory RL (1987). *The Oxford Companion to the Mind*. (Oxford: Oxford University Press).
12 Harvey W (2000). Taking concise history and symptoms. *Optician* **219**(5741), 20–26.
13 Helms DB and Turner JS (1981). *Exploring Child Behavior*. (New York: Holt, Rhinehart and Wislon).
14 Bowlby J (1998). *Attachment and Loss: 1, Attachment*. (London: Hogarth Press).
15 Sroufe LA and Waters E (1977). Attachment as an organisational construct. *Child Dev.* **48**, 1184–1199.
16 Harvey W (2001). Hand-held autorefractors: A comparative trial of their uses in paediatric screening. *Optician* **222**(5815), 20–22.
17 Giltrow-Tyler F (1990). *Children's Visual Problems, Module 3: Partially Sighted Children*. (Oxford: Radcliffe Medical: Press).

Appendix 1: Ocular Embryology

Chris Wigham

It is estimated that 5 per cent of births have a recognisable 'abnormality' that arises from a failure of the normal developmental processes in the embryo.[1] A significant proportion are abnormalities of the eye and its adnexa.[2] The purpose of this Appendix is twofold. Firstly, it aims to provide a basic understanding of the development of the embryo and concentrates on the events that form the eyes and their adnexa. Secondly, it attempts to utilise this foundation material to consider the causes of ocular developmental abnormality and review the clinical assessment and management of developmental abnormalities.

Principles of embryonic development

'In the beginning...' is a single cell (the diploid zygote) formed by fusion of the (haploid) sperm and ovum. What happens next? If each cell divides at the same rate (*Figure A1.1*, scenario A), a blob of cells is produced that quickly dies from lack of nutrition. However, if cells divide and, importantly, die at carefully controlled rates (*Figure A1.1*, scenario B), a 'normal' healthy human results.

The control of division and death in the embryo is a complex process that involves a number of genes and their gene products [such as the homeobox genes that programme cell differentiation, genes that code for the production of chemical signals (growth factors) and receptors that enable cells to communicate], and cell adhesion molecules that enable cells to act together to establish complex multicellular structures.[3,4] The result of all this programming and signalling is that individual cells are directed to follow particular paths of development, to become specialised in their activity and to act co-operatively in the assembly of cellular aggregates that we call tissues, organs and, ultimately, humans.

Many millions of these control steps and/or events take place in the formation of a fully formed human, and of course these developmental events do not stop at birth, but continue into adulthood. As might be expected in such a fabulously intricate dance, 'missed steps' can, and do, occur by any one of a number of mechanisms. A cell may not divide, it may not divide at the correct time, a message may not be sent or received or it may be sent at the wrong time, or cells may fail to join and act together.[5,6] The unfortunate outcome of these 'errors' is a developmental abnormality that results in a defect in form or function. The errors that occur early in gestation, between days 1–30, tend to be the most catastrophic. This is the period in which the major organs are induced, including the eyes, and during which the embryo is most susceptible. It is perhaps fortunate that most of these severely damaged embryos spontaneously abort. Whereas 5 per cent of live births are considered to have an abnormality, the actual number of abnormalities is much higher than this. It is estimated that only 50 per cent of conceptions survive to birth; the majority of these losses result from catastrophic developmental abnormalities.[1] In view of the complexity of these developmental events, it is amazing that the populace is so apparently 'normal'. In reality, we are most likely not. It is highly probable that most of us have a developmental abnormality, but fortunately it is so minor as to pass unnoticed. The concept of the 'normal' human should, perhaps, be held with this in mind.

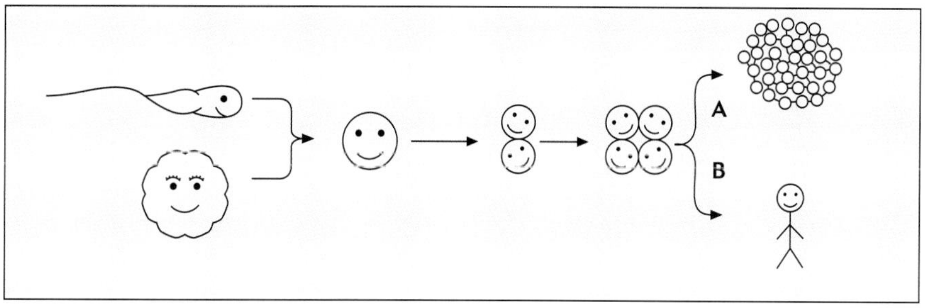

Figure A1.1
Human development, from beginning to completion

Development of the embryo

As early as the eight-cell stage in the development of the embryo, differences in cell behaviour can be recognised, with each cell 'switched' to follow a particular developmental path. These paths are seen in subsequent divisions, as particular cells migrate to form the basic germ layers of the embryo, the ectoderm, mesoderm and endoderm (*Figure A1.2*). This process of germ layer formation is called gastrulation, and is the first time at which the cells act co-operatively. The germ layers now continue to develop in a pattern that is remarkably similar between species, in which the ectoderm forms nervous tissue and skin, the mesoderm forms muscle and connective tissue and the endoderm forms gut structures and some glands.[5]

The first real sign of the future human and the body line is seen with the differentiation of a group of ectoderm cells into neural ectoderm. This differentiation occurs under the prompting of a special set of mesoderm cells, the notochord, which lie just underneath the ectoderm. Rapid growth of neural ectoderm produces two hillocks along the full length of the embryo (*Figure A1.3*). With the fusion of these hillocks a tube of cells, the neural tube, is formed that develops into the central nervous system and, as is evident later, provides many of the structures of the eye.[7] Cells of the neural tube (and surface ectoderm) at the 'head' end now divide furiously to form an anterior enlargement that becomes somewhat isolated from the rest of the embryo – the future brain. Any abnormal development of this anterior neural tube results in major abnormalities of the brain and head structures.

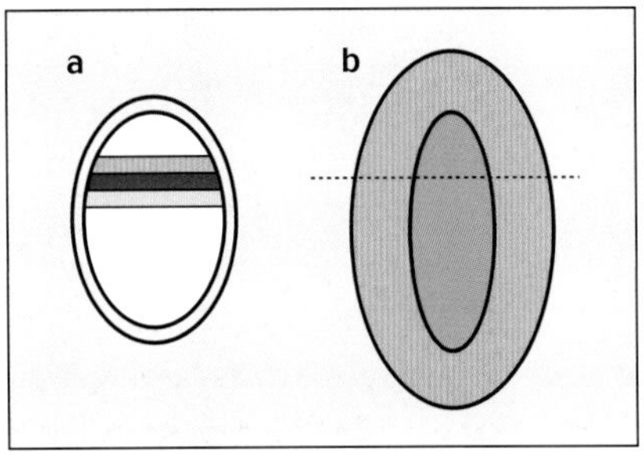

Figure A1.2
(a) The embryo at approximately 14 days. The three germ layers are evident in the germ plate: ectoderm (blue), mesoderm (red) and endoderm (green). (b) A view of the germ plate from above, showing the position of the prospective neural ectoderm (orange) within the ectoderm (blue). The dashed line indicates the point of section used in Figure A1.3 (a–d)

Interestingly, even in such severely damaged embryos, eye structures may still form. These abnormal eyes can fuse to form a cyclopean eye, or partially fuse as in synophthalmos.[8] The vast majority of these severely malformed embryos spontaneously abort – none survive.

As the neural tube fuses, a group of cells bud off its dorsal surface to form neural crest cells. These neural crest cells have a number of vital roles. One is to help fill the space between the ectoderm and neural tube (embryological 'packing material'). These space-filling neural crest cells are called mesenchyme (to note their similarity in function to mesoderm) and differentiate into muscles and connective tissues in the head region. Whereas the precise contribution of neural crest and true mesoderm to the production of head and eye structures is still a subject of debate, neural crest mesenchyme is now believed to be the major contributor to the formation of eye structures.[9,10]

As the neural tube at the head end continues to grow, three segments become identifiable; these become the fore, mid and hind brain (*Figure A1.4*). From the anterior part of the fore brain (telencephalon), the cerebral hemispheres develop. From the posterior portion (diencephalon), the eyes and thalamus form. The mid-section forms midbrain, and the hind-section becomes cerebellum, medulla and brain stem.

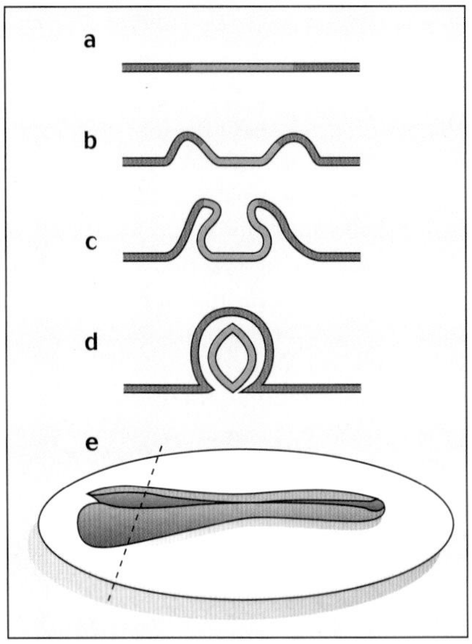

Figure A1.3
The embryo from days 14 to 21. (a) The ectodermal component of the neural plate (as in Figure A1.2). (b) The formation of hillocks. (c) Extension of the hillocks provides the first signs of the neural tube. (d) Fusion of the apical edges of the hillocks frees the neural tube. (e) Top view of the plate showing the embryo. The neural tube has fused, except at the head and tail region. The dashed line indicates the point of section used in Figure A1.5

Viewing the brain as a straight tube can help to identify the origins of the cranial nerves. Cranial nerves 1 and II originate from the fore brain, III and IV from midbrain (IV arises from the dorsal side) and all the remaining nerves from the hind brain. Flexion of the tube and overgrowth of the telencephalon to surround the other brain components provide the adult structure and, interestingly, bring the prospective eyes closer to the cranial nerves that will supply them.[5]

The key stages are summarised in *Table A1.1*.

The eyes and adnexa

A bulge on either side of the diencephalon provides the first sign of the future eye (*Figure A1.5*). Continued bulging produces a 'ball' (the optic vesicle) on a 'stick' (the optic stalk) from which the eye develops. This step also provides the first example of the origins of developmental abnormality in the eye. A failure of the diencephalon to bulge produces an embryo with no eyes (i.e., anophthalmos).[8] Why bulging should fail to occur is considered later, but both

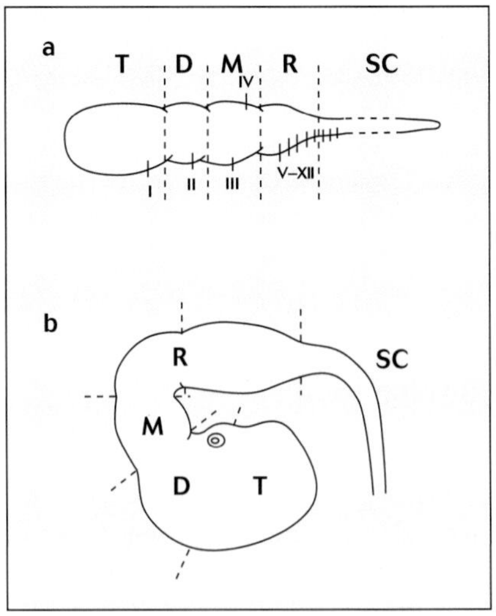

Figure A1.4
The anterior neural tube (prospective brain at 3–4 weeks). (a) Differentiation of the major components of the brain has begun. T, telencephalon; D, diencephalon; M, mesencephalon; R, rhombencephalon; SC, spinal cord. The points of origin of the cranial nerves are noted (I to XII). (b) Flexure has taken place, to move the diencephalon and mesencephalon closer. Overgrowth of the telencephalon surrounds the other brain structures

environmental and genetic causes are suggested. Each vesicle now comprises an extended neural tube enclosed within the surface ectoderm, and the mesenchyme occupies the space between.

Retina (gross structure)

An inwards invagination and/or dimpling of the vesicle gives rise to the optic cup, and the neural ectoderm folds back on itself to form two layers. The outer layer (adjacent to the ectoderm) develops pigment and becomes the retinal pigment epithelium (RPE).[11] The inner layer becomes the neural retina. As the inwards folding continues, the two layers eventually come into contact, but they do not fuse. This lack of fusion (no intercellular junctions) helps explain why in retinal detachment the separation is usually between the RPE and neural retina.

A number of abnormalities can be traced to this stage in development. Atrophy of the optic vesicle again produces anophthalmos. Failure to invaginate produces a congenital cystic eye (a thin-walled fluid-filled cyst that occupies the orbit) instead of an eye. Incomplete invagination leads to congenital retinal non-attachment. The inductive processes that cause the vesicle to fold inwards are not yet fully dissected. However, of interest is that if the neuro-ectodermal part of the vesicle fails to make 'contact' with the correct surface area of the ectoderm, a miniature but otherwise normal eye (microphthalmos) can result.[8]

Lens

The component of surface ectoderm that invaginates into the optic cup forms a ball of epithelial cells that become the lens (*Figure A1.6*). The first step in lens development is the secretion of a basement membrane by the epithelial cells; this will be the lens capsule. When activated by growth factors released from the developing retina, the epithelial cells closest to the retina elongate to fill the vesicle cavity.[12] These are the primary lens fibre cells. Secondary lens fibres arise from epithelial cells all around the equator, which bud off and elongate. As they elongate they run to the posterior pole between the capsule and primary fibre bases and to the anterior pole between the primary fibres and the anterior epithelial cells.

Table A1.1 Key stages of embryo development

Around 5 per cent of live births are considered to have some form of recognisable abnormality
Cell behaviour differences occur as early as the eight-cell stage
Germ-layer formation is called gastrulation
Ectoderm forms nerve tissue and skin
Mesoderm forms muscle and connective tissue
Endoderm forms gut and some glandular tissue
Neural ectoderm, under the influence of the mesoderm notochord, forms the neural tube
Anterior neural tube forms the brain
Three regions of anterior neural tube develop:
forebrain comprises the anterior telencephalon (cerebral hemispheres) and posterior diencephalons (thalamus and eyes)
mid-section forms the midbrain
hind-section forms the cerebellum, medulla and brainstem

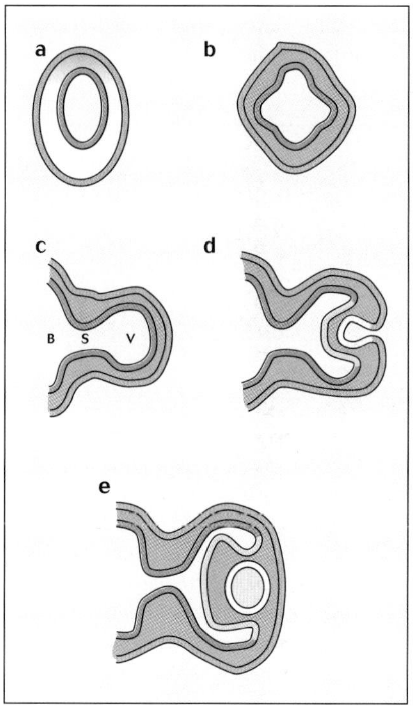

Figure A1.5
Formation of the optic vesicle and optic cup. (a) The neural tube is complete (orange) and enclosed within surface ectoderm (blue). Neural crest cells (pink) are being formed from the dorsal surface of the tube. (b) The outwards bulge of the diencephalon wall is just beginning. (c) The optic vesicle is formed (V), and connected to the brain (B) by the optic stalk (S). (d) Invagination of the vesicle has begun and the neural ectoderm of the tube becomes bilayered. The outer layer (orange) becomes retinal pigment epithelium (RPE), and the inner layer (yellow) becomes neural retina. The surface ectoderm also invaginates, and the cells that are enclosed (light blue) become the lens. Mesenchyme has spread to fill the space between the ectoderm and neural ectoderm. (e) The cup is complete. Prospective RPE and neural retina approach and soon contact. The primordial lens cells are now free of the surface ectoderm

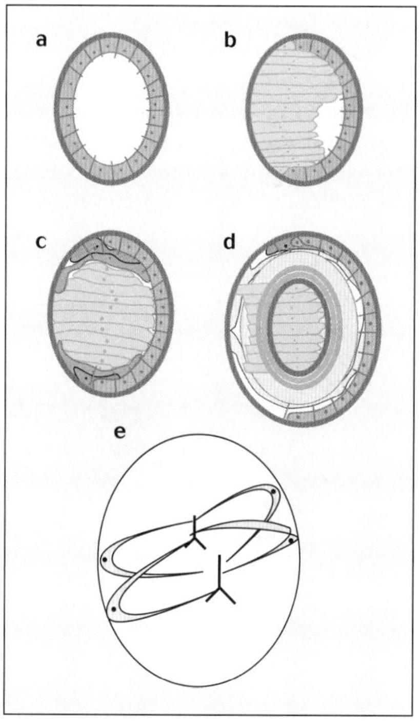

Figure A1.6
Lens development. (a) Lens epithelial cells secrete a basement membrane that becomes the capsule. (b) Posterior epithelial cells extend towards the front to occupy the space within the ball of cells. These are the primary lens fibre cells. (c) The first set of equatorial epithelial cells elongate to surround the primary fibres. These, in turn, are enclosed by the second set. (d) More secondary fibre cell layers are laid down and compress the early cells towards the centre. (e) Viewed from the front, each individual fibre cell (four shown here) can be seen to extend from the posterior to the anterior pole. The points at which cells meet at the front and back are called sutures (Y-shaped structure). By spreading the junctions in this way the scatter of axial light is minimised

In this way, the primary fibres are enveloped by the first set of secondary fibres and, in turn, each subsequent secondary fibre layer enclose its predecessor. Repetition of this process puts down layer-upon-layer of lens fibre cells in a process that does not end until death. The junctions at which the secondary fibre cells meet, at the anterior and posterior poles (the optical axis), have the potential to scatter light. To minimise this effect, the fibre cells have slightly different lengths, which has the effect of spreading the junctions, and these now form just-visible lines known as sutures.[13] The failure of surface ectoderm to invaginate into the cup, under the stimulus of the adjacent neuroectoderm cells, produces an aphakic eye. Failure of the primary lens fibres to elongate and the abnormal deposition of lens fibre proteins (crystallins) produces lens abnormalities and cataract.[12,14–16]

Failure of the lens stalk to disintegrate and release the ball of epithelial cells into the cup causes abnormal development of a number of anterior segment structures, referred to as Peter's anomaly. The cornea and angle structures are particularly affected, which leads to opacities and congenital glaucoma.[17,18] One aspect of the invagination to form the optic cup that is important, but often difficult to conceptualise, is that the 'dimpling' is not uniform over the full 360° of the cup. A helpful analogy is to consider the vesicle as a balloon. If a fist is pushed into the balloon, a uniform cup or depression is produced and encloses the fist. However, to nourish the tissues within the depression (lens and neural retina), blood vessels need to grow from the main section of the developing embryo, along the optic stalk and around the rim of the cup. Axons that grow from the developing ganglion cells on the inside of the cup have to follow a similar path to reach the brain (i.e., the lateral geniculate nucleus). To make access and exit easier, nature has chosen not to use a fist, but the edge of a flat hand to invaginate the vesicle. The effect is to produce a cup or depression that is almost complete, except for the position of the hand, where now there is a deep groove (*Figure A1.7*).

The deep groove is termed the optic fissure and provides a 'short cut' into and out of the cup. The short cut is only temporarily available, however, and the edges of the fissure soon fuse to complete the cup.[19] The cells that form the optic stalk now support and surround the vessels and axons to form the optic nerve. Failure of the fissure to close results in an absence of cup structures in the inferior nasal field. These absences are known as retinal, ciliary and iris colobomas.[8,9]

Retina (fine structure)

Almost from the start of invagination, the retina begins its differentiation (*Figure A1.8*). The outer cells of the cup (prospective RPE) lay down pigment. The inner cup cells (prospective neural retina) divide repeatedly to form a dense cellular area closest to the RPE, with an acellular zone adjacent to the basement membrane (prospective inner limiting membrane, ILM). By week seven the inner retina has formed two layers (inner and outer neuroblastic layers, INB and ONB) separated by an acellular area (transient layer of Chievitz). The INB forms ganglion cells (in the ganglion cell layer, GCL) the axons of which, seeking to exit the fissure before it closes, form the nerve fibre layer (NF). Cells at the inner margin of the ONB now migrate inwards to meet cells at the outer margins of the INB. The result is an acellular divide (inner and outer plexiform layers, IPL and OPL) on the inner and outer aspects of what is now the inner nuclear layer and home to the cell bodies of the amacrine, bipolar, horizontal and Müller cells. The cells that remain in the ONB become the cell bodies of the photoreceptors (the outer nuclear layer, ONL). The cilia extended by these cell bodies become the photoreceptor outer segments (PR).

Although the pattern of retinal cells is evident by 28 weeks, the final arrangement is not complete until a few months after birth. In this intervening period the fovea is formed by lateral displacement of the inner retinal components, the outer segments elongate and the peripheral retina extends to accommodate the growing eyeball.[7,8]

Developmental abnormalities of the retina can occur, for example, when the neural retina does not invaginate completely, when a disorganised retina (retinal dysplasia) is produced[20] and when pigment fails to develop and abnormal foveal structures result.[21]

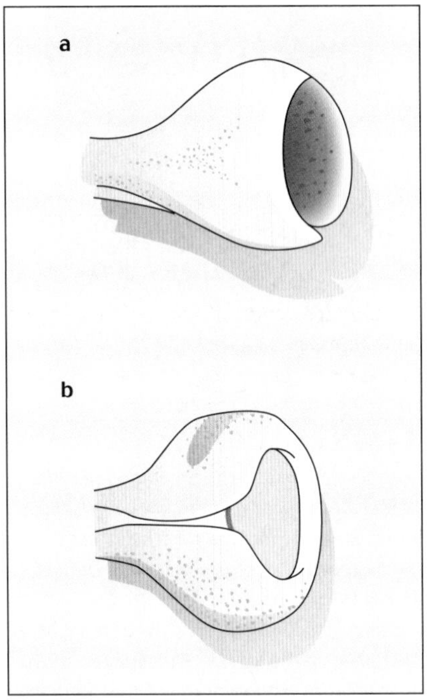

Figure A1.7
The neuro-ectodermal component of the optic cup illustrating the position of the optic fissure. (a) The prospective RPE and neural retina are shown. The position of the fissure, slightly nasal and inferior, can be seen. (b) A view from the underside showing the position of the lens (blue) at the mouth of the cup, and the fissure through which the hyaloid artery and ganglion cell axons are to pass

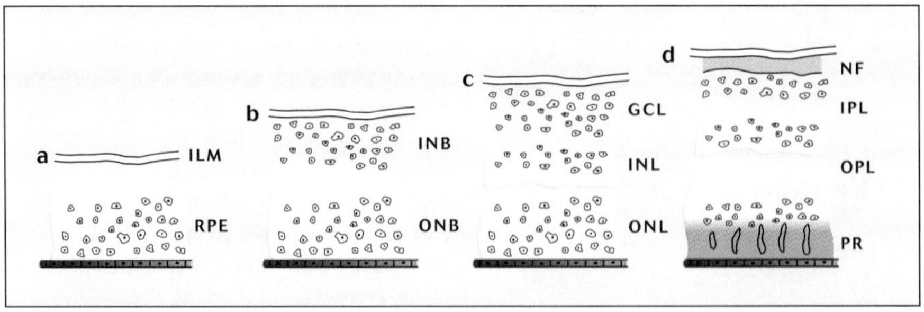

Figure A1.8
Development of the retina. (a) Cells of the inner layer of the optic cup have multiplied to form a layer 6–7 cells thick. (b) Cells migrate through the 'empty' zone towards the basement membrane (ILM) to form the inner and outer neuroblastic layers (INB, ONB). (c) Cells migrate from both blastic layers towards the centre to form the inner nuclear layer (INL). 'Empty' areas either side fill with cell processes and become the plexiform layers (IPL, OPL), and the INB produces ganglion cells to form the germ cell layer (GCL). (d) Finally, the cells in the outer nuclear layer (ONL) put out a cilium from which the outer segments develop to form the photoreceptors (PR), and the ganglion cells put out their axons, which run across the retina surface to form the nerve fibre layer (NF)

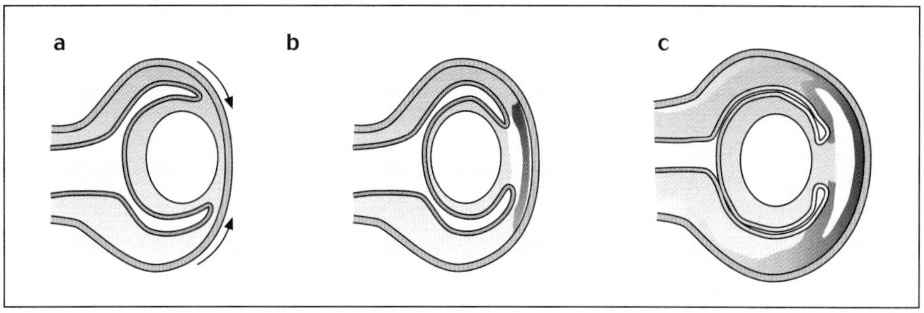

Figure A1.9

Formation of cornea and angle. (a) Mesenchyme between the rim of the cup and surface ectoderm migrates between lens and surface ectoderm. (b) Sedimentation of this mesenchyme on the surface ectoderm (now the corneal epithelium) forms corneal endothelium and then stroma. Adjacent cells are breaking down to form the prospective anterior chamber. (c) The rim of the cup is now extending forwards between the mesenchyme and anterior lens surface. The anterior chamber is deepening and moving peripherally to form the angle

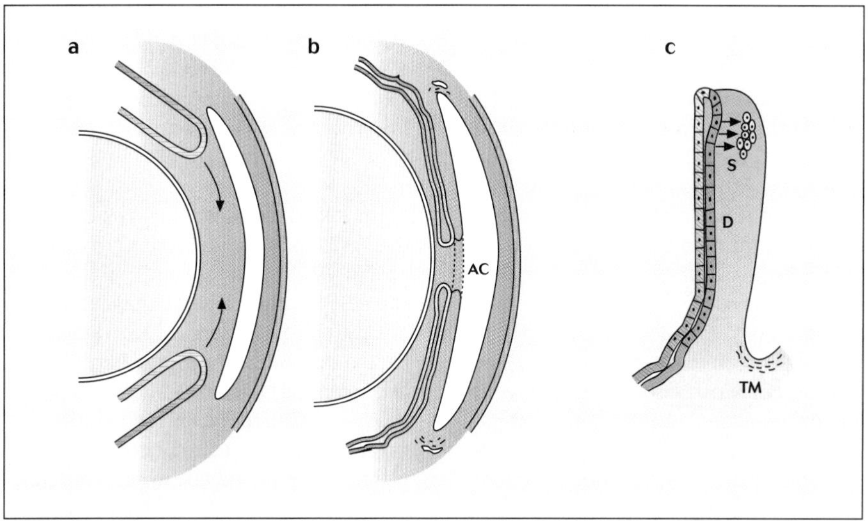

Figure A1.10

Development of the iris. (a) The rim of the cup extends forwards between the face of the lens and the mesenchyme. (b) Mesenchyme that sediments onto the surface of the iris forms the iris stroma. The disintegration of mesenchyme enlarges the anterior chamber (AC). Where the cornea and iris meet, mesenchyme now forms the structures of the outflow pathway. (c) Cells now bud off the pigmented iris epithelium near the tip. These cells settle in the stroma to form the sphincter muscle (S). These same cells, but not in the tip region, become the dilator (cells adjacent to the dark line, labelled D). The trabecular mesh (TM) and other components of the aqueous drainage path are now formed from mesenchyme cells at the junction of cornea and iris, the angle

Anterior structures

While structures are developing at the back of the embryonic eye, significant changes occur at the front of the eye (*Figure A1.9*). Corneal epithelium develops from ectoderm in front of the opening to the cup. Corneal stroma and endothelium form from mesenchyme that migrates in waves from the periphery into the space between the corneal epithelium and lens, before sedimenting onto the epithelium. At the same time, adjacent mesenchyme cells (those cells mid-way between the developing cornea and lens) break down to form a cavity; this is the prospective anterior chamber. The controlled apoptosis (i.e., programmed cell death) of mesenchyme continues towards the periphery and contributes to the overall process of angle formation and establishment of the aqueous drainage path. The thin layer of mesenchyme that remains in front of the lens becomes vascularised by the hyaloid circulation and forms the pupillary membrane. As shown later, the pupillary membrane contributes to iris formation. Failure of the cornea and angle to develop properly can produce a variety of abnormalities (e.g., Peter's anomaly and the Axenfeld–Rieger syndrome) and cause congenital glaucoma.[8,10,20,22]

Uvea, vitreous and sclera

Cup cells divide at the rim of the neuro-ectodermal, which causes the rim to extend forwards between the front surface of the lens and the pupillary membrane. This extended rim forms the epithelial components of the iris and ciliary body, which, like the rest of the neuro-ectodermal cup, is bilayered. The outermost layer, which is an extension of and therefore continuous with the RPE, is pigmented. The inner layer is continuous with the neural retina and unpigmented, except in the iris, where it develops pigment to increase the effectiveness of the light barrier. Mesenchyme that sediments onto the ciliary epithelium forms the ciliary muscle and stroma (*Figure A1.10*). The pupillary membrane that attaches to the iris epithelium forms the iris stroma. The rare exception to the rule that muscles develop from mesodermal tissue is demonstrated twice in the iris. Firstly, cells bud off the pigmented epithelium near the tip of the rim to settle in the adjacent stroma; these become the iris sphincter. Secondly, these same pigmented epithelial cells (except for those close to the rim) lay down contractile proteins and act together as the dilator muscle.[7,8] The failure, or partial failure, of the rim to develop results in either a complete absence of iris structures (i.e., aniridia) or a rudimentary stump. This abnormality is often associated with failure of the pupillary membrane to atrophy, glaucoma (caused by blockage of the trabecular mesh) and cataracts. Failure of the dilator muscle to form produces a small pupil (i.e., microcoria).[11]

Around the outside of the neuro-ectodermal cup, and beneath the surface ectoderm, a vascular bed is formed from mesenchyme (*Figure A1.11*). The bed connects to branches of the ophthalmic artery (the long and short posterior ciliary arteries) and provides for the needs of developing external eye structures. Later, these vessels contribute to the vasculature of the choriocapillaris, choroid and anterior segment. Mesenchyme within the optic cup forms another vascular bed and primary vitreous. This intra-cup vascular bed is supplied by a branch of the ophthalmic artery (the hyaloid artery) that enters the cup through the optic fissure. In later weeks, as the hyaloid vasculature disintegrates, small branches bud out from the hyaloid artery at the point where it enters the eyeball. These buds extend across the surface of the developing reti-

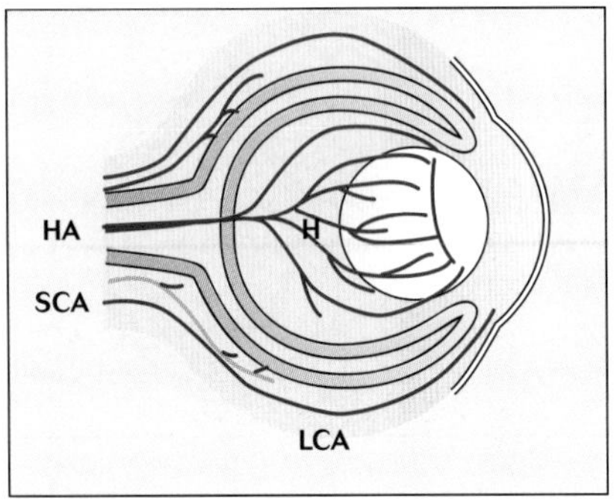

Figure A1.11
Early vasculature of the eye. The interior of the cup is supplied by the hyaloid artery (HA) and its associated vessels (H). Structures outside the cup are supplied by the long ciliary arteries (LCA) in the anterior portion and short ciliary arteries (SCA) for the remainder

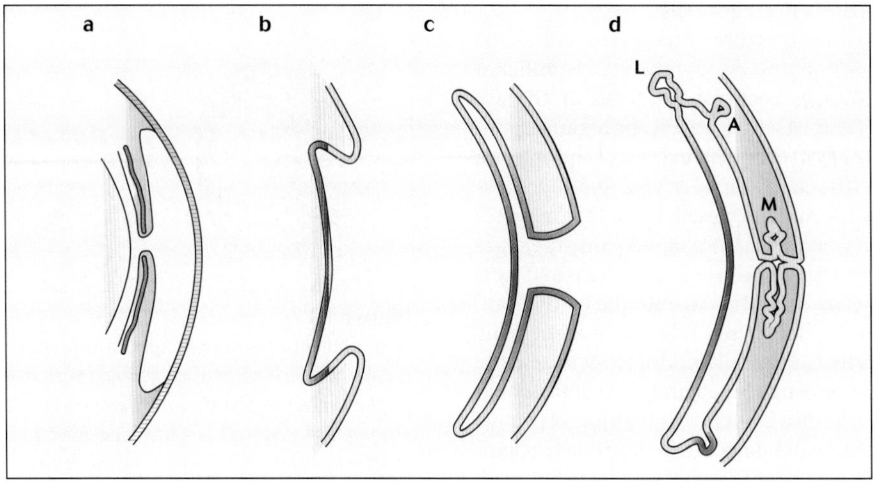

Figure A1.12
Development of the lids. (a, b) Surface ectoderm both superior and inferior to the cornea becomes folded to form two ridges. (c) The ridges elongate and move towards each other. (d) The ridges meet and fuse. Prior to birth these ridges (lids) separate again to form the palpebral aperture. Epithelial cells that invade the lid stroma (pink) at the lid margins form the meibomian glands (M). In a similar way, the accessory glands (A) are formed in the tarsal zone. Epithelial cells that form a pit in the fornix zone extend to enter the prospective orbital space and become the lacrimal gland (L)

na to become the central retinal circulation. At the same time, secondary vitreous is secreted by mesenchyme and compresses the primary vitreous and remains of the hyaloid vasculature into a thin column that runs from the retina to the back surface of the lens, called Cloquet's canal.[7,8,9,11]

Failure of the hyaloid vasculature and primary vitreous to break down can lead to persistent hyperplastic primary vitreous and its associated problems of cataract, abnormal ciliary development and the formation of a fibrovascular mass between the retina and lens, called leucocoria.[9,20] Incomplete disintegration of the hyaloid vasculature can leave vessel remains in Cloquet's canal and sometimes a small papilla on the disc surface.[11] Collagen secreted by the mesenchyme cells that surround the neuro-ectodermal cup forms the sclera. As sclera is laid down, a group of mesoderm cells invade it to become the extraocular muscles. Between the developing sclera and RPE, mesenchyme and the external vasculature combine to form the choroid. Abnormal melanin formation in the choroid (and elsewhere in the eye) results in a hypopigmentary abnormality.[22]

Adnexa

The ectoderm (epithelium) peripheral to the cornea is now induced to form two simple folds. These folds become the eyelids (*Figure A1.12*). As they extend, they come together and fuse. Before birth they separate to form the palpebral aperture. The meibomian and accessory glands of the lids form from lid epithelial cells that migrate into the lid stroma. The lacrimal gland is formed by an epithelial invasion of the prospective orbital space by epithelial cells at the apex of the fold, the prospective tarsal conjunctiva.[23] Where the developing palpebral apertures meet on the nasal side, buds of the developing lacrimal canaliculi insert into the palpebral margin. These buds connect to a groove in the frontal (facial) ectoderm, formed by the developing maxillary process, to form the lacrimal drainage path. Lid abnormalities can result from, for example, a failure of the lids to separate fully (ankyloblepharon), incorrect insertion of the levator (ptosis) or short lids that prevent the palpebral aperture from closing completely (microblepharon).

The above provides a description of the major steps in eye development. A more detailed description can be found from texts cited. An approximate chronology for these major events is given in *Table A1.2*. As can be seen, the major steps are all but complete within the first 12 weeks. Abnormalities that occur after this time are, as a result, less devastating and are usually localised to a specific tissue.

Table A1.2 A chronology of eye formation

Age of embryo (weeks)	*Size of embryo (mm)*	*Ocular structure*
3	2.5	Bulge in diencephalon wall
4	3.5	Optic vesicle
4.5	7	Optic cup
5	8	Lens vesicle, RPE, corneal epithelium, primary vitreous
5.5	10	Hyaloid artery and nerve fibres in fissure
6	13	Commencement of neural retina differentiation
6.5	15	Lens vesicle cavity filled with primary fibre cells
6.75	18	Corneal endothelium
7.5	20	Ganglion axons reach LGN, corneal stroma
7.75	25	Sclera sediments
8.5	30	Secondary vitreous forms
12	50	Hyaloid vasculature disintegrated
16	90	Iris and ciliary processes form, sphincter just evident
24	200	Retina components complete, choroid formed, iris dilator present
32	280	Trabecular mesh and angle complete
36	400	Retinal vasculature complete, iris fully pigmented, pupillary membrane disintegrates

Development of abnormality

Having described the developmental steps that form the eye, it is now possible to focus on the 'errors' in these processes, and the ocular abnormalities that result. The cause of the 'error' and subsequent abnormality can be recognised at different levels. Many abnormalities are known to have genetic origins that can be dominant or recessive, as discussed in Chapters 2 and 3.[8,23,24]

Many abnormalities have a teratogenic cause that results from the effects of viruses, chemicals, radiation and so on. Others have no identifiable cause. Whatever the cause, the effect can be considered at the cell and molecular level. However, only in recent years has it become possible to identify the nature of these cellular and subcellular events. A useful insight as to the general mechanisms of development can be gained by observing the processes whereby neural ectoderm folds to become the neural tube and whereby the lens vesicle becomes separated from the surface ectoderm stalk to lie free within the optic cup. Change in cell shape and co-operativity between cells to form new structures require the deposition of intracellular proteins, particularly cytoskeletal proteins (such as microtubules and microfilaments), and the formation of intercellular adhesions and junctions. In neuro-ectodermal cells that are to form the neural tube, microtubules are seen to arrange themselves along the long axis of the cell and microfilaments to arrange themselves in circles at the apical margins of the cell. When the filaments contract, because of the cytoskeletal proteins, the effect is a change in cell shape that initiates the fold. Adding drugs that inhibit the formation of these cytoskeletal proteins (cytochalasin A and colchicine), prevents the folding and development of the neural tube.[1]

When the optic vesicle invaginates, the surface ectoderm (lens placode) sinks into the cup to form a ball of epithelial cells, which remain attached by a stalk. Detachment of the ball requires the stalk cells to die and disintegrate. As these are young healthy cells, their death must be a positive act, so particular genes within the cell that control cell death (apoptosis) are activated. The 'switch' that activates apoptosis genes could be many things, however molecules such as transforming growth factor β (TGF-β, a growth factor) have been implicated.[17] How cells are induced and/or instructed to produce these biological switches (growth factors) and how particular cells (the stalk cells) are targetted demonstrates further levels of complexity that are yet to be described and discovered.

However, it is possible now to see how the genetic or teratogenic cause of the abnormality may be manifest. An abnormal gene might encode a defective structural protein or receptor. A teratogen might exert an effect directly on a particular protein or indirectly by affecting gene expression. The most serious of ocular abnormalities, anophthalmia, has an incidence in some parts of the world of 0.5 per cent of conceptions (most of these embryos are lost). The geographical variation in its incidence suggests that it could have an environmental cause. However, it also shows patterns of inheritance that demonstrate genetic origins. Whatever the origin of the effect, the action might be a mechanism similar to that described above, such that the failure of the diencephalon wall to bulge results from a failure of the cells to lay down structural proteins, or possibly the teratogen affects the deposition.

Clearly, recent advances in cell biology, molecular biology and molecular genetics are bringing us much closer to resolving the origins of developmental abnormalities, as well as the mechanisms of their action. It is highly likely that in the years to come these advances may offer possible interventions, perhaps through genetic manipulation, to eliminate or replace defective genes or by the direct application of factors that regulate or modify cell development and are targetted at particular cell populations.

References

1 Gilbert SF (1988). *Developmental Biology*, Second Edition. (Sunderland, MA: Sinauer Associates).
2 McKeown T (1976). Human malformations: An introduction. *Br Med Bull*. **32**, 1–3.
3 Muller WA (1997). *Developmental Biology*. (New York: Springer Verlag).
4 Homeobox Genes Database. www.mssm.edu/molbio/hoxpro/new/hox-pro00.html.
5 O'Rahilly R and Muller F (1992). *Human Embryology and Teratology*. (New York: Wiley–Liss).
6 Wiggs JL (1995). *Molecular Genetics of Ocular Disease*. 1995. (New York: Wiley–Liss).
7 Bron AJ, Tripathi RC and Tripathi BJ (1997). *Wolff's Anatomy of the Eye and Orbit*, Eighth Edition. (Edinburgh: Chapman Hall Medical).
8 Duane TD and Jaeger EA (1986). *Biomedical Foundations of Ophthalmology*, Volume 1. (London: Harper and Row).
9 Forrester J, Dick A, McMenamin P and Lee P (1996). *The Eye: Basic Sciences in Practice*. (New York: Saunders).
10 Bahn CF, Falls HF, Varley GA, *et al*. (1964). Classification of endothelial disorders based on neural crest origin. *Ophthalmology* **91**, 558–563.
11 Pearson AA (1974). *The Development of the Eye*. (Alexandria: American Academy of Ophthalmology and Otolaryngology).
12 Schulz MW, Chamberlain CG, de Longh RU and McAvoy JW (1993). Acidic and basic FGF in ocular media and lens: Implications for lens polarity and growth patterns. *Development* **118**, 117–126.
13 Hogan MJ, Alvarado JA and Weddell JE (1971). *Histology of the Human Eye: An Atlas and Textbook*. (London: Saunders).
14 Tasman J and Jaeger EA (1991). *Duane's Clinical Ophthalmology*. (New York: Lippincott).
15 Graw J (199). Cataract mutations and lens development. *Prog Retina Eye Res*. **18**, 235–267.
16 Van Dijk J (2001). Rubella handicapped children: An everlasting problem. www.tr.wou.edu/dblink/VANDIJK10.htm.

17 Ozeki H, Ogura Y, Hirabayashi Y and Shimada S (2001). Suppression of lens stalk apoptosis by hyaluronic acid leads to faulty separation of the lens vesicle. *Exp Eye Res.* **72**, 63–70.
18 Beebe DC and Coates M (2000). The lens organises the anterior segment: Specification of neural crest cell differentiation in the avian eye. *Dev Biol.* **220**, 424–431.
19 Ozeki H, Ogura Y, Hirabayashi Y and Shimada S (2000). Apoptosis is associated with formation and persistence of the embryonic fissure. *Curr Eye Res.* **20**: 367–372.
20 Trachimowicz RA (1994). Review of embryology and its relation to ocular disease in the pediatric population. *Optom Vis Sci.* **71**, 154–163.
21 Boissy RE and Nordlund JJ (1997). Molecular basis of congenital hypopigmentary disorders in humans: A review. *Pig Cell Res.* **10**, 12–24.
22 Shields MB, Buckley E, Klintworth GK and Thresher R (1985). Axenfeld–Rieger syndrome. A spectrum of developmental disorders. *Surv Ophthalmol.* **29**, 387–409.
23 Makarenkova HP, Ito M, Govindarajan V, *et al.* (2000). FGF10 is an inducer and Pax6 a competence factor for lacrimal gland development. *Development* **127**, 2563–2572.
24 Renie WA (1986). *Goldberg's Genetic and Metabolic Eye Diseases.* (New York: Little, Brown and Co).

Appendix 2: Genetics and the Eye

Richard Armstrong

Approximately 4000 genetic diseases or syndromes are known to affect humans, 33 per cent of which involve the eye.[1] In addition, of the cases of blindness caused by disease, 75 per cent occur in individuals under 15 years of age and approximately 50 per cent of these are hereditary.

Hereditary factors are involved in several of the most important diseases of the eye. These include cataract, in which both the development and age of onset may be inherited,[2] and glaucoma, in which 90 per cent of non-environmental cases of open-angle glaucoma may be linked to mutant genes. In addition, diabetic retinopathy and retinitis pigmentosa[3] may be linked to mutant genes; the latter exhibits a particularly complex pattern of inheritance. Recent advances in molecular genetics have enabled some of the genes associated with these ocular diseases to be identified, the precise location of these genes on specific chromosomes to be determined, and the effects of defects in these genes to be studied. These advances are likely to have a profound impact on the classification, diagnosis and, ultimately, treatment of ocular disorders that affect children.

This appendix and Chapter 8 describe the basic elements of genetics necessary to understand the new advances and the impact that these advances may have on the study and treatment of ocular disease in children. This appendix firstly describes the patterns of inheritance of human characteristics, how they are transmitted between the generations and the structure of chromosomes. It then describe how deoxyribose nucleic acid (DNA) was discovered to be the chemical constituent of genes, the structure and replication of DNA and how proteins are made within cells. The effect of mutations in the genes and how the activities of genes are regulated is also described.

Mendel's experiments

Genetics is the study of the characteristics (such as form, shape, function or disease) of individuals that are inherited (i.e., passed from one generation to another). It is important to understand the basis of inheritance, what exactly is inherited and how these inheritable 'factors' are passed from one generation to another.

We know today that the transmission of characteristics in human families can, in many circumstances, be described by quite simple rules. These rules were first worked out by an Augustinian monk and contemporary of Charles Darwin, Gregor Mendel, in the 1860s. Much of Mendel's work was carried out using plants, especially pea plants. It is relatively easy to carry out breeding experiments with such plants, because the pollen of one plant is simply placed on the ovary of the other. In addition, the peas that the plants produce differ from each other in distinct ways; for example, they may be smooth or wrinkled, yellow or green.

As an illustration of Mendel's work, consider the experiment described in *Figure A2.1*, published by Mendel in 1866. Plants that produce round peas were mated or crossed with those that produced wrinkled peas. All the pea plants resulting from this cross (which Mendel termed the F1 generation) had round peas; the wrinkled characteristic had apparently disappeared. Mendel then crossed random pairs of plants from the F1 generation to obtain a second generation (F2). In the F2 generation, however, plants that produced wrinkled peas reappeared, but were, on average, less numerous than those that produced round peas. Indeed, in repeated experiments the plants that produced

Parents	Round peas (AA)	x	Wrinkled peas (aa)
F1 generation		Round peas (Aa)	
F2 generation		Pollen	
		A or a	
	A	AA (Round)	Aa (Round)
Eggs	or		
	a	Aa (Round)	aa (Wrinkled)

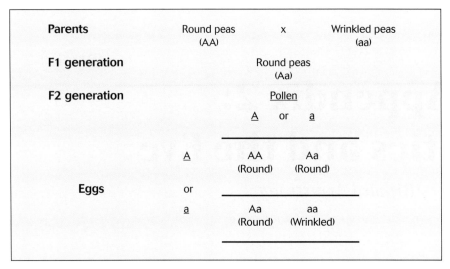

Figure A2.1
An example of Mendel's experiments

round peas were nearly always three times as frequent as those that produced wrinkled peas. Mendel tried several different types of cross based on seven distinctive characteristics of the pea plants, such as yellow versus green peas, but obtained essentially the same results. The 3:1 ratio that Mendel observed in the F2 generation appeared to be a fundamental property of the mating and the transmission of the characteristics.

A number of facts can be deduced from this experiment. Firstly, some 'factor' must have been transmitted from parent to offspring so that the round and wrinkled characteristics could be inherited. Mendel was one of the first individuals to suggest that 'factors', which were called genes by Wilhelm Johannsen some 30 years after Mendel, were passed from the parental plants to the young plants in the sex cells, the pollen and eggs. Secondly, not all the characteristics are equivalent, as some types are more important than others; for example, although one parent had round peas and the other wrinkled peas, all the F1 plants produced by crossing these parents had round peas. Mendel concluded that the round characteristic was 'dominant' to the wrinkled characteristic, such that, when both characteristics are present in the same individual, only the effect of the dominant characteristic is observed.

The results of Mendel's experiment can be explained if it is assumed that a factor, or gene, represents the round characteristic (A) and a gene represents the wrinkled characteristic (a), and that each cell of the parent plants, with the exception of the sex cells, contains two copies of the relevant gene (*Figure A2.1*). The pollen and the eggs only contain a single copy of each gene as a result of the process of meiosis (described in a later section). On crossing the original plants, the F1 plants have the genetic constitution, or 'genotype', 'Aa'. All of these plants produce round peas because the round characteristic is dominant to the wrinkled characteristic. If two of the F1 plants are now crossed, we have a more complex situation because each plant produces two different types of pollen and eggs, which contain either the 'A' or 'a' gene and, therefore, there are four possible combinations of matings (*Figure A2.1*).

If each mating occurs at approximately the same frequency, then the 3:1 ratio in the F1 generation can be explained. Hence, the importance of Mendel's experiments was that it suggested the means by which characteristics could be transmitted between parents and their offspring and enabled rules to be devised to describe this process of transmission. Mendel published his principles of heredity in 1866, but their importance was not recognised until 1900. These principles are now regarded as the foundation of the study of inheritance.

Cell division

Genes for many thousands of human characteristics are carried on threads called chromosomes, located within the nucleus of each cell. In fact, each somatic cell (i.e., all cells other than sex cells), which have a nucleus, contains the genetic information to produce a complete individual.[4]

Each type of organism has a constant number of chromosomes, usually an even number because, through the sperm and egg, the offspring receive one complete set of chromosomes. A species has a particular number of chromosomes, but this is not sufficient to identify a species since several different organisms may have the same chromosome number. Although chromosomes had been discovered almost a century earlier, the number of chromosomes in human cells was not determined until 1956. With the exception of the sex cells, which have one complete set of chromosomes, humans have a total of 46 chromosomes in each somatic cell; two complete sets of 23. Chromosomes are not normally visible within the nucleus of the cell, however, except when cell division takes place. Consequently, cells must be induced to divide in order to observe and study chromosomes.

Mitosis

All cells in the body pass through a cell cycle. Prior to cell division, there is a phase of cell growth (G1 phase) followed by a phase in which the genes are duplicated (S phase). This is followed by a second phase of growth (G2 phase), after which the cell divides into two by a process known as mitosis. During mitosis, two identical cells are produced, each cell with exactly the same genes as the parent. For descriptive purposes, mitosis is often divided into five phases, but the process is essentially continuous (*Figure A2.2*). The nucleus prior to cell division is said to be in 'interphase'; the chromosomes are not visible and it is assumed that the chromosomal threads are spread throughout the nucleus.

During 'prophase' the chromosomes become visible for the first time and appear as double-thread structures, each of which is termed a chromatid; the double threads result from the duplication of genes during interphase. The chromatids are joined at a single location along their length by a common centromere. The membrane around the nucleus disappears and the chromatids, which are now shorter and thicker, become located in the centre of the cell (a stage termed 'metaphase'). A spindle of protein fibres appears and the chromatids become attached to it by means of the centromere. The centromere splits and the pairs of chromatids separate and move towards opposite poles of the cell ('anaphase'). During 'telophase' the chromatids arrive at opposite ends of the cell, a new nuclear membrane forms around each new set of chromosomes, they become less distinct and the cell returns to interphase.

Mitosis in the lens of the eye

The best place to see mitosis in the eye is in the cells of the lens. The lens of the eye is derived from the surface ectoderm cells, which overlie the optic vesicle. Histologically, the mature lens is composed of three portions – the capsule, epithelium and lens cells. The capsule helps the lens to acquire nutrients from the aqueous fluid, since it is the only body tissue not in direct contact with blood vessels. The zonular fibres are also inserted into the lens and their action helps to mould the shape of the lens during accommodation. The epithelial cells are large and cuboidal, with a large spherical nucleus.

Mitosis takes place within these cells at the equator of the lens and new cells are consequently added to the lens; the new cells elongate to form the lens fibres. The lens itself is composed of these lens fibres, which are organised into densely packed lamellae. During development, the cells lose their nucleus and become specialised for the production of special lens proteins called crystallins.

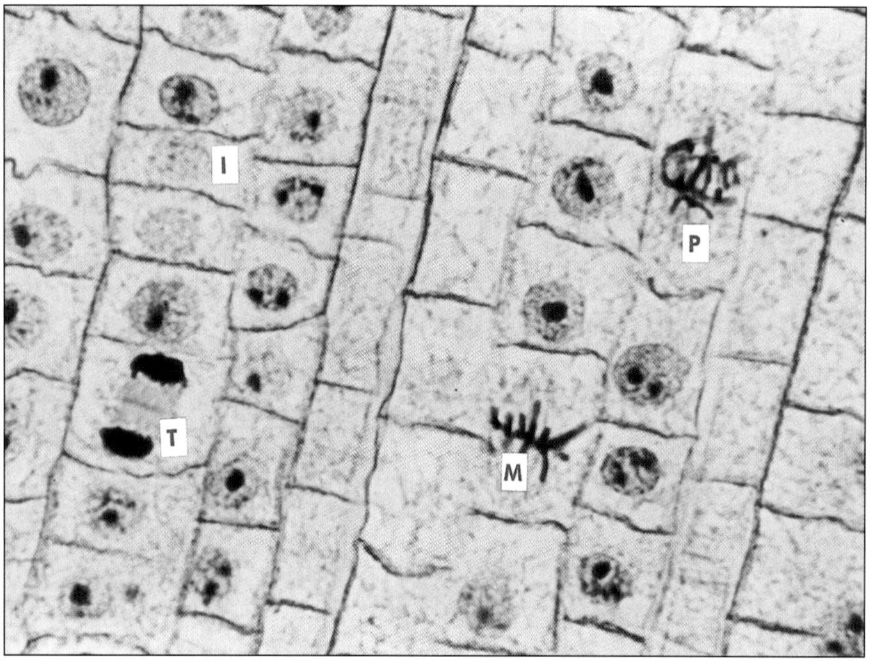

Figure A2.2
Stages in cell division by mitosis (I, interphase; P, prophase; M, metaphase; T, telophase)

Meiosis

A different process of cell division, however, takes place in the cells that are precursors to the sperm and egg. The human chromosome number of 46 remains constant from one generation to the next. To prevent the doubling of chromosomes, which would occur at each fertilisation, the number are reduced to half in the sex cells by a process called meiosis. Hence, although each somatic cell contains two complete sets of chromosomes – the maternal and paternal chromosomes inherited from the parents – the sperm and eggs only contain one complete set.

In addition, during meiosis each maternal chromosome pairs with its homologous partner, the corresponding paternal chromosome, and the two exchange genes by crossing-over (*Figure A2.3*). This process introduces variability into the sex cells, since some sex cells have chromosomes with genes from both parents. Sex cells that possess chromosomes with genes from both parents are said to contain 'recombinants'. Whether or not recombinants of a particular pair of parental genes occurs depends on how close the genes are on the chromosome. If two genes are at either ends of the chromosome, it is almost certain that meiosis will result in recombinants. If two genes are very close together (i.e., side by side on the same chromosome), it is much less likely that recombinants will be formed, since a cross-over point would have to occur precisely between the two genes. This fact is the basis of 'linkage analysis', one of the most important ways to determine where genes are located on chromosomes.

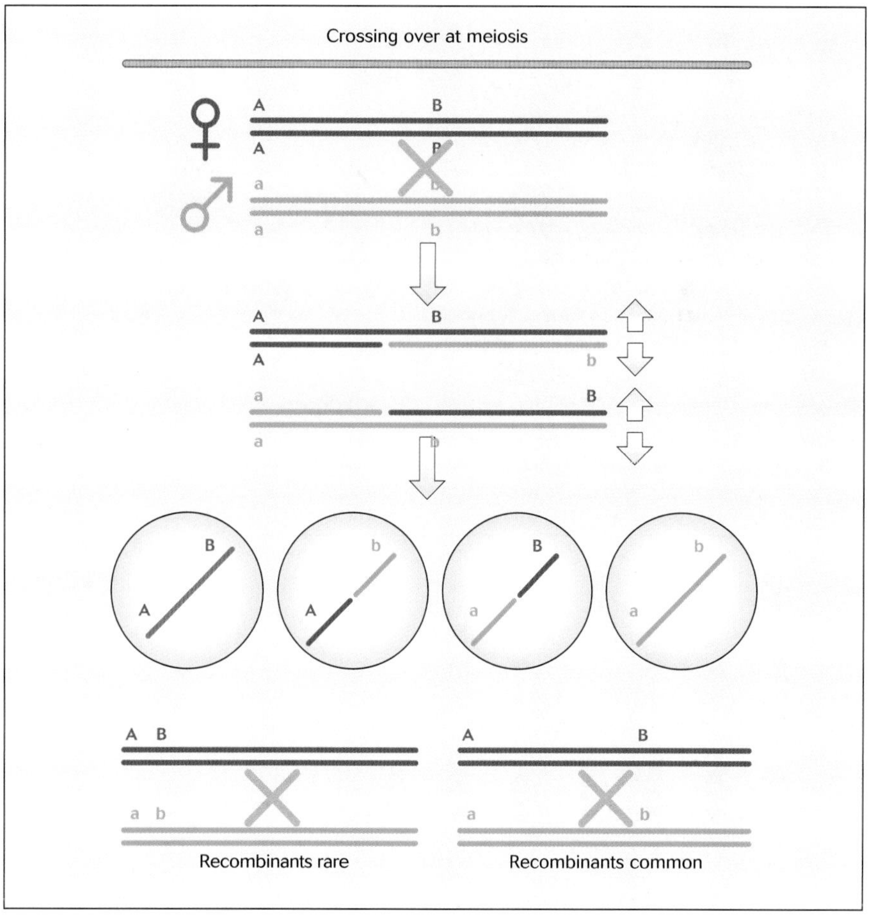

Figure A2.3
Crossing over at meiosis in the cells that are precursors to the sperm and egg. Homologous chromosomes, each of which is doubled, pair and exchange genes by crossing over between the inner strands. This results in some sex cells with the genes in new combinations (e.g., Ab and aB), which are termed recombinants

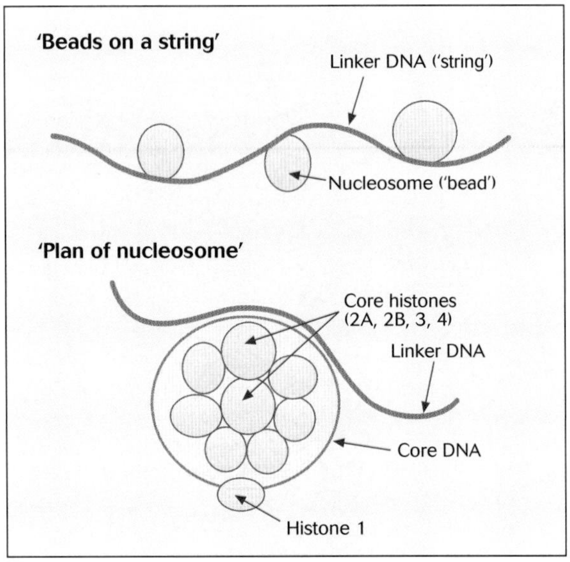

Figure A2.4
Structure of chromosomes. During the interphase each chromosome consists of a long, thin thread with nucleosomes connected by DNA ('beads on a string'). Each nucleosome is composed of proteins (histones) with the DNA coiled around them

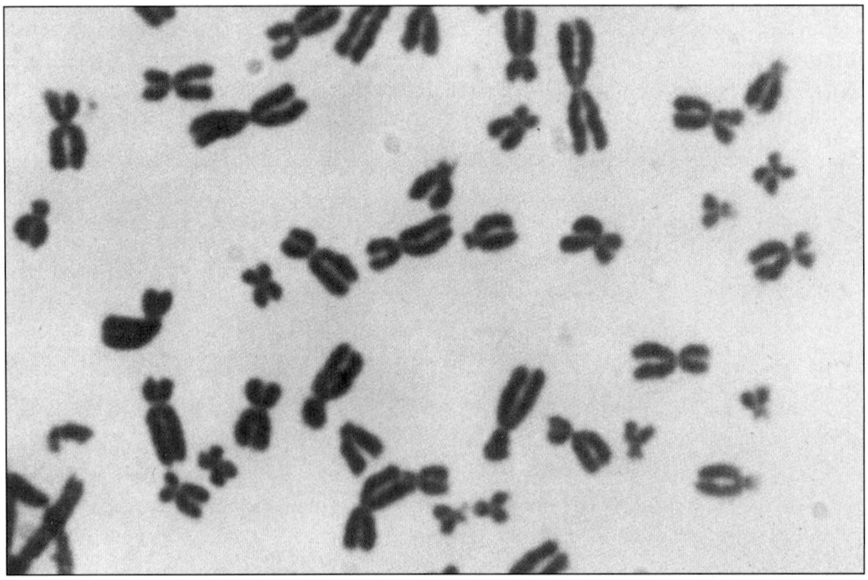

Figure A2.5
A preparation of human chromosomes

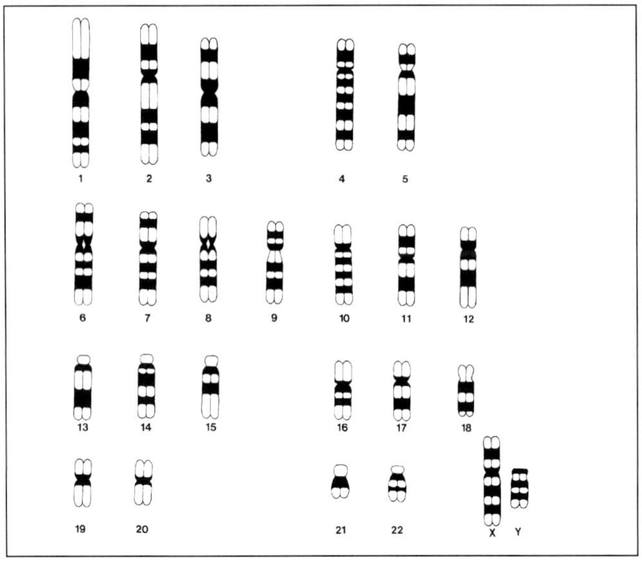

Figure A2.6
Human 'karyotype'

Chromosomes

Structure of chromosomes

Consideration of the processes of mitosis and meiosis raises two important questions. Firstly, what happens to the chromosomes after cell division is complete and, secondly, why are chromosomes only visible during cell division? Chemical analysis of chromosomal material, termed chromatin, reveals it to be composed of DNA, a small amount of ribonucleic acid (RNA) and two sets of proteins, the most important of which are called histones.

A good model of a chromosome, as it exists during interphase, is that it resembles 'beads on a string' (*Figure A2.4*). Each bead is called a nucleosome, the fundamental unit of the chromosome; adjacent nucleosomes are connected by the 'string' called 'linker DNA'.[5,6] The structure of an individual nucleosome, which resembles an ellipsoid disk, reveals that the histones provide the physical support for the DNA. Nine histones are present, with histone 1 on the outside of the nucleosome to provide support and two each of histones 2A, 2B, 3 and 4 located on the inside with the 'core DNA' wrapped around them.

When the cell prepares for cell division, the chromosomes begin to shorten and coil up like a spring; in fact, the ultimate length of a chromosome during cell division is approximately 10,000 times shorter than it is at interphase. The nature of the folding is unclear, but the fibres are believed to be wound in on themselves to form a helix with six nucleosomes per turn. Some regions become more tightly coiled than others, which leads to the characteristic banded appearance of the chromosomes (see *Figure A2.6*); the light areas represent less tightly coiled regions than the dark bands. The banding pattern is unique to each chromosome and provides one of the means used to identify chromosomes. The bands do not correspond with individual genes, however, and it is likely that several genes correspond to each band.

The human karyotype

A preparation of human chromosomes (*Figure A2.5*) shows that they vary in size, shape and the position of the central constriction, the centromere. The standard method used to present such a preparation is as a 'karyotype', in which the chromosomes are presented in order of size and centromere location (*Figure A2.6*).

A preparation of human chromosomes reveals that 22 pairs are perfectly matched in shape and size, known as the 'autosomes'. The remaining two chromosomes are known as the sex chromosomes and determine gender; the female has two matched X chromosomes and the male has a single X and a Y chromosome. The Y chromosome is considerably smaller than the X and, compared with the X chromosome, actually contains relatively few genes. The presence of the centromere divides a chromosome into two arms. When the arms are of unequal length, the short arm is designated 'p' and the long arm 'q'; the short arm is positioned uppermost in a karyotype. If the arms are of equal length, the 'p' and 'q' arms are based on the banding pattern. Regions on the arms of the chromosome are identified by numbers arranged in ascending order outwards from the centromere along the short and long arms.

Since, with the exception of the sex cells, each cell of our bodies contains two complete sets of chromosomes, each cell also contains two copies of each individual type of gene. As Mendel discovered, genes may exist in alternative forms, called 'alleles'. The round and wrinkled characteristics of Mendel's peas are the alleles of a gene that determine the surface characteristics of the pea. If a gene exists in alternative forms and an individual carries two identical alleles of a gene, let us say AA, the individual is described as homozygous for that gene. By contrast, if an individual carries two different alleles, say Aa, then the individual is said to be heterozygous. In addition, because of the dominance relationships between alleles, it may not be possible to distinguish an individual with genotype AA from one with Aa, since in both cases only the effect of allele A is actually observed. Hence, it is necessary to distinguish between the phenotype of an individual, that is how the genes actually manifest themselves, and the 'genotype', the genes present in the individual.

Abnormal numbers of chromosomes

Occasionally, individuals are born who do not have the normal 46 chromosomes, but who either lack a chromosome or have an increased number of chromosomes. The most familiar example of this phenomenon is Down's syndrome,[7] in which individuals are born with a number of physical and physiological differences compared with the normal. Individuals with Down's syndrome often have a short stature, characteristic head shape, eyelids and face, and may show a degree of mental retardation. Most Down's individuals have 47 chromosomes in each cell, with an extra copy of chromosome 21, and hence the condition is often referred to as trisomy-21. Down's syndrome arises as a result of a problem during the process of meiosis, in which the homologues of chromosome 21 fail to separate after pairing and the exchange of genes. The result is that some of the sex cells have two copies of chromosome 21, and hence three copies of chromosome 21 result after fertilisation. Down's individuals may develop several ocular problems during their lives.

A similar failure of chromosomes to separate after pairing at meiosis can also affect the sex chromosomes. In Turner's syndrome, individuals are born with only a single X chromosome and no Y chromosome (designated XO) and, phenotypically, appear short in stature with broad chests and with webs of skin that join the neck and shoulders. Such individuals physically resemble females, but are sterile and possess no viable ovaries. In contrast, in Klinefelter's syndrome individuals possess two X chromosomes and a Y (designated XXY) and, phenotypically, show a combination of male and female characteristics with long legs and breasts, but with male genitals.

Patterns of inheritance

The genes carried on our chromosomes determine the shape and form of our bodies and control the biochemical and physiological processes within our cells. Genes, however, exhibit a variety of different forms of inheritance that depend on whether they are dominant or recessive and whether they are located on an autosome or on a sex chromosome. Some genes are not even located within the nucleus of the cell, and such genes exhibit a quite different pattern of inheritance, termed 'mitochondrial inheritance'.

Autosomal dominant inheritance

If a characteristic is determined by a dominant gene located on an autosome, the characteristic is said to display 'autosomal dominant inheritance'. Individuals who manifest an autosomal dominant trait are usually heterozygotes since there is often a disadvantage associated with the presence of dominant genes.

An example of a human trait determined by dominant genes is blood group. Blood group is determined by three alleles of gene I (IA, IB, IO), with IA and IB being dominant to IO. By contrast, IA and IB are 'equivalent' to each other, or 'codominant'. Hence, individuals inherit two of these alleles from their parents, which results in blood group A if they inherit one or two copies of IA, blood group B if they inherit one or two copies of IB, and blood group AB if they inherit IA and IB. Individuals of blood group O carry two copies of the gene IO.

There are approximately 1900 dominantly inherited characteristics in humans. Some of these genes cause autosomal dominant disorders that may not be expressed in an individual. Consequently, an individual may inherit an autosomal dominant disorder and pass it on to the next generation; such individuals are known as 'dominant carriers'. In addition, some autosomal dominant disorders are not manifest in an individual until later in life. Examples of autosomal dominant disorders that affect the eye include aniridia, retinoblastoma,[8] certain forms of optic atrophy and retinitis pigmentosa.[3]

Autosomal recessive inheritance

If a characteristic is determined by a recessive gene located on an autosome, the characteristic is said to display 'autosomal recessive inheritance'. For a recessive characteristic to be displayed in the phenotype, the individual must be homozygous for the recessive allele (i.e., 'aa'). Hence, autosomal recessive disorders are relatively uncommon, since heterozygotes that display one normal and one abnormal gene carry the defective gene, but do not display its effects.

A good example of an autosomal recessive disorder is albinism, which is characterised by an inability of the cells to make the pigment melanin. Hence, the skin and hair are light in colour, with little coloration in the iris of the eye. Several ocular disorders are determined by this type of inheritance, including certain forms of retinitis pigmentosa[3] and Stargardt's disease.

Sex-linked inheritance

Thomas Morgan, working in the 1900s on the fruit fly *Drosophila*, discovered that some characteristics, such as eye colour, are associated with the sex of the fly. The female, being XX, transmits one X chromosome to each of her male and female offspring. A male, however, can only transmit an X chromosome to his female offspring. This results in a pattern of inheritance distinctly different from that of autosomal disorders. In addition, the X chromosome carries a full complement of genes, but the Y chromosome carries relatively few genes, two of the best-known being the H-Y antigen,[9] which determines the presence of certain antigens in the male, and the testicular determining factor (TDF).

A male obtains his Y chromosome from his father and his X chromosome from his mother. Consequently, a male displays the effects of a recessive gene inherited on the

X chromosome from his mother, since there are relatively few dominant genes on the Y chromosome to counter their effect.

A classic X-linked disease is haemophilia, in which the blood does not clot because of the lack of a gene for one of the clotting agents. Some forms of baldness in men are also inherited as a sex-linked gene. A relatively common ocular X-linked recessive disorder is red–green colour blindness, in which the majority of individuals affected are male and the characteristic is passed from mothers to sons. Another example is congenital juvenile retinoschisis.

It is now believed some genes are common between the X and Y chromosomes and so crossing over can occur between the short arms of the two sex chromosomes, and thus these genes (known as holandric genes) can be transmitted from fathers to sons.

Mitochondrial inheritance

A further form of 'sex linked' inheritance, but markedly different in its genetic determinants, is associated with the female line of inheritance. Such forms of inheritance are associated with genetic determinants that code for mitochondria, which are cellular organelles responsible for vital intracellular energy conversion. Mitochondria have their own DNA, which (compared with nuclear DNA) demonstrates a unique form, mutation rate and inheritance pattern.

Human beings inherit mitochondrial DNA, and therefore any defective genes, by acquisition of mitochondria from the female egg. Mitochondria are considered to be autonomous organelles, and hence many investigators speculate that they are 'enslaved bacteria'. The autonomous nature of mitochondria, particularly their potentially different rates of replication and absence of obvious DNA segregation, results in near-random incorporation of mitochondria and associated DNA within developing ova. Individuals born to a mother with mitochondrial genetic determinants associated with a disease characteristic may therefore show marked phenotypic variation that ranges from individuals with only marginally compromised mitochondrial function to individuals with few effective mitochondria.

What are genes made of?

One of the first discoveries that led ultimately to the recognition of DNA as the substance of genes was made by Freidrich Miescher in 1869. He found that cell nuclei contained a unique chemical constituent, which he called nuclein. A further advance was made in the 1920s, when it was discovered that human chromosomes were largely made up of two substances, two types of proteins (the most important of which were termed histones) and a sugar (DNA), either of which could constitute the genetic material.

One piece of evidence that suggested DNA was the more likely constituent was obtained in 1924. It was discovered that the somatic (non-sex) cells of the body had exactly twice the amount of DNA as the sex cells, the sperm and the egg. Since the sex cells have exactly half the genes of the somatic cells through meiosis, this observation was a strong indication that DNA made up the genetic material. In 1944, the first proof that DNA was the material of genes was discovered. DNA was extracted from dead bacteria and used to transfer certain 'factors' from bacteria that did not possess a capsule to those with a capsule.[10] Transfer of such 'factors' was believed to be the prime function of the genetic material.

Conclusive evidence that DNA was the substance of the genes was found in the 1950s by Alfred Hershey and colleagues in experiments that involved viruses. A virus is a sub-microscopic particle that causes a variety of diseases in humans, including several that affect the eye.[11] A virus particle comprises a protein shell (capsid), which encloses the nucleic acid, so viruses are composed of essentially the same substances as human chromosomes. Viruses lack a cellular structure and therefore do not possess organelles, such as mitochondria, which would provide the energy for replication. As a consequence, viruses have to invade living cells to reproduce.

Certain viruses, called bacteriophages or phages, invade bacterial cells to replicate; it was the study of this process that provided conclusive evidence that DNA was the substance of the genes (*Figure A2.7*). Each phage particle is composed of a head region, which contains the nucleic acid, surrounded by protein. In addition, there is an ensheathed tail with attachment fibres at its base. The phage particles attach themselves to the surface of the bacterial cell and inject their DNA into the host cell through the tail. Only the virus DNA actually enters the bacterial cell. Within the cell, new phage DNA and the proteins that make up the capsid are replicated. The various constituents are then assembled and the cell bursts open to release the new phage particles. The importance of this experiment was that phage DNA was injected into the bacterium and was able to instruct the cell to make specific proteins, exactly as genes were assumed to do in normal cells.

Structure of DNA

In the 1950s, a chemical structure for DNA was proposed by Watson and Crick in Cambridge, work that built on the pioneering studies in X-ray diffraction at King's College, London, by Franklind and Wilkins.

It was suggested that DNA is built from simple units called nucleotides, which are strung end-to-end in a long thread.[12] A single nucleotide (*Figure A2.8*) is made up of three parts: a type of sugar (deoxyribose) composed of five carbon atoms in a ring, a phosphate group and a nitrogen-containing base. There are four types of nucleotides with different variations in the nitrogen base; the sugar and phosphate group remain constant. Two of the nucleotides, called adenine and guanine, have bases with a double-ring structure,

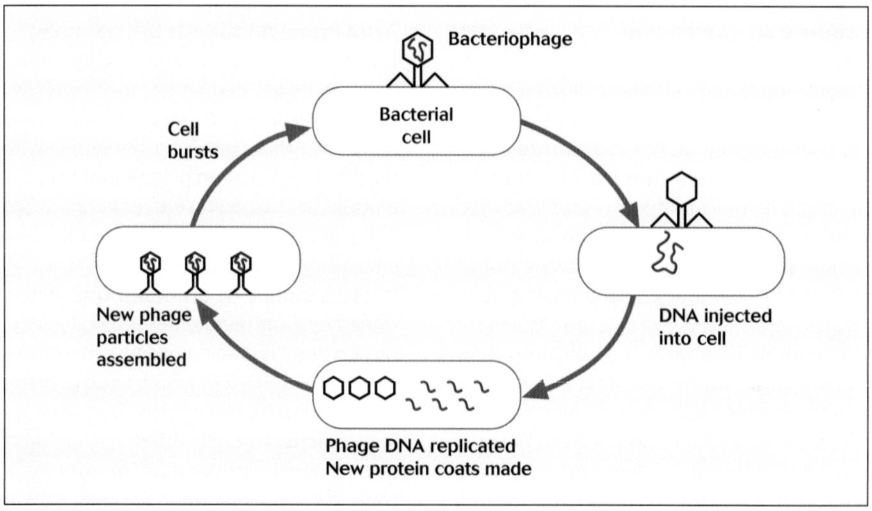

Figure A2.7
Replication of a bacteriophage virus within a bacterial cell

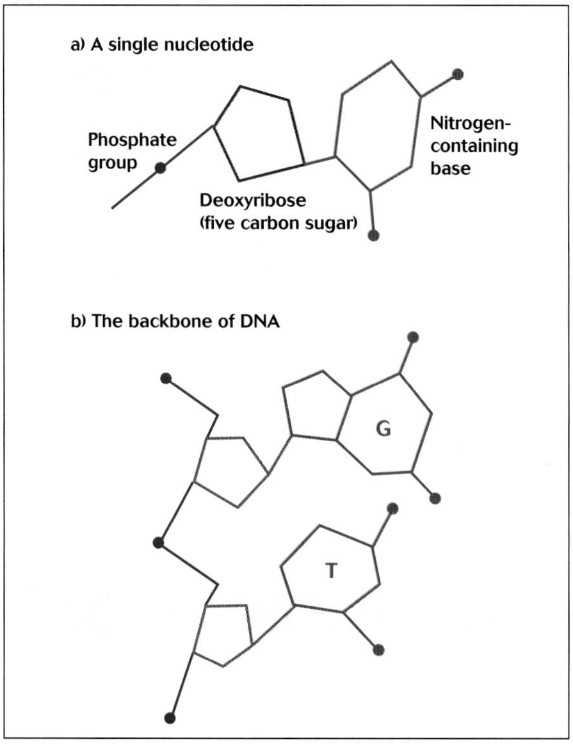

Figure A2.8
(a) Structure of a single nucleotide. (b) Attachment of two nucleotides to form a single chain of DNA (G, guanine-containing nucleotide; T, thymine-containing nucleotide)

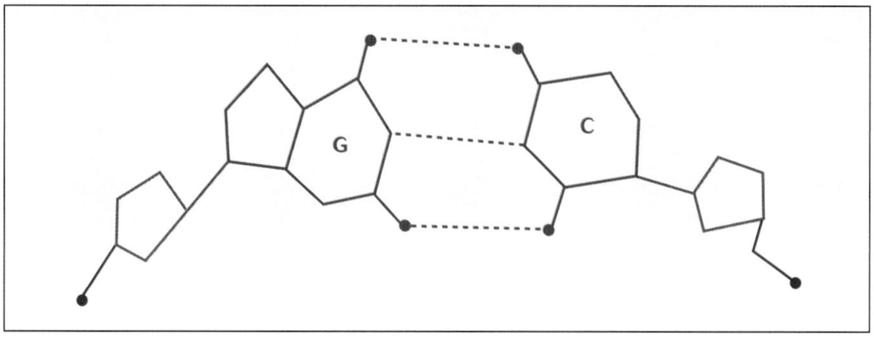

Figure A2.9
Attachment of two strands of nucleotides to form the 'double helix' of DNA (G, guanine-containing nucleotide; C, cytosine-containing nucleotide)

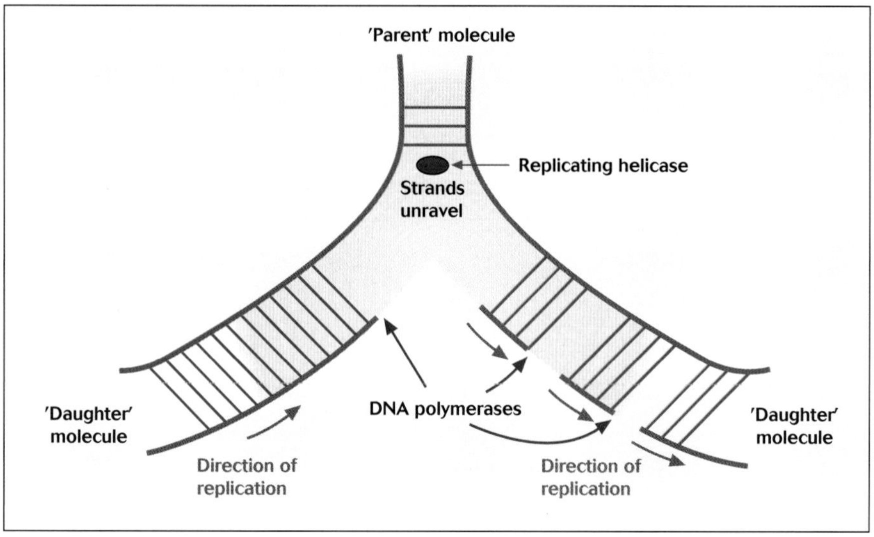

Figure A2.10
Replication of DNA

while the remaining two, called cytosine and thymine, comprise single rings. In the DNA molecule itself, the sugar of one nucleotide is attached to the phosphate group of the next nucleotide in the sequence. Watson and Crick demonstrated that the DNA molecule consist of two such strands of nucleotides helically wound around each other – hence the term double helix – with the bases pointing to the inside of the molecule (*Figure A2.9*). The two strands are held together by weak chemical bonds between the respective bases.

There is an exact relationship, however, between the sequence of bases on each strand, since an adenine-containing nucleotide on one strand always binds to a thymine-containing nucleotide on the second or complementary strand, as determined by Irving Chargaff in 1947. Similarly, a guanine-containing nucleotide always binds to a nucleotide that contains cytosine. Two important conclusions can be drawn from this structure. First, because the two strands of nucleotides are only weakly joined, it is relatively easy to separate them into two single strands of DNA. Second, because there is an exact relationship between the bases on each strand, the sequence on the second strand is complementary to that on the first, so if one is known, the other can be identified. Both of these facts are important in the development of molecular genetics and are discussed in Chapter 8.

Replication of DNA

One of the most important features of Watson and Crick's model is that it suggests how the DNA molecule could produce copies of itself.[13] It is essential that any proposed structure for DNA should have this feature since it is well known that genes replicate themselves during interphase before cell division takes place, as discussed above.

It was Watson and Crick who suggested that DNA replication occurred in a 'semi-conservative manner', by which they meant that each daughter molecule consisted of one strand from the original parent DNA and one newly synthesised strand. Essentially, the two strands of DNA unravel and each individual strand is used as the basis or 'template' to synthesise a second complimentary strand of DNA (*Figure A2.10*). DNA synthesis, however, proceeds differently in relation to each of the original parent strands. On one strand, synthesis proceeds in a direction towards the point of unravelling, new nucleotides being added to

Table A2.1 Examples of various different types of proteins important in the eye

Type of protein	*Example*	*Location*
Structural	Collagen, crystallins	Stroma of cornea, crystalline lens
Transport	Haemoglobin	Blood vessels
Receptor	Rhodopsin	Photoreceptor cells
Protective	Antibodies	Blood vessels
Contractile	Actin, myosin	Eye muscles

the end of the new strand. By contrast, on the complimentary strand, small sections of new DNA are synthesised, but in the opposite direction (i.e., away from the point of unravelling), and these are joined up later to form a complete strand. A number of enzymes are involved in this process, including a replicating helicase, which unravels the strands, various DNA polymerases (termed α, β, γ and δ) that join nucleotides together, and a DNA ligase that joins up already synthesised segments of DNA.

DNA code

DNA is a code that contains the instructions to the cell on how to build a protein. Proteins are vital to the functioning of all living cells, and an illustration of this importance to the structure and function of the eye is shown in *Table A2.1*. Proteins are incorporated into the structure of the cells of the eye, enable the eye to move, have a transport function, act as receptors and protect the eye from infection. Hence, by controlling the manufacture of such proteins, DNA influences every aspect of the structure and function of cells. A protein is a specific linear combination of 20 commonly found amino acids joined together by peptide bonds to form an amino acid chain or polypeptide. A single protein may contain as few as 50 or as many as several hundred amino acids.

DNA is the code that determines the sequence of amino acids (i.e., the DNA sequence of a gene corresponds to the order of the amino acids in a protein). Three sequential nucleotides, called a 'sense codon', provide the code for each amino acid; the sequence thymine–cytosine–adenine (TCA), for example, is the code for serine, and cytosine–adenine–thymine (CAT) is that for valine. Hence, the sequence TCACAT is an instruction to the cell to join serine to valine as one stage in the manufacture of a protein. Each protein is therefore specified by a certain number of nucleotides, which is called a 'cistron'. Some codons are not used to incorporate amino acids into protein and are called 'nonsense codons'. These codons are often used to indicate stopping points or 'chain termination', thus informing the cell that the manufacture of a particular protein is complete.

How proteins are made in the cell

Proteins are not assembled in the nucleus of the cell, but in the cytoplasm. Consequently, the DNA code for the protein is transferred to a more mobile molecule, called messenger RNA (mRNA), which can transfer the message to the cytoplasm. In the nucleus, the portion of DNA that represents the gene unravels and is used as the template to manufacture mRNA, a process called transcription. Transcription of the genetic information contained in DNA is also known as 'gene expression'. mRNA is one of three types of RNA involved in protein synthesis and is a single-stranded molecule that differs from DNA in that the base uracil replaces thymine. Many genes do not consist of continuous stretches of DNA, but of coding regions called 'exons', which provide the code for the appropriate protein, separated by DNA sequences, called introns, which do not. Transcription incorporates the DNA code represented by the exons only. Some regulatory DNA sequences have been found within the introns of a gene,[14] but it is thought unlikely that introns are involved in the process of gene expression. Several enzymes are involved in the process of transcription, including three types of RNA polymerase.

Within the cytoplasm, each amino acid constituent of the protein is attached to a short piece of nucleic acid called transfer RNA (tRNA), which has the function of carrying the amino acids from the cytoplasm to the sites of protein synthesis. The protein itself is assembled on a ribosome, a small particle abundant in the cytoplasm of cells. Another type of RNA, called ribosomal RNA (rRNA), is an integral part of the ribosome and appears to be important in holding together the ribosome, mRNA and tRNA. The mRNA becomes attached to the ribosome at one end (*Figure A2.11*),

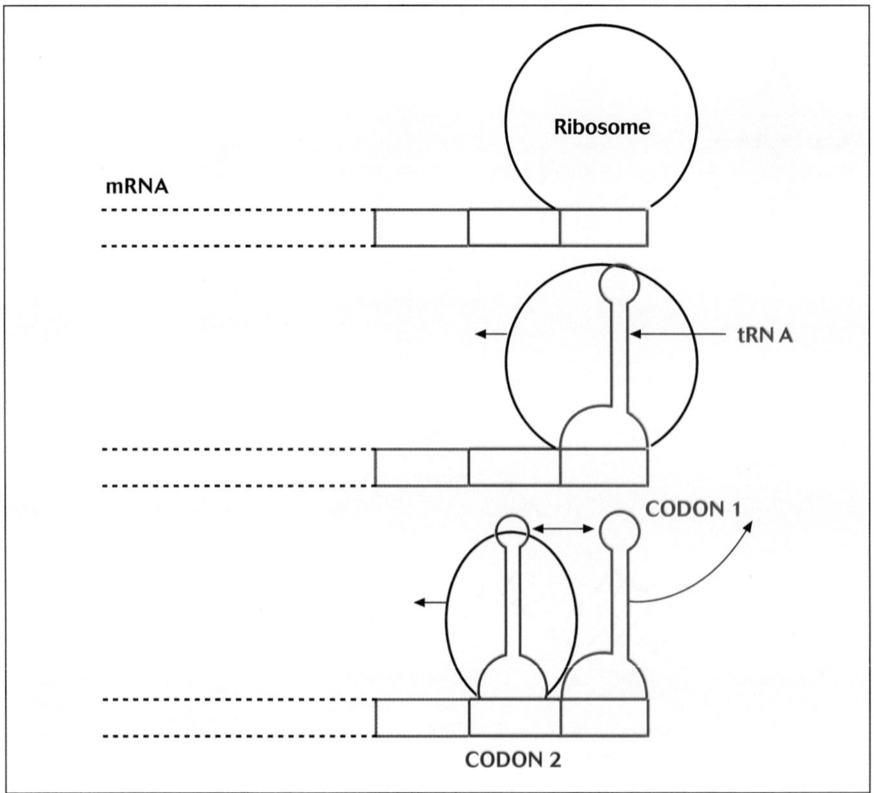

Figure A2.11
Translation of the message: the manufacture of a protein

which enables the first amino acid in the sequence to bind to the mRNA by its appropriate tRNA. The ribosome moves along the mRNA one codon at a time. At each codon, the appropriate amino acid is able to bind and is joined to the growing chain of amino acids until protein synthesis is complete. Many ribosomes may translate the same message into protein at the same time, and the process in humans is relatively rapid, with a new amino acid being added to the chain each second.

Gene mutations

There may be inaccuracies in the translation of a message and either no protein or an altered form of the protein may be made. Most of these problems result from changes or mutations of the gene. Some understanding of the effect of mutations in the DNA of genes is necessary to predict and understand their impact within cells (*Figure A2.12*).

Studies suggest that many of the mutations responsible for ocular disease are 'substitutions'. In such a mutation, a single base or nucleotide is replaced within a DNA molecule by another. Hence, only one of the three nucleotides within a codon, the unit responsible for coding an individual amino acid, is altered. A mutation of this nature is not as potentially disruptive as an insertion of one or more base pairs into the DNA of the gene. For example, an insertion of two base pairs in the GTPase regulator gene (RPGR) has been suggested in the X-linked form of retinitis pigmentosa.[15] This type of insertion induces a 'frame shift', which results in a greatly modified and prematurely shortened protein with little, if any, natural function.

Substitution mutations associated with ocular disease are commonly 'missense mutations', the alteration of one base within a codon, which gives rise to a protein that differs by only a single amino acid (i.e., a glycine replacement for arginine). Missense mutations of this nature may have variable consequences. Those mutations that give rise to the substitution of a similar amino acid within a protein, such as valine for alanine, result in little modification. However, other substitutions may be of greater consequence and significantly compromise protein function. A further two types of substitution are less common, but are potentially more disruptive than missense mutations. In one form, a codon is modified by base substitution from one coding for an amino acid, such as glutamate, to a stop or termination codon. Such a mutation may also be termed a null mutation or 'nonsense mutation', and frequently results in a shortened protein with little natural function. A similar type of mutation has been identified in the gene for retinoblastoma in several families.[8] In addition to nonsense mutations, 'splice site mutations' have been recognised. These mutations may also be extremely disruptive and require some knowledge of gene organisation to comprehend their impact. As described above, genes are composed of introns, which are not responsible for protein coding, and exons, which are responsible for the order of amino acid incorporation into proteins. A base substitution in a splice site, a region that separates an exon from an intron, can disrupt such a site and give rise to the incorporation of intron DNA into protein synthesis. As introns may comprise 90 per cent of a human gene, any resultant protein is likely to have very different characteristics to its natural counterpart.

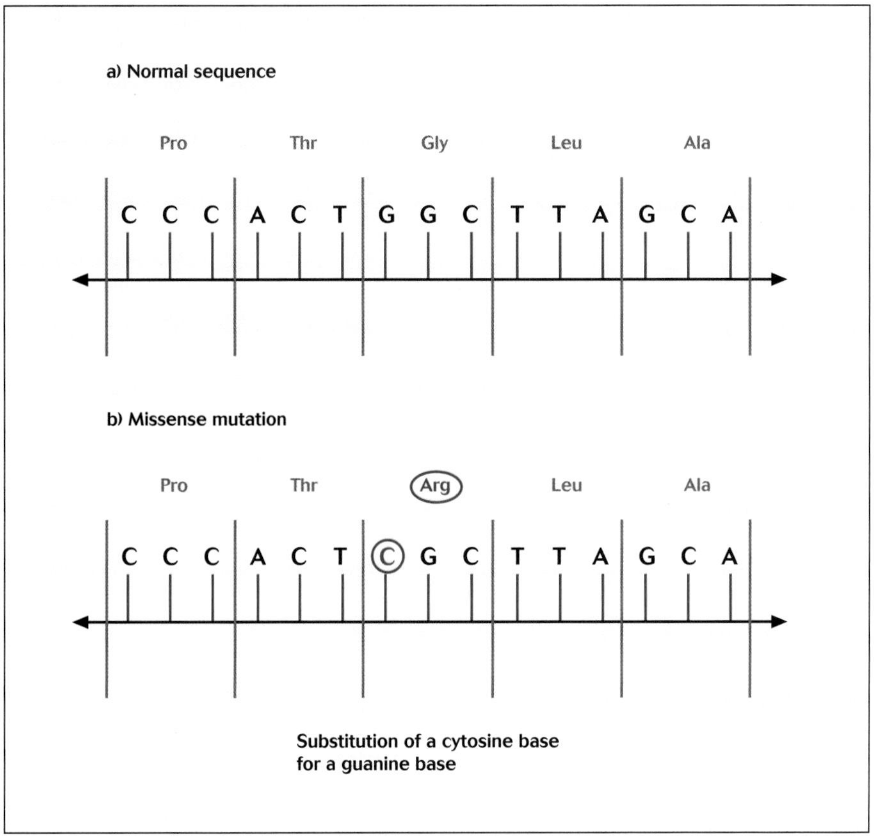

Figure A2.12
An example of a gene mutation

Gene regulation

All of the cells of the body contain the same population of genes. By providing the codes to make essential proteins, genes influence all aspects of the structure and function of the cells. The body, however, contains a large number of different types of cell, each with a particular structure and many with a unique or specialised function (e.g., a neuron has a completely different appearance and function to a liver cell). In addition, in the retina of the eye many different types of cell are present, including photoreceptor cells that contain the photopigments and initiate the process of vision, various types of neuron that process the signals of the photoreceptor cells before conveying the information to the brain, and the pigment epithelial cells. Hence, what determines the structure and function of these cells if they all contain the same genes? The answer is that a particular cell only utilises a proportion of its available genes.

Different populations of genes are active in each type of cell and, by manufacturing a particular group of proteins, determine the form and ultimate function of that cell. For this process to work efficiently, however, there must be a way to switch genes off and on, and so regulate the activities of genes.

If a gene is prevented from making a protein it can essentially be regarded as 'switched off'. As discussed above, the synthesis of a protein involves two stages, namely transcription (in which the DNA code is transferred to mRNA) and translation (which involves the manufacture of the protein on a ribosome in the cytoplasm). Gene regulation could occur either at the translation or at the transcription stage, but in most cases genes are regulated at the transcription stage (i.e., the DNA code is not transferred to mRNA).

Gene regulation of the haemoglobin molecule

Studies of the haemoglobin molecule, a protein with the specialised function of transporting oxygen and carbon dioxide within the blood stream, are particularly important in the study of gene regulation. Haemoglobin is a complex molecule, which (in humans) comprises a number of polypeptide chains termed α, β, γ, δ and ε. The polypeptide chains that make up the molecule, however, vary at different stages of the embryo and in the early months of life. Prior to birth, the main constituents of haemoglobin are two 'α' and two 'γ' chains, but after birth two 'α' and two 'β' chains predominate. In addition, the 'ε' chain is only present during early embryonic stages, while the 'δ' chain is only present after birth. Hence, studies of the haemoglobin molecule suggest that there must exist regulatory genes that switch synthesis from one group of genes to another during the early months of life.

Gene regulation in bacteria

Studies of the bacterium *Escherichia coli* provided the first evidence of a possible mechanism of gene regulation and resulted in the theory known as 'The Operon Theory'.[16] In certain bacteria, the genes that code for the enzymes necessary for the manufacture of the sugar lactose are normally switched off. If lactose is present in the culture medium in which the bacteria grow, however, the genes are switched on and the bacteria can manufacture lactose. A key feature of this mechanism is the presence of a regulatory gene (or R-gene) that codes for a regulatory protein. Several genes are actually involved in the process of making lactose (*Figure A2.13*), however, including a promoter gene (P-gene), an operator gene (O-gene), the R-gene and the genes that make the relevant enzymes.

When no lactose is present in the medium, the regulatory protein binds to the DNA at the region of the O-gene. This prevents the enzyme RNA polymerase from binding to the P-gene, an essential step in switching on the genes for lactose. As a consequence, the genes for lactose remain switched off. By contrast, if lactose is present in the medium, it interacts with the regulatory protein and prevents it from binding to the site of the O-gene. This allows the RNA polymerase to bind to the P-gene and the unrepressed O-gene allows the attachment of RNA polymerase to the transcript region and hence the genes for lactose are switched on. The essential point about this mechanism is that it depends on the shape of the regulatory protein. It has a precise molecular shape that allows it to bind, like pieces of a jigsaw puzzle, to the region of the DNA that contains the O-gene. When lactose is added, however, it binds to the regulatory protein, which alters its shape sufficiently so that it no longer fits the site of the O-gene. Although initially studied in bacteria, operon-like transcriptional control was found recently in human cells.

Gene regulation and disease

Gene regulation may be involved in one of the most important types of disease in humans, namely malignant disease or cancer. Some forms of cancer may have a genetic basis, which may involve the regulation of genes that control the rate of cell division. A demonstration of this was made in an experiment first carried out in 1982, which showed that if a particular piece of DNA, which originated from bladder cancer cells, was injected into normal tissue culture cells, the normal cells began to divide in a chaotic and uncontrolled manner and became cancerous. The particular piece of DNA that has this transforming function is known as an 'oncogene'; it is an abnormally mutated form of a 'proto-oncogene', differing from it by a single nucleotide (point mutation). Hence, the normal gene may control cell growth and division, while the abnormal gene lacks this ability to control growth, such that cancer may be the consequence. Oncogenes, however, may exert their effects by several different mechanisms. In some cases, the presence of the oncogene results in 'amplification' of the proto-oncogene (i.e., the proto-oncogene is replicated until it is present in many copies). This results in the accumulation of the normal gene product of the proto-oncogene within the cell (i.e., a regulatory protein that may cause the cell to become cancerous).

Another way that genes may result in malignant disease is the invasion of a cell by a retrovirus. Retroviruses only contain a single strand of RNA, but within the cell a double-stranded complementary DNA is synthesised using the virus RNA as a template. This piece of viral DNA may become incorporated into the DNA of the

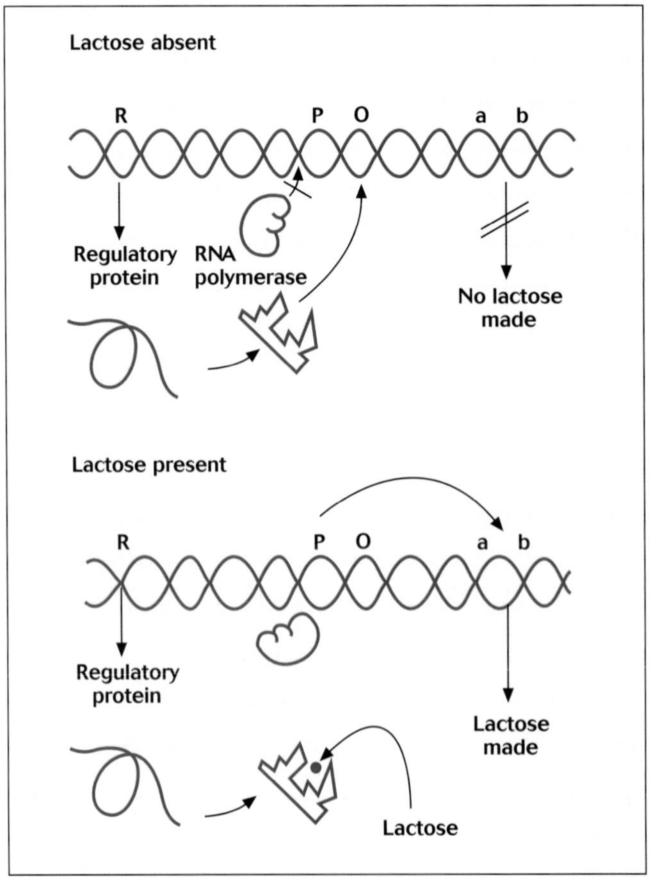

Figure A2.13 *Gene regulation according to the 'Operon theory' (R, regulatory gene; P promoter gene; O, operator gene; a, b, genes that make the enzymes for lactose)*

chromosomes of the host. If this happens at a site close to that of a proto-oncogene, cancer may be the result. Retroviruses are believed to cause certain forms of leukaemia in humans, and suspected that they cause others.

Summary

In this chapter, we describe the patterns of inheritance of human characteristics, and show how they are transmitted between generations. Many characteristics are transmitted according to relatively simple rules first worked out by Mendel. The various patterns of inheritance of human traits, including autosomal dominant and recessive, sex-linked and mitochondrial inheritance, each give rise to a distinct pattern of characteristics in subsequent generations. In addition, we describe the structure of the chromosomes that carry the genes that determine human characteristics. Normally, chromosomes are composed of thin threads ('beads on a string'), but during cell division they become much shorter and thicker and can be studied readily.

We also introduce basic concepts of genetics that relate to DNA and show, firstly, how it was established that DNA was the genetic material. By the 1950s, a structure for DNA had been proposed which showed how genes could replicate themselves. The basis of the DNA code was then worked out and it was demonstrated how the basic unit of the code, the sense codon, provided the code for an amino acid and that the sequence of codons in the DNA corresponded to the sequence of amino acids in a protein. The manufacture of a protein is a two-stage process that involves three types of RNA. During transcription, the DNA code is transferred to mRNA, which enables the code to be transferred to the cytoplasm. During translation, amino acids attached to tRNA molecules are brought to the ribosomes and attached in a chain to form the protein. Occasionally, this process may go wrong as a result of a mutation within a gene and either no protein or an altered form of the protein may be made, which results in the disruption of cell function and possible disease. In each type of cell with a specialised function, different populations of genes are active and, as a consequence, the activities of genes have to be regulated. In addition, defects in gene regulation may play an important role in human disease, and particularly in the development of cancer.

References

1 Stine GJ (1989). *The New Human Genetics*. (Dubuque; WC Brown).
2 Armstrong RA and Smith SN (2000). The genetics of cataract. *Optom Today* **Nov 17**, 33–35.
3 Armstrong RA (2000). The rod photoreceptor ABCR gene and its significance in ocular disease. *Optician* **220**, 19–24.
4 Steward FC (1970). From cultured cells to whole plants: The induction and control of their growth and morphogenesis. *Proc Roy Soc (Lond)* **B175**, 1–30.
5 Thomas JO (1984). The higher order structure of chromatin and histone H1. *J Cell Sci*. **1**, S1–S20.
6 Eissenberg JC (1985). Selected topics in chromatin structure. *Ann Rev Genet*. **19**, 484–536.
7 Armstrong RA and Carroll H (1996). Neurological and ocular abnormalities in patients with Down's syndrome. *Optom Today* **Feb 26**, 22–24.
8 Armstrong RA and Smith SN (1999). Retinoblastoma and the new genetics. *Optom Today* **Mar 12**, 43–47.
9 Simpson E (1987). Separation of the genetic loci for the H-Y antigen and for testis determination on human Y chromosome. *Nature* **326**, 876–878.
10 Avery OT, MacLeod CM and McCarty M (1944). Studies on the chemical nature of the substance inducing transformation of pneumoccocal types. *J Exp Med*. **79**, 37–158.

11 Armstrong RA (2000). Microbiology of the eye. *Ophthalmic Physiol Opt*. **20**, 429–441.
12 Watson JD and Crick FHC (1953). Molecular structure of nucleic acids: A structure for dcoxyribose nucleic acid. *Nature* **171**, 737–738.
13 Watson JD and Crick FHC (1953). Genetical implications of the structure of deoxyribonucleic acid. *Nature* **171**, 964–967.
14 Caskey TC (1987). Genetic therapy: Somatic gene transplants. *Hosp Pract*. **22**, 181–198.
15 Armstrong RA and Smith SN (1999). Retinitis pigmentosa and the new genetics. *Optom Today*, **Dec 17th**, 26–32.
16 Jacob F and Monod J (1961). Genetic regulatory mechanisms in the synthesis of proteins. *J Mol Biol*. **3**, 318–338.

Multiple Choice Questions

There is one answer per question; the answers are given in the next section.

Chapter 1

1 Which of the following is *not* a function that can be measured with a visual evoked potential (VEP) technique?
A Visual acuity;
B Contrast sensitivity;
C Stereopsis;
D Convergence;
E Colour vision.

2 How long does complete myelination of the nerve fibres take in the normal infant?
A 4–6 months;
B 2 years;
C 1 year;
D 4 years;
E 9 months.

3 Which value is a generally accepted estimate of visual acuity at 6 months of age?
A 1 cycle per degree (cpd);
B 2–5cpd;
C 6cpd;
D 12cpd;
E 18cpd.

4 The young infant does not control accommodation accurately because of:
A A lack of sensory stimulus as a result of a large depth of focus;
B Immaturity of the ciliary muscle;
C A lack of ability to converge;
D Poor contrast sensitivity;
E The presence of hypermetropia.

5 Which of the following functions is present at birth?
A Stereopsis;
B Vertical saccades;
C Vestibulo-ocular reflex;
D Accommodation;
E Trichromacy.

6 At 6 months of age in the normal infant, which of the following has matured to adult levels?
A Visual acuity measured by preferential looking;
B myelination of the nerve fibres;
C Astigmatism;
D Smooth pursuit movements;
E Contrast sensitivity measured by VEP.

7 The cones in the newborn infant retina are thought to limit visual acuity because they are:
A Packed too closely together;
B Too narrow;
C Too long;
D Not closely packed together;
E Absent.

8 At 2 months of age an infant:
A Has no colour perception;
B Has gross fusion;
C Demonstrates monocular OKN to a temporal-ward stimulus;
D Can accurately follow a fast-moving target with smooth movements;
E Can discriminate between red and green.

9 Emmetropisation is thought to occur because of:
A Passive growth of the eye;
B Spectacle correction of refractive error;
C An active feedback mechanism;
D Combination of A and B;
E Combination of A and C.

10 Children with strabismus tend to:
A Develop myopia;
B Develop increasing hypermetropia;
C Show emmetropisation;
D Initially become myopic, and then emmetropise;
E Initially become hyperopic, and then emmetropise.

11 Most children are born with:

A 1.00D of against-the-rule astigmatism that shifts to with-the-rule after 5 years;
B No astigmatism that increases to 1.00D against-the-rule by 5 years;
C 1.00D with-the-rule astigmatism that changes to against-the-rule by 5 years;
D 1.00D against-the-rule astigmatism that remains unchanged by 5 years;
E 1.00D with-the-rule astigmatism that decreases to no astigmatism by 5 years.

12 Visual acuity measured with VEP first reaches adult values by:

A 2–3 months;
B 6–8 months;
C 12 months;
D 18 months;
E 3 years.

Chapter 2

1 Which statement is correct? Congenital myopia is:

A The most common aetiology of myopia;
B More common than congenital high hyperopia;
C More likely to occur in premature infants with retinopathy of prematurity (ROP) than those without it;
D Likely to regress;
E Often associated with esophoria.

2 Which of the following statements is true?

A There is no association between increased incidence of astigmatism and prematurity;
B Less than 10 per cent of children aged between 6 and 15 years of age are myopic;
C Exophoria is a risk factor in the development of juvenile myopia;
D In most ethnic groups twice as many girls than boys are born myopic;
E Juvenile myopia is more common than congenital myopia in developing countries.

3 Prematurity has *not* been shown to be associated with:

A Increased incidence of myopia;
B Increased incidence of astigmatism;
C Increased incidence of strabismus;
D Maternal alcohol use during pregnancy;
E Albinism.

4 Which of the following statements is true:

A Idiopathic nystagmus is often associated with high astigmatism;
B Strabismus affects 1 per cent of children;
C Congenital exotropia has an increased incidence in premature infants;
D Albinos are just as likely to have strabismus as other children;
E Congenital cortical cataracts usually require surgery.

5 Which of the following is *not* a risk factor for the development of amblyopia:

A Strabismus;
B High astigmatism;
C Unilateral congenital cataract;
D Marked ptosis;
E Optic disc drusen.

6 Which of the following is *not* a common aetiology of congenital cataract:

A Rubella;
B Retinoblastoma;
C Heredity;
D Steroid use in pregnancy;
E Down's syndrome.

7 Which of the following statements is true?

A Retinoblastoma occurs in 0.5 per cent of children;
B There is no genetic link in retinoblastoma;
C Congenital toxoplasmosis does not have systemic effects;
D Toxoplasmosis occurs through infestation with the intestinal roundworm of cats and dogs;
E Retinopathy of prematurity may lead to retinal detachment.

8 Which of the following statements is *not* true?

A Epicanthus is associated with squints;
B Duane's retraction syndrome is caused by an intraocular muscle malinsertion;
C A chorioretinal scar at the macula may lead to strabismus;
D Blepharitis in children most commonly results from *Staphylococcus aureus* infection;
E Cleft palate is associated with an increased incidence of optic disc anomalies.

9 Which of the following statements is *not* true?

A Around 5–8 per cent of males have a colour vision anomaly;
B A female can have an X-linked colour vision defect only if her father and his father both also have the same;
C A protanope may confuse red with black or dark brown;
D A deuteranope may confuse green with red or orange;
E About 4–5 per cent of all boys have deuteranomalous trichromacy.

10 Which of the following is *not* true of anomalous trichromats?

A They may pass the City University Colour Vision Test;
B They may have problems entering certain professions;
C They will match any red–green mix with yellow on a Nagel anomaloscope;
D They account for the majority of hereditary colour vision defects;
E They affect less than 1 per cent of females.

11 Which of the following is true of blue (tritan) colour-vision defects?
A They are more likely to be inherited than acquired;
B Inherited tritan defects are sex linked;
C The incidence of inherited tritan defects is around 0.005 per cent;
D Acquired defects occur most often through congenital cataract;
E They are the most severe form of colour-vision defect.

12 Which statement is true?
A The City University Test is the most sensitive colour-vision test;
B The City University Test has been shown to differentiate between the two types of dichromacy more effectively than the Ishihara Test;
C Ishihara plates with paths of dots to trace have been shown to be very effective;
D The first plate in the Ishihara Test identifies dichromats;
E The Nagel anomaloscope is the most commonly used colour-vision test in clinical practice.

Chapter 3

1 The repeatability of an acuity test:
A Relates to how long the test takes to perform;
B Reflects how complex a measure of acuity it is;
C Is only relevant in preferential looking tests;
D Reflects how variable the results it produces are;
E Is only relevant in letter-matching tests.

2 The most useful test in optometric practice with which to assess the visual acuity of young infants is:
A Preferential looking;
B Visual evoked potentials (VEPs);
C Letter matching;
D Picture naming;
E Stycar balls.

3 Which of the following statements is *not* true? Persistent interocular acuity differences:
A Are unlikely to affect normal visual development;
B Can be detected by monocular acuity testing;
C Are not the norm in childhood;
D May be the result of uncorrected anisometropia;
E Should be investigated further.

4 Which of the following statements is *not* true? Visual acuity (VA) maturation occurs as a result of:
A Maturation in size and shape of photoreceptors;
B Development of cortical connections and processes;
C Improved control of eye movements and accommodation;
D Increase in pupil size;
E Improved organisation of photoreceptors.

5 VEPs provide:
A A subjective test of resolution acuity;
B An objective test of resolution acuity;
C A subjective test of recognition acuity;
D An objective test of recognition acuity;
E An objective test of detection acuity.

6 Resolution acuity tests should only be used in preference to recognition acuity tests when:
A A child is intellectually or physically unable to perform a recognition test;
B A child has strabismic amblyopia;
C A child is not able to name letters or pictures;
D A child has a visual impairment;
E A 'crowded' acuity is required.

7 Which of the following is *not* a recognition acuity test?
A LH symbols;
B Kay picture test;
C Cardiff acuity test;
D Sonksen–Silver acuity system;
E Illiterate E.

8 Which of the following is *not* a resolution acuity test?
A Keeler acuity system;
B LH symbols;
C Cardiff acuity test;
D VEP test;
E Teller acuity cards.

9 Near VA is affected by accommodative function. Considering this association, which of the following statements is *not* true?
A A child's near VA can be assessed using the near Kay picture test;
B Accommodative function is usually ample in childhood;
C Accommodation in childhood may be reduced by neurological impairment;
D Children with visual impairment may have reduced accommodative function;
E Children's near VA can only be assessed when they are able to read.

10 A significant difference in acuity as measured by the LogMAR acuity test is:
A One letter;
B Two letters;
C Three letters;
D Four letters;
E 0.05 logMAR.

11 The LogMAR acuity test provides:
A Uncrowded measures of recognition acuity only;
B Uncrowded measures of resolution acuity only;
C Crowded measures of recognition acuity only;
D Uncrowded and crowded measures of recognition acuity;
E Uncrowded and crowded measures of resolution acuity.

12 According to Salt *et al.* (1995; see Chapter 3 references for full details), adult levels of acuity (6/6) may not be measured by letter-naming or -matching tests until:
A 2 years of age;
B 3 years of age;
C 4 years of age;
D 5 years of age;
E 6 years of age or older.

Chapter 4

1 Which of the following is *not* true? Accommodation should be relaxed in the following techniques:

A Static retinoscopy;
B Cycloplegic retinoscopy;
C Dynamic retinoscopy;
D The Mohindra technique;
E Autorefractor use.

2 Which of the following combinations would be suitable to use on a 3-year-old child undergoing his or her first cycloplegic refraction?

A One drop 0.5 per cent proxymetacaine followed, after 5 minutes, by one drop 1 per cent cyclopentalate;
B One drop 0.5 per cent cyclopentalate;
C Two drops 1 per cent tropicamide instilled at 5 minute intervals;
D 1 per cent atropine instilled twice a day for 3 days prior to examination;
E Two drops 0.5 per cent cyclopentalate instilled immediately after each other.

3 Which of the following statements is *not* true?

A Atropine should not be used in infants under the age of 3 months;
B A tonus allowance is not needed when atropine is used;
C Atropine is a muscarinic antagonist;
D Use of atropine can produce mydriasis that lasts for up to a fortnight;
E Use of atropine can cause a reduction in the effectiveness of a patient's sweat glands.

4 Which statement is true?

A A typical dynamic lag of accommodation can be 1.50D;
B Residual accommodation with the use of cyclopentalate is typically 2D;
C When performing a cycloplegic examination, retinoscopy should not commence until the accommodation has fallen below 2D;
D If the Mohindra technique is used, a 2D allowance must be made to account for the 50cm working distance;
E An allowance must be made for the working distance when performing dynamic retinoscopy.

5 Which of the following is *not* advisable when refracting an infant under 3 months of age?

A The Mohindra technique;
B A 'ret' or lens rack;
C Dynamic retinoscopy;
D Performing retinoscopy while the child is asleep;
E A cycloplegic refraction using 1 per cent tropicamide.

6 Giving a prescription is necessary:

A If anisometropia is 0.50DS;
B If astigmatism of 1.50DC is found in a child 12 months of age;
C In a 1-year-old child whose prescription is R –0.75DS, L –0.75DS;
D In an accommodative esotrope of age 2.5 years;
E If a dynamic lag of accommodation of 1D is found.

7 Dynamic retinoscopy:

A Measures refractive error;
B Can highlight the presence of astigmatism;
C Should be performed monocularly;
D Must be performed from a fixed working distance;
E Uses an accommodative target at 6m.

8 Which statement is *not* true? When accommodation takes place:

A The ciliary muscle contracts;
B The lens becomes more convex;
C The ciliary muscle has been stimulated by acetylcholine;
D The tonus of the ciliary muscle alters;
E The focus point of the eye may 'lag' behind the position of the object of interest.

9 Instilling a cycloplegic agent:

A Can help a practitioner to perform the Mohindra technique;
B Can be facilitated by the use of a local anaesthetic;
C Can produce miosis, which lasts longer than the cycloplegia;
D Always leaves a small amount of residual accommodation;
E Results in an increase in the power of the crystalline lens.

10 Which of the following is *not* true? The Mohindra technique:

A Works better in scotopic conditions;
B Works better monocularly;
C Requires a known level of accommodation to be present;
D Can induce myopia;
E Can be performed while the infant is feeding.

11 Tonic accommodation:

A Is not thought to be dependent on refractive error;
B Is abolished by the use of 1 per cent cyclopentalate;
C Must be assumed to be the level of accommodation present for the results of the Mohindra technique to be reliable;
D Is about 2.50D;
E Cannot be abolished fully.

12 Which of the following is *not* true? Anisometropia:

A May not be permanent if demonstrated at birth;
B May be found to be of different amounts when a cycloplegic is used, compared with when a cycloplegic is not used;
C Should always be corrected fully in cases where a correction is deemed clinically necessary;
D Is only significant at levels of over 1.50DS;
E Is of less concern in myopic children.

Chapter 5

1 Which statement is true?

A Myopia has a high prevalence in all Asian populations;
B The prevalence of myopia is greater in Caucasian than in Chinese populations;
C The prevalence of myopia in Eskimos increased by over 50 per cent in one generation;
D Both A and C;
E Both A and B.

2 The prevalence of myopia in Caucasian children at 6 years of age is approximately:

A 30 per cent;
B 6 per cent;
C 15 per cent;
D 25 per cent;
E 2 per cent.

3 The odds ratio for developing myopia if both parents are myopic is:

A 3;
B 2;
C 4;
D 6;
E 8.

4 The heritability of refractive error has been reported to be:

A 0.25;
B 0.33;
C 0.82;
D 0.73;
E 0.50.

5 Which of the following is false? Myopia has been found to have an association with:

A Parental history of myopia;
B Higher intelligence levels;
C Increased use of visual display units;
D Chinese race;
E Occupation.

6 Which of the following is *not* true? Juvenile onset myopia is:

A Correlated with an increase in axial length;
B Correlated with a steeper cornea;
C The most common aetiology of myopia;
D Likely to progress;
E Likely to have a parental history of myopia.

7 Which of the following is *not* associated with high myopia?

A Down's syndrome;
B Congenital stationary night blindness;
C Microspherophakia;
D Stickler's syndrome;
E Diabetes.

8 Which statement regarding use of bifocal or multifocal spectacle lenses in reduction of myopia progression is true:

A The rationale for using bifocal or multifocal lenses stems from myopes who have an increased lag of accommodation during near work;
B The use of bifocal or multifocal lenses results in reduction of retinal blur at near;
C The use of bifocal or multifocal lenses results in reduction of accommodative demand;
D Combination of A and C;
E Combination of A, B and C.

9 The COMET study is investigating the reduction of myopia progression with:

A Contact lenses;
B Bifocal spectacle lenses;
C Multifocal spectacle lenses;
D Pirenzepine;
E Atropine.

10 Antimuscarinics are believed to reduce myopia progression by:

A Reducing the accommodative demand;
B Their action on the ciliary muscle and iris;
C Their action on M1 receptors in the retina;
D Their action on M4 receptors in the retina;
E All of the above.

11 The CLAMP study is investigating the reduction of myopia progression with:

A Contact lenses;
B Bifocal lenses;
C Multifocal spectacle lenses;
D Pirenzepine;
E Atropine.

12 Interventions to reduce myopia progression in humans have included:

A Timolol;
B Atropine;
C Contact lenses;
D Multifocal spectacle lenses;
E All of the above.

Chapter 6

1 What is the percentage volume of the eye at birth with respect to its adult value?

A 25 per cent;
B 40 per cent;
C 50 per cent;
D 75 per cent;
E 100 per cent.

2 In humans, ocular dominance columns are thought to develop over what period in early life?

A 6 years;
B 6 months;
C 6 days;
D 6 weeks;
E Fully developed at birth.

3 **Smooth pursuit and head tracking are known to reach full maturity by:**
A 6 months;
B 6 weeks;
C 2 months;
D 5 months;
E None of the above.

4 **Stereoacuity has been shown to improve up to what age?**
A 6 months;
B 6 years;
C 5 years;
D 18 years;
E No improvement seen from levels at birth.

5 **Heterotropia caused by unilateral blindness in an adult is most likely to be:**
A Exotropia;
B Esotropia;
C Cyclotropia;
D Both A and B;
E Hypertropia.

6 **A wide interpupillary distance tends towards which phoria?**
A Exophoria;
B Esophoria;
C Cyclophoria;
D Hypophoria;
E Hyperphoria.

7 **The most likely explanation for Duane's retraction syndrome is:**
A Thickening of the lateral rectus muscle;
B Fibrosis of the lateral rectus muscle tendon;
C Abnormal connection between the facial nerve and the lateral rectus;
D Sixth nerve palsy;
E Abnormal misdirection of a branch of the third nerve that supplies the medial rectus to the lateral rectus.

8 **Which of the following is *not* a typical feature of oculocutaneous albinism?**
A Loss of melanin;
B Nystagmus;
C Fewer fibres decussate at the optic chiasm;
D Photophobia;
E Incomplete foveal differentiation.

9 **Spasmus nutans:**
A Does not resolve with time;
B Is a horizontal nystagmus accompanied by head nodding;
C Is a double levator palsy;
D May result from dorsal midbrain defects;
E Typically presents between 3 and 18 years.

10 **Which of the following cranial nerves is *not* affected by Moebius syndrome:**
A Facial;
B Abducent;
C Accessory;
D Glossopharyngeal;
E Hypoglossal.

11 **Which of the following is *not* a feature of third nerve aberrant regeneration?**
A Elevation of the upper lid on down gaze;
B Abduction of the affected eye on attempted up gaze;
C Pupil constriction on adduction;
D Retraction of the globe on attempted up or down gaze;
E The mechanism for the regeneration is uncertain.

12 **The most common acquired ocular motor nerve palsy is that of:**
A IVth;
B IInd;
C IIIrd;
D VIth;
E VIIth.

Chapter 7

1 **Persistent epicanthal folds may give the impression of:**
A Exotropia;
B Superior oblique overaction;
C Inferior oblique overaction.
D Exophoria;
E Superior oblique underaction.

2 **The term associated phoria refers to:**
A The movement seen under the cover in the cover test;
B The phoria measured by a Maddox rod;
C The phoria measured in a fully compensated heterophoria;
D The size of prism needed to align the nonius strips on a fixation disparity unit;
E The phoria found in increased levels in dyslexia.

3 **Binocular vision recovery to a base-out prism may be demonstrated:**
A From birth;
B At 6 months of age;
C Only in amblyopes;
D Not before 6 years of age;
E After the plasticity period.

4 **Which of the following is *not* a stereopsis test?**
A TNO;
B Titmus;
C Lang;
D Frisby;
E Base-out prism.

5 **Which *one* of the statements about abnormal retinal correspondence (ARC) is true?**
A Bagolini lens streaks cross through the light target, even though strabismus is present if ARC is harmonious;
B Lightly ingrained ARC is stable and unchanging;
C The angle of esodeviation increases as a fixation point is moved towards the nose in ARC;
D Lang's two-pen test is a quantitative assessment of ARC;
E Patients with deeply ingrained ARC need occlusion therapy.

6 Which of the following represents a suitable period of occlusion for a 15-month-old infant?
A 10 minutes daily;
B 30 minutes daily;
C 4 hours daily;
D Full time;
E 6 hours daily.

7 Which of the following is *not* necessarily a contraindication to occlusion therapy?
A Reversal amblyopia;
B Intractable diplopia;
C Psychological distress;
D Decompensating heterophoria;
E Age of the patient.

8 Partial occlusion refers to:
A The use of intermittent occlusion;
B The use of occlusion for a short period;
C The use of an opaque occluder;
D The use of a translucent occluder of variable density;
E Use of a hand-held occluder.

9 Penalisation refers to:
A Total occlusion by optical means;
B Cycloplegia;
C Reduction of acuity by occlusion;
D Partial occlusion by optical means;
E The preferred method of management when loss of binocular control is feared.

10 Penalisation may be carried with all the following except:
A Modified contact lens prescription in front of the fixating eye;
B Fogging lens in front of the fixating eye;
C Modified prescription lenses in front of the fixating eye;
D Frosted lens in front of the fixating eye;
E Atropine in the fixating eye.

11 Which might be appropriate for the management of convergence excess?
A Negative addition segment;
B Convergence exercises;
C Exercising negative relative accommodation;
D Exercising positive relative convergence;
E Positive addition segment.

12 Which of the following is and/or are unlikely to help a near exophoria?
A Flipper lenses;
B Stereograms;
C Exercising negative relative accommodation;
D Exercising positive relative accommodation;
E Flipper prisms.

Chapter 8

There are no questions for Chapter 8.

Chapter 9

1 The critical period for visual development:
A Lasts throughout childhood;
B Is the same as the sensitive period;
C Is identical for all visual modalities;
D Spans the first 10–16 weeks of infancy;
E Has no bearing on congenital cataract management.

2 Amblyopia:
A Affects 20 per cent of the population;
B Can be classified into two different subgroups;
C Can be treated by atropine penalisation of the fellow eye;
D Does not occur in myopic anisometropia;
E Is never bilateral.

3 With regard to cataract morphology:
A Anterior polar cataracts are associated with a poor visual prognosis;
B Bilateral lamellar cataracts require early surgical intervention;
C Nuclear cataracts are usually managed by providing appropriate refractive correction;
D Sutural cataracts are often visually insignificant;
E Posterior lenticonus can be steroid induced.

4 In the post-operative management of infants with congenital cataracts:
A Minimal occlusion therapy is usually needed after unilateral cataract surgery;
B Early optical correction is critical;
C Aphakic glaucoma always occurs within weeks of surgery;
D Vitreous wicks can be managed conservatively;
E Strabismic amblyopia is unusual in bilateral cases.

5 In non-organic visual loss:
A There is a gender bias towards boys;
B Severe visual loss is usually associated;
C Referral is usually instigated by an optometrist;
D There is no association with social conflict;
E The visual prognosis is usually poor.

6 In retinopathy of prematurity (ROP):
A Premature babies born at or less than 31 weeks gestational age are at risk of ROP;
B Uncontrolled oxygen administration is currently the main cause of ROP;
C Infants at risk of ROP undergo screening by neonatologists;
D Infants with stage 1 and stage 2 ROP can be discharged safely;
E ROP is treated by laser photocoagulation of neovascular tissue.

7 In treated ROP:
A Laser treatment is always successful in restoring normal visual function;
B Children can be discharged safely from further follow-up;
C Normal emmetropisation is usually observed;
D The retina recovers to give a normal appearance;
E Intracerebral haemorrhage may result in reduced vision despite a fundus of normal appearance.

8 With regard to the incidence of retinoblastoma:
A It is more common in girls than in boys;
B Strabismus is the most common presenting feature;
C It has a worldwide incidence of approximately one in 20,000;
D Hereditary forms usually present at 6 years of age;
E Most tumours are inherited.

9 Regarding the management of retinoblastoma:
A Children with retinoblastoma are best managed by external beam irradiation;
B Patients show greatest survival when treated by a team of ophthalmologists and oncologists at their nearest hospital;
C External beam radiation is applied if the tumour is shown to have invaded the optic nerve head after the eye is enucleated;
D Examination of the parents is not required in unilateral retinoblastoma;
E Younger siblings of an affected patient should be entered into a screening programme that involves examinations under anaesthesia.

10 Which of the following is *not* associated with direct blunt trauma to the eye?
A Posterior embryotoxon;
B Lens dislocation;
C Cataract;
D Retinal commotio;
E Hyphaema.

11 With regard to retinal haemorrhages after shaken-baby syndrome:
A Pre-retinal haemorrhages disappear most quickly;
B Intracranial bleeding always coexists;
C They may provide a clue as to the timing of injury;
D Superficial retinal haemorrhages disappear completely within 24 hours;
E Their pathogenesis is very well understood.

12 Which of the following is *not* associated with shaken-baby syndrome?
A Intraretinal haemorrhages;
B Perimacular folds;
C Subdural haemorrhage;
D Vitreous haemorrhage;
E Angioid streaks.

Chapter 10

1 Duane's retraction syndrome (DURS) is normally caused by:
A VIth cranial nerve palsy;
B Anomalous blood supply to the lateral rectus muscle;
C Aplasia of the VIth cranial nerve nucleus;
D Absent lateral rectus muscle;
E An acquired brainstem tumour.

2 Which of the following is *not* a feature of Moebius syndrome?
A Absence of pectoralis major muscle;
B Loss of corneal sensation;
C Corneal ulceration;
D Entropion;
E Hypermetropic astigmatism.

3 In the congenital fibrosis of extraocular muscle (CFEOM) syndromes:
A The replacement of striated muscle with fibrous collagenous tissue is characteristic;
B Surgery does not usually improve head posture;
C The forced duction test reveals normal passive movement of the eye;
D Squint surgery restores normal ocular movements;
E The condition shows relentless progression.

4 Which of the following statements concerning double elevator palsy (DEP) is correct?
A DEP is so-called because of the apparent paralysis of the upper eyelid levator palpebrae superioris muscle and the superior rectus muscle;
B The involved eye is always hypotropic;
C DEP is not compatible with normal binocular function;
D An absent Bell's phenomenon is a regular feature;
E Acquired DEP may be caused by a brain tumour.

5 Which of the following statements concerning neuromuscular disorders is correct?
A Transient congenital myasthenia gravis is caused by maternal transfer of antibodies to acetylcholine;
B Myotonic dystrophy is a mitochondrial disorder;
C All cases of congenital myasthenia resolve by 12 weeks;
D In CFEO muscle biopsy reveals fibrosis of the extraocular muscles;
E Progressive external ophthalmoplegia can be associated with heart defects.

6 Which of the following is true in anterior segment dysgenesis?
A The presence of posterior embryotoxon results in a 50 per cent risk of glaucoma;
B Rieger syndrome is associated with dental anomalies;
C Iridogoniodysgenesis anomaly results from mutations in the CYP1B1 gene;
D Axenfeld anomaly results in an abnormal pupil;
E Glaucoma does not develop until the end of the first decade.

7 Which of the following is true in Peter's anomaly?
A It is always unilateral;
B Cataract is not a feature;
C Surgical management is straightforwards;
D There is a defect in the posterior cornea;
E Glaucoma is not an associated feature.

8 In sclerocornea, which of the following is correct?
A The cornea is always totally opaque;
B Both eyes are usually affected symmetrically;
C Malformation syndromes may be associated;
D The cornea has a steep curvature;
E Visual behaviour of affected children is good.

9 Which of the following is true in primary trabecular dysgenesis (primary congenital glaucoma)?
A It is usually autosomal dominant in inheritance;
B Affected eyes typically exhibit high hypermetropia;
C Surgical success rates are poor;
D Corneal clouding is a feature;
E Anisometropia is uncommon.

10 Which of the following is true of aniridia?
A Only the anterior segment of the eye is affected;
B Glaucoma is rarely associated;
C If cataract occurs it is always an insignificant anterior polar opacity;
D The underlying gene defect is in PAX6;
E All affected children are at risk of Wilms' tumour.

11 Which of the following is true in microphthalmia and anophthalmia?
A The axial length of the eye is one standard deviation below (the mean of) age-matched normal eyes;
B In simple microphthalmia, only the anterior segment is abnormal;
C In anophthalmia there is always complete absence of ocular tissue;
D Microphthalmia may arise from a variety of genetic mechanisms;
E Coloboma is not associated with microphthalmia.

12 Which of the following statements concerning albinism is correct?
A Nystagmus worsens with age;
B The fovea is normal;
C Iris transillumination is unique to albinism;
D There are three main autosomal recessive forms of oculocutaneous albinism (OCA);
E Visual evoked potentials are unhelpful in making the diagnosis.

Chapter 11

1 Which of the following statements is *not* correct? Spectacle frames selected for children should:
A Ensure an anatomically correct fit;
B Place the lenses correctly in front of the eyes;
C Be comfortable, stable and not damage the forming nasal features;
D Not inhibit the natural development of the nasal structure;
E Be made using components designed for adult frames.

2 Which of the following statements is *not* correct? When comparing the main features of a spectacle frame designed for a child with one designed for an adult, the:
A Crest height is larger;
B Frontal angle is larger;
C Splay angle is larger;
D Frontal width is smaller;
E Angle of side is smaller.

3 With reference to the development of children's facial measurements, which of the following is *not* correct?
A Crest height becomes more negative with age;
B Bridge projection becomes more positive with age;
C Frontal angle reduces with age;
D Splay angle reduces with age;
E Head width increases with age.

4 With reference to children's facial measurements, which of the following statements is *not* correct?
A Children's faces do not grow at a steady rate;
B Children's facial structures differ in proportion from those of adults;
C A child's nose alters considerably during development;
D Only two dimensions remain practically unchanged – the angle of crest and the apical radius;
E The facial measurements of Afro-Caribbean children do not significantly differ from those of Caucasian children.

5 With reference to the facial measurements of children with Down's syndrome, which of the following statements is *not* correct?
A Down's syndrome children show a slight, but insignificant, increase in crest height with age;
B The bridge projection in Down's syndrome appears to increase with age;
C Children with Down's syndrome have frontal angles that are smaller than normal and splay angles that are larger than normal;
D Older Down's syndrome children have interpupillary distances that are smaller than normal;
E The head width of a Down's syndrome child is larger than normal in younger children, but smaller than normal in older children.

6 Which type of bridge is most suitable for an infant or toddler?
A A keyhole bridge;
B An adjustable pad bridge with large nose pads;
C A 'w' bridge;
D A regular bridge with a low crest height and a negative bridge projection;
E A regular bridge with a high crest height and a positive bridge projection.

7 With reference to spectacle frame measurements, which of the following statements is *not* correct?
A Crest height is defined as the distance, measured in the assumed spectacle plane, between the lower limbus and the nasal crest;
B The careful selection of crest height can be used to control the vertical position of a frame;
C Bridge projection is defined as the horizontal distance between the assumed spectacle plane and the eyelashes in their most projecting position;
D The careful selection of bridge projection can be used to control the horizontal position of a frame;
E Bridge height is synonymous with crest height.

8 With reference to the Comoframe, which of the following statements is *not* correct?
- A It can be used by older children to reduce the risk of facial and ocular trauma during sporting activities;
- B It can be used during the treatment of amblyopia by occlusion;
- C It can be used to correct infantile aphakia;
- D It is available as a trial frame for the refraction of young babies;
- E It is most suited for general paediatric dispensing.

9 With reference to polycarbonate, which of the following statements is *not* correct?
- A Polycarbonate has a high impact resistance;
- B Polycarbonate does not warp, chip or discolour with age;
- C Polycarbonate has a relatively high refractive index ($n_d = 1.586$) with a relatively high V-value ($V_d = 47$);
- D Polycarbonate is one of the lightest lens materials available;
- E Polycarbonate absorbs UV radiation below 380nm.

10 With reference to polycarbonate, which of the following statements is correct?
- A Compared with CR39 or glass, the surface quality of polycarbonate is excellent;
- B The V-value of polycarbonate is high and does not cause visual problems when viewing off-axis;
- C Polycarbonate has a scratch resistance equivalent to that of spectacle crown glass;
- D Surface coatings reduce the impact resistance of polycarbonate;
- E Polycarbonate has limited use in practice because it is available only in a white, single-vision form.

11 To achieve an appropriate fit a particular patient requires a frame with a 2° pantoscopic tilt. In primary gaze, the pupil centres correspond with a point 2mm above the horizontal centre line. The optical centres of the correcting lens should be placed:
- A 2mm above the horizontal centre line;
- B 1mm above the horizontal centre line;
- C On the horizontal centre line;
- D 1mm below the horizontal centre line;
- E 2mm below horizontal centre line.

12 Which of the following is correct. Specialist lenses are available for use in cases of:
- A Convergence weakness exophoria;
- B Accommodative esotropia;
- C Non-accommodative esotropia;
- D Hyperphoria;
- E Incyclophoria.

Chapter 12

1 Contact lenses should be fitted only if:
- A The child wants lenses;
- B The parents want the child to have lenses;
- C Slit-lamp examination can be carried out;
- D Combination of A and C;
- E Combination of B and C.

2 A child who wants contact lenses, but who is too nervous, can be helped towards wearing them by:
- A Telling them they look better in lenses;
- B Everting the eyelids;
- C Having the parent instil artificial tears for a few weeks;
- D Instilling drops in the practice;
- E Making a follow-up appointment many months ahead.

3 Which of the following is true?
- A Most children can be fitted with RGP lenses;
- B Children should not be fitted with RGP lenses;
- C It is inadvisable to use local anaesthetic drops when fitting children with RGP lenses;
- D RGP lenses should always be the first choice when fitting children;
- E RGP lenses are more uncomfortable for children than for adults.

4 Which of the following is correct?
- A An eye with unilateral ametropia always does well with a contact lens;
- B Orthokeratology works better on children under 10 years of age;
- C Fitting RGP lenses has been proved to retard myopia progression;
- D High myopes do well with lenses because the image becomes magnified.
- E Patching always improves the vision in a unilaterally hypermetropic eye.

5 Which is correct?
- A Aphakes have better acuity in spectacles;
- B Aphakes have better acuity in contact lenses;
- C Aphakes have a wider field of vision in spectacles;
- D Combination of A and C;
- E Combination of B and C.

6 Contact lenses may need to be fitted together with IOLs in infants because:
- A Bifocal IOLs are not yet available;
- B The IOL may decentre in infants;
- C There is post-operative astigmatism;
- D The power of the IOL is initially too high;
- E The power of the IOL is initially too low.

7 Which of the following is incorrect about silicone rubber lenses?
- A The first trial lens should be 0.2mm steeper than K;
- B The first trial lens should be approximately 0.7mm more than horizontal visible iris diameter (HVID);
- C They have very high oxygen permeability;
- D They are useful in children with dry eyes;
- E They cannot be made with an ultraviolet inhibitor.

8 Which of the following is correct about RGP lenses in infants?
- A They should be fitted with increased edge clearance;
- B They should not be fitted if the lids are squeezed tightly;
- C They should be fitted 3mm smaller than HVID;
- D They should only be fitted under a general anaesthetic;
- E They cannot be made with an ultraviolet inhibitor.

9 Which of the following is incorrect?
A Children with nystagmus have difficulty seeing with RGP lenses;
B Patients with Marfan's syndrome have flat corneas;
C Lenses that fit a microphthalmic aphakic infant may fit an adult microphthalmic aphake;
D Nanophthalmic eyes can have prescriptions of more than +20DS;
E Buphthalmic eyes tend to be more sensitive than normal.

10 Which of the following is correct?
A Tinted lenses help congenital aniridics to see better;
B Albinos always see better if their astigmatism is corrected;
C Cosmetic iris lenses improve the cosmesis in cases of unilateral coloboma;
D Reducing the amount of light that enters the eye improves the visual acuity in albinos;
E Patients with achromatopsia always see better with a red tint.

11 Aphakic patients cannot be fitted with silicone hydrogel lenses because:
A They are too expensive;
B The material is too rigid;
C They are not manufactured in the necessary parameters;
D They need replacing too often;
E They do not correct enough astigmatism.

12 Which of the following is *not* true?
A Microphthalmic corneas show worst neovascularisation;
B Lipid leakage can lead to amblyopia in a young eye;
C Aphakic eyes should have their intraocular pressure checked regularly;
D As the aphakic eye grows, the contact lens radius increases and the power decreases.
E Infants have a high blink rate.

Chapter 13

1 Blind and partially sighted registration statistics for the UK are compiled from data supplied by which of the following organisations?
A WHO;
B DoH;
C Local authority social services departments;
D Local Education Authorities;
E RNIB.

2 The proportion of children on school rolls in England with statements of special educational need (SEN) is approximately:
A 0.31 per cent;
B 3.1 per cent;
C 20 per cent;
D 31 per cent;
E 60 per cent.

3 Specialist support services for the schooling of children with visual impairment (VI) are usually arranged by:
A A general practitioner;
B An orthoptist;
C An ophthalmologist;
D A qualified teacher of the visually impaired (QTVI);
E A school nurse.

4 Which of the following statements about the low vision assessment of a child with VI is false?
A Assessment of accommodative function is important;
B Assessment of reading function with words or sentences on a log scale is preferable;
C Assessment of refraction is rarely helpful, since most children with VI are emmetropic;
D Assessment of binocular status can be valuable;
E Assessment of contrast sensitivity (CS) can help predict 'real world' functioning.

5 Which of the following statements about the 'Hiding Heidi' test is false?
A The response to the test can be either verbal, pointing or based on preferential looking;
B The test measures chromatic CS;
C Contrast levels on the cards are 1.25 per cent, 2.5 per cent, 5 per cent, 25 per cent, 50 per cent and about 100 per cent;
D The test employs a low-contrast face stimulus;
E The test may be used on younger children or in cases where comprehension for a letter-based CS test is difficult.

6 For the fluent reading of text with a print size of N10, a child is likely to require a minimum near visual acuity threshold of:
A N5;
B N6;
C N8;
D N10;
E N20.

7 Which of the following statements about magnification devices to help with reading in childhood VI is false?
A When using a stand magnifier, high emergent vergence is often necessary;
B A wide range of magnification is available with stand magnifiers;
C When prescribing a high reading addition, the estimated add equals the working distance (in dioptres) minus half the amplitude of accommodation;
D When dispensing a reading addition in bifocal format, the segment should usually be placed at the lower pupil margin;
E The limited magnification provided by bar and bright-field magnifiers makes these devices unsuitable in most instances.

8 Which of the following statements about telescopic devices is false?
A A spectacle-mounted full-field telescope may be useful for copying from the blackboard;
B A handheld telescope may assist an older child with independent travel;
C Binoculars are often easier for a younger child to handle;
D A bioptic telescope offers the potential for both distance spotting with magnification and unmagnified orientation through the spectacle carrier lens;
E Telescopes are sometimes rejected in the classroom because they are considered too conspicuous.

9 Adaptations in the classroom that may be of value to a child with VI include which of the following?
A A reading stand or angled desk;
B Large print;
C Local task lighting;
D Black felt tip pens for writing;
E All of the above.

10 A CCTV or other electronic aid for a child with VI is most likely to be funded by which one of the following organisations?
A The Local Social Services Department;
B The Local Education Authority (LEA);
C National or local charities;
D Employment Services;
E Hospital Eye Service.

11 Which of the following statements about prescribing a tint for a child with VI is false?
A A tint of about 15 per cent light transmission factor (LTF) removes the presence of discomfort glare in most cases;
B A tint with selective short-wavelength attenuation can be useful in selected cases;
C A red-free green tint is helpful in children with cone dystrophy;
D The Corning CPF photochromic lenses are yellow, amber or red in colour;
E Transitions photochromic lenses can be used in selected cases.

12 With respect to the provision of reports after a paediatric low vision assessment, which of the following is false?
A The content of the report should include details on visual function;
B The report should try to link visual function to relevant examples of functional vision;
C The qualified teacher of the visually impaired should receive a copy of the report;
D Consent to release patient information is not required where a child is under 16 years of age;
E The report should make recommendations on the use of spectacles and low vision devices, adaptive equipment, lighting and glare control.

Chapter 14

1 Which of the following conditions has been identified by the National Screening Committee (NSC) as having the potential to cause severe vision defect?
A Strabismus;
B Glaucoma;
C Anisometropia;
D Astigmatism;
E Myopia.

2 The aim of the neonatal fundus screen in premature and babies with low birth weight is to detect retinopathy of prematurity (ROP) at which stage?
A Stage one;
B Stage two;
C Stage three;
D Stage four;
E Stage five.

3 Before what pre-term age do babies automatically qualify for ROP screen?
A 26 weeks;
B 29 weeks;
C 30 weeks;
D 31 weeks;
E 36 weeks.

4 The NSC recommends that examination of red reflex should be undertaken perinatally before what age?
A 4 weeks;
B 5 weeks;
C 7 weeks;
D 8 weeks;
E 11 weeks.

The correct answer is C. The NSC have recommended red-reflex assessment before 7 weeks, together with an assessment of visual behaviour and detection of squint.

5 Absence of red reflex may indicate the presence of:
A Congenital cataract;
B Strabismus;
C Amblyopia;
D Keratoconus;
E Microphthalmia.

6 Congenital cataracts occur in:
A 1 in 1000–2000 births;
B 1 in 4000 births;
C 1 in 8000 births;
D 1 in 9000 births;
E 1 in 10,000 births.

7 Sure Start is the government initiative to:
A Provide new health centres;
B Introduce new premises for screening programmes;
C Integrate health education and family support;
D Introduce localised screening programmes;
E Expand vision screening within schools.

8 The NSC recommends that the only screening to be carried out before the age of 4 years should be that for:

A Media opacities and ROP;
B Glaucoma and media opacities;
C Media opacities and amblyopia;
D Amblyopia;
E Strabismus.

9 The advantage of school entry screening is:

A The potential for 100 per cent coverage;
B All children can read by this age;
C School nurses can perform the screen;
D It is the ideal age to detect media opacities;
E Parents comply fully with any advice based on findings.

10 LogMAR-based vision tests are preferential to Snellen-based tests because:

A Pre-literate children can perform the test;
B The test is portable;
C The scoring system has linear progression;
D They are cheaper;
E They measure CS function.

11 What percentage of boys have red–green colour vision deficiency?

A 0.5 per cent;
B 5 per cent;
C 8 per cent;
D 0.002 per cent;
E 20 per cent.

12 One of the benefits of the identification of colour vision deficit is:

A Appropriate career choice advice;
B Early detection permits early treatment;
C Use of coloured overlays may assist reading;
D Warning of a future inability to drive;
E Identifies the need for special training.

Chapter 15

1 According to the Denver Developmental Screening Test, a child might be expected to respond to voices from others by what age?

A From birth;
B At 3 months of age;
C At 5–6 months of age;
D At 12 months of age;
E At 24 months of age.

2 Most researchers believe a child to be capable of using two or more related words by what age?

A At 3 months of age;
B At 6 months of age;
C At 12 months of age;
D At 20–24 months of age;
E At 36 months of age.

3 Which of the following communication development milestones is least reliant on visual input?

A Interpersonal communication;
B Response to aural cues;
C Group interaction;
D Distance correspondence;
E Orientation relative to another.

4 Which of the following behaviours may indicate the need for assessment by a speech-language specialist?

A Lack of response to others talking by 1 month of age;
B Inability to follow simple instructions by 10 months of age;
C Inability to understand simple questions by 12 months of age;
D Inability to use simple sentences by 3 years of age;
E Inability to be understood by a stranger at 12 months of age.

5 The percentage of early learning estimated to be based upon visual input is what?

A 10–20 per cent;
B 20–40 per cent;
C 50–60 per cent;
D 60–80 per cent;
E 80–90 per cent.

6 Which of the following statements concerning eidetic imagery is correct?

A It is a result of progressive semantic-processing development;
B It is most likely found in adults;
C It is exclusive to autistic children;
D It becomes less significant as semantic processing develops;
E It is related to the concentration of photoreceptors in the retina.

7 Which of the following might be inappropriate to establishing the best environmental orientation for a child patient?

A Informal surroundings;
B Greeting before entering the consulting room;
C A white coat;
D Use of new equipment, provided it is introduced appropriately;
E Slow and fluent movement.

8 Which of the following actions might *not* be appropriate when examining an 8-month-old patient?

A Addressing the child as well as the parent;
B Lots of music and bright pictures to relax the child;
C Keeping individual procedures as brief as possible;
D Making the appointment outside a natural feeding time;
E Gathering information from a parent or guardian prior to the consultation.

9 'Stranger fear' is classically associated with which age group?

A Birth to 9 months of age;
B 9 months to 3 years of age;
C 3–5 years of age;
D 5–11 years of age;
E 11–18 years of age.

10 A parent wishes to know the outcome of an assessment of their 17-year-old daughter. Which of the following is correct?

A Until 18 years of age a parent has full access to child health records;
B A child has no rights under the Data Protection Act;
C After his or her 16th birthday, the patient needs to give consent for details of the examination to be passed on;
D A parent has no access to their children's medical records;
E The parent needs to consult the general practitioner for permission.

11 Pronoun confusion and excessive questioning may be a result of what?

A Excessive questions by carers earlier in life;
B An inability to cope with impairment;
C A signal of mental instability;
D A result of previous assessment being not detailed enough;
E A sign of poor vision.

12 Which specialised language might be most appropriate for a deaf–blind child?

A British Sign Language;
B Paget;
C Makaton;
D Lip-reading;
E Hands-on signing.

Multiple Choice Answers

For convenience, the questions are repeated here.

Chapter 1

1 Which of the following is *not* a function that can be measured with a visual evoked potential (VEP) technique?

A Visual acuity;
B Contrast sensitivity;
C Stereopsis;
D Convergence;
E Colour vision.

The correct answer is D. VEP technique has been used extensively to assess vision development in infants. Results have been reported for all functions except convergence.

2 How long does complete myelination of the nerve fibres take in the normal infant?

A 4–6 months;
B 2 years;
C 1 year;
D 4 years;
E 9 months.

The correct answer is B. The myelination of the visual pathway is not complete until around 2 years of age, and prior to that neural transmission may be impaired, which in turn limits visual acuity and contrast sensitivity.

3 Which value is a generally accepted estimate of visual acuity at 6 months of age?

A 1 cycle per degree (cpd);
B 2–5cpd;
C 6cpd;
D 12cpd;
E 18cpd.

The correct answer is C. In their widely quoted paper, Banks and Salapatek (1978; see Chapter 1 references for full details) give the value of visual acuity as 6cpd at 6 months of age.

4 The young infant does not control accommodation accurately because of:

A A lack of sensory stimulus as a result of a large depth of focus;
B Immaturity of the ciliary muscle;
C A lack of ability to converge;
D Poor contrast sensitivity;
E The presence of hypermetropia.

The correct answer is A. Any small errors in accommodation can be tolerated by the small infant eye because the depth of focus alleviates the need for accuracy.

5 Which of the following functions is present at birth?

A Stereopsis;
B Vertical saccades;
C Vestibulo-ocular reflex;
D Accommodation;
E Trichromacy.

The correct answer is C. The vestibulo-ocular reflex is present at birth.

6 At 6 months of age in the normal infant, which of the following has matured to adult levels?

A Visual acuity measured by preferential looking;
B myelination of the nerve fibres;
C Astigmatism;
D Smooth pursuit movements;
E Contrast sensitivity measured by VEP.

The correct answer is D. Smooth pursuit movements mature to adult levels by 6 months of age. All the other functions have a longer developmental period.

7 The cones in the newborn infant retina are thought to limit visual acuity because they are:

A Packed too closely together;
B Too narrow;
C Too long;
D Not closely packed together;
E Absent.

The correct answer is D. The infant cones are shorter, broader and less densely packed in a lattice than are the adult cones.

8 At 2 months of age an infant:

A Has no colour perception;
B Has gross fusion;
C Demonstrates monocular OKN to a temporal-ward stimulus;
D Can accurately follow a fast-moving target with smooth movements;
E Can discriminate between red and green.

The correct answer is E. Infants can demonstrate colour discrimination (i.e., dichromacy) at 2 months of age.

9 Emmetropisation is thought to occur because of:

A Passive growth of the eye;
B Spectacle correction of refractive error;
C An active feedback mechanism;
D Combination of A and B;
E Combination of A and C.

The correct answer is E. Emmetropisation is thought to occur as a result of two processes, an active feedback mechanism that 'guides' the refractive state and a passive genetically predetermined process of normal eye growth.

10 Children with strabismus tend to:

A Develop myopia;
B Develop increasing hypermetropia;
C Show emmetropisation;
D Initially become myopic, and then emmetropise;
E Initially become hyperopic, and then emmetropise.

The correct answer is C. Research has shown that children who develop strabismus demonstrate either increasing hypermetropia or no change in refractive error.

11 Most children are born with:

A 1.00D of against-the-rule astigmatism that shifts to with-the-rule after 5 years;
B No astigmatism that increases to 1.00D against-the-rule by 5 years;
C 1.00D with-the-rule astigmatism that changes to against-the-rule by 5 years;
D 1.00D against-the-rule astigmatism that remains unchanged by 5 years;
E 1.00D with-the-rule astigmatism that decreases to no astigmatism by 5 years.

The correct answer is A. The mean value of 1.00D against-the-rule astigmatism at birth shifts to a prevalence of with-the-rule astigmatism after 5 years.

12 Visual acuity measured with VEP first reaches adult values by:

A 2–3 months;
B 6–8 months;
C 12 months;
D 18 months;
E 3 years.

The correct answer is B. Visual acuity measured by VEP has a faster maturation than preferential looking visual acuity, and reaches adult values at 6–8 months.

Chapter 2

1 Which statement is correct? Congenital myopia is:

A The most common aetiology of myopia;
B More common than congenital high hyperopia;
C More likely to occur in premature infants with retinopathy of prematurity (ROP) than those without it;
D Likely to regress;
E Often associated with esophoria.

The correct answer is C. The incidence of congenital myopia is greatest in premature children with ROP.

2 Which of the following statements is true?

A There is no association between increased incidence of astigmatism and prematurity;
B Less than 10 per cent of children aged between 6 and 15 years of age are myopic;
C Exophoria is a risk factor in the development of juvenile myopia;
D In most ethnic groups twice as many girls than boys are born myopic;
E Juvenile myopia is more common than congenital myopia in developing countries.

The correct answer is D. Girls are twice as likely as boys to be born myopic. Prematurity is associated with an increased incidence of astigmatism, 15–30 per cent of children of age 6–15 years are myopic, esophoria is a risk factor in the development of juvenile myopia and congenital myopia is more common than juvenile myopia in developing countries.

3 Prematurity has *not* been shown to be associated with:

A Increased incidence of myopia;
B Increased incidence of astigmatism;
C Increased incidence of strabismus;
D Maternal alcohol use during pregnancy;
E Albinism.

The correct answer is E. Prematurity has not been shown to be associated to albinism.

4 Which of the following statements is true:

A Idiopathic nystagmus is often associated with high astigmatism;
B Strabismus affects 1 per cent of children;
C Congenital exotropia has an increased incidence in premature infants;
D Albinos are just as likely to have strabismus as other children;
E Congenital cortical cataracts usually require surgery.

The correct answer is A. Strabismus affects between 3 and 5 per cent of children, congenital esotropia is more common in premature infants, strabismus is much more common in albinos and congenital cortical cataracts do not normally affect vision significantly.

5 Which of the following is *not* a risk factor for the development of amblyopia:

A Strabismus;
B High astigmatism;
C Unilateral congenital cataract;

D Marked ptosis;
E Optic disc drusen.

The correct answer is E. Optic disc drusen is not a risk factor for the development of amblyopia.

6 Which of the following is *not* a common aetiology of congenital cataract:
A Rubella;
B Retinoblastoma;
C Heredity;
D Steroid use in pregnancy;
E Down's syndrome.

The correct answer is B. Retinoblastoma is not a common aetiology of congenital cataract.

7 Which of the following statements is true?
A Retinoblastoma occurs in 0.5 per cent of children;
B There is no genetic link in retinoblastoma;
C Congenital toxoplasmosis does not have systemic effects;
D Toxoplasmosis occurs through infestation with the intestinal roundworm of cats and dogs;
E Retinopathy of prematurity may lead to retinal detachment.

The correct answer is E. Retinoblastoma occurs in 0.005 per cent of children and 6 per cent of all cases have a positive family history. Congenital toxoplasmosis may be associated with severe brain damage or convulsions. Toxocariasis is caused by infestation with the intestinal roundworm of cats and dogs.

8 Which of the following statements is *not* true?
A Epicanthus is associated with squints;
B Duane's retraction syndrome is caused by an intraocular muscle malinsertion;
C A chorioretinal scar at the macula may lead to strabismus;
D Blepharitis in children most commonly results from *Staphylococcus aureus* infection;
E Cleft palate is associated with an increased incidence of optic disc anomalies.

The correct answer is A. Epicanthus is associated with pseudosquints.

9 Which of the following statements is *not* true?
A Around 5–8 per cent of males have a colour vision anomaly;
B A female can have an X-linked colour vision defect only if her father and his father both also have the same;
C A protanope may confuse red with black or dark brown;
D A deuteranope may confuse green with red or orange;
E About 4–5 per cent of all boys have deuteranomolous trichromacy.

The correct answer is B. A female can only be colour defective if both her father and her mother's father are also colour defective.

10 Which of the following is *not* true of anomalous trichromats?
A They may pass the City University Colour Vision Test;
B They may have problems entering certain professions;
C They will match any red–green mix with yellow on a Nagel anomaloscope;
D They account for the majority of hereditary colour vision defects;
E They affect less than 1 per cent of females.

The correct answer is C. Only total protanopes and deuteranopes match any red–green mix with yellow.

11 Which of the following is true of blue (tritan) colour-vision defects?
A They are more likely to be inherited than acquired;
B Inherited tritan defects are sex linked;
C The incidence of inherited tritan defects is around 0.005 per cent;
D Acquired defects occur most often through congenital cataract;
E They are the most severe form of colour-vision defect.

The correct answer is C. With an incidence of 0.005 per cent, tritan defects are rarely inherited.

12 Which statement is true?
A The City University Test is the most sensitive colour-vision test;
B The City University Test has been shown to differentiate between the two types of dichromacy more effectively than the Ishihara Test;
C Ishihara plates with paths of dots to trace have been shown to be very effective;
D The first plate in the Ishihara Test identifies dichromats;
E The Nagel anomaloscope is the most commonly used colour-vision test in clinical practice.

The correct answer is B. The City University Test is more effective than the Ishihara Test at differentiating between the two types of dichromats, but it is not as sensitive to anomalous trichromacy. The first plate in the Ishihara Test should be seen by all who are tested.

Chapter 3

1 The repeatability of an acuity test:
A Relates to how long the test takes to perform;
B Reflects how complex a measure of acuity it is;
C Is only relevant in preferential looking tests;
D Reflects how variable the results it produces are;
E Is only relevant in letter-matching tests.

The correct answer is D. Repeatability relates to the variability of a measurement technique.

2 The most useful test in optometric practice with which to assess the visual acuity of young infants is:
A Preferential looking;
B Visual evoked potentials (VEPs);
C Letter matching;
D Picture naming;
E Stycar balls.

The correct answer is A. Infants can be assessed using either preferential looking or VEPs, but VEP techniques are not generally available in optometric practice.

3 Which of the following statements is *not* true? Persistent interocular acuity differences:
A Are unlikely to affect normal visual development;
B Can be detected by monocular acuity testing;
C Are not the norm in childhood;
D May be the result of uncorrected anisometropia;
E Should be investigated further.

The correct answer is A. Interocular acuity differences are not normal and impair normal visual development, as the eye with poorer vision becomes amblyopic if not treated appropriately.

4 Which of the following statements is *not* true? Visual acuity (VA) maturation occurs as a result of:
A Maturation in size and shape of photoreceptors;
B Development of cortical connections and processes;
C Improved control of eye movements and accommodation;
D Increase in pupil size;
E Improved organisation of photoreceptors.

The correct answer is D. If pupil size increases it is more likely to make VA worse, but it changes little in the period during which VA matures most rapidly. The other options are all true.

5 VEPs provide:
A A subjective test of resolution acuity;
B An objective test of resolution acuity;
C A subjective test of recognition acuity;
D An objective test of recognition acuity;
E An objective test of detection acuity.

The correct answer is B. VEPs are objective and the stimuli used are grating or checkerboard resolution acuity tests. A subjective test involves the subject telling the examiner what he or she can see, or matching the stimulus to a key card.

6 Resolution acuity tests should only be used in preference to recognition acuity tests when:
A A child is intellectually or physically unable to perform a recognition test;
B A child has strabismic amblyopia;
C A child is not able to name letters or pictures;
D A child has a visual impairment;
E A 'crowded' acuity is required.

The correct answer is A. Resolution acuity tests are less sensitive than recognition tests. They tend to overestimate acuity in visual impairment and in strabismic amblyopia. If a child cannot name letters, then he or she may be able to letter match, but very young children and infants do not have the intellectual or physical ability to do this. Resolution tests do not provide a crowded acuity.

7 Which of the following is *not* a recognition acuity test?
A LH symbols;
B Kay picture test;
C Cardiff acuity test;
D Sonksen–Silver acuity system;
E Illiterate E.

The correct answer is C. The Cardiff acuity test is a preferential looking test that estimates resolution acuity.

8 Which of the following is *not* a resolution acuity test?
A Keeler acuity system;
B LH symbols;
C Cardiff acuity test;
D VEP test;
E Teller acuity cards.

The correct answer is B. The LH symbols are a naming or matching recognition test.

9 Near VA is affected by accommodative function. Considering this association, which of the following statements is *not* true?
A A child's near VA can be assessed using the near Kay picture test;
B Accommodative function is usually ample in childhood;
C Accommodation in childhood may be reduced by neurological impairment;
D Children with visual impairment may have reduced accommodative function;
E Children's near VA can only be assessed when they are able to read.

The correct answer is E. Letter- and picture-matching tests are available for near vision testing so children can be assessed before they are able to read.

10 A significant difference in acuity as measured by the LogMAR acuity test is:
A One letter;
B Two letters;
C Three letters;
D Four letters;
E 0.05 logMAR.

The correct answer is D. Four letters (0.1 LogMAR) is a significant difference. Smaller differences may be ascribed to variability in test–retest measurements rather than to a real difference in acuity measures.

11 The LogMAR acuity test provides:
A Uncrowded measures of recognition acuity only;
B Uncrowded measures of resolution acuity only;
C Crowded measures of recognition acuity only;
D Uncrowded and crowded measures of recognition acuity;
E Uncrowded and crowded measures of resolution acuity.

The correct answer is D. The LogMAR acuity test is a letter-matching acuity test that comes in both crowded and isolated letter formats, and thus enables uncrowded and crowded measures of recognition acuity.

12 According to Salt *et al.* (1995; see Chapter 3 references for full details), adult levels of acuity (6/6) may not be measured by letter-naming or -matching tests until:
A 2 years of age;
B 3 years of age;
C 4 years of age;
D 5 years of age;
E 6 years of age or older.

The correct answer is E. Testing a large group of children with the Sonksen–Silver letter matching test, measured acuities of 6/6 were only achieved by 90 per cent of children when they were aged 6 years or older.

Chapter 4

1 Which of the following is *not* true? Accommodation should be relaxed in the following techniques:
- A Static retinoscopy;
- B Cycloplegic retinoscopy;
- C Dynamic retinoscopy;
- D The Mohindra technique;
- E Autorefractor use.

The correct answer is C. Dynamic retinoscopy requires the accommodation to be in an active state, by use of a near target, so its effectiveness can be measured.

2 Which of the following combinations would be suitable to use on a 3-year-old child undergoing his or her first cycloplegic refraction?
- A One drop 0.5 per cent proxymetacaine followed, after 5 minutes, by one drop 1 per cent cyclopentalate;
- B One drop 0.5 per cent cyclopentalate;
- C Two drops 1 per cent tropicamide instilled at 5 minute intervals;
- D 1 per cent atropine instilled twice a day for 3 days prior to examination;
- E Two drops 0.5 per cent cyclopentalate instilled immediately after each other.

The correct answer is A. 0.5 per cent cyclopentalate and 1 per cent tropicamide do not produce adequate cycloplegia in a 3-year-old child, while the use of atropine is only advised if 1 per cent cyclopentalate does not produce satisfactory cycloplegia. Use of a local anaesthetic prior to the instillation of cyclopentalate can help reduce the stinging felt.

3 Which of the following statements is *not* true?
- A Atropine should not be used in infants under the age of 3 months;
- B A tonus allowance is not needed when atropine is used;
- C Atropine is a muscarinic antagonist;
- D Use of atropine can produce mydriasis that lasts for up to a fortnight;
- E Use of atropine can cause a reduction in the effectiveness of a patient's sweat glands.

The correct answer is B. A tonus allowance of the order of 1DS is needed when atropine is used, as use of this drug completely abolishes the tonus of the ciliary muscle.

4 Which statement is true?
- A A typical dynamic lag of accommodation can be 1.50D;
- B Residual accommodation with the use of cyclopentalate is typically 2D;
- C When performing a cycloplegic examination, retinoscopy should not commence until the accommodation has fallen below 2D;
- D If the Mohindra technique is used, a 2D allowance must be made to account for the 50cm working distance;
- E An allowance must be made for the working distance when performing dynamic retinoscopy.

The correct answer is C. For cycloplegic refraction results to be the most accurate, maximum cycloplegia for the drug used must be reached before retinoscopy takes place.

5 Which of the following is *not* advisable when refracting an infant under 3 months of age?
- A The Mohindra technique;
- B A 'ret' or lens rack;
- C Dynamic retinoscopy;
- D Performing retinoscopy while the child is asleep;
- E A cycloplegic refraction using 1 per cent tropicamide.

The correct answer is E. 1 per cent tropicamide is only thought to produce adequate cycloplegia in patients in their late teens or older.

6 Giving a prescription is necessary:
- A If anisometropia is 0.50DS;
- B If astigmatism of 1.50DC is found in a child 12 months of age;
- C In a 1-year-old child whose prescription is R –0.75DS, L –0.75DS;
- D In an accommodative esotrope of age 2.5 years;
- E If a dynamic lag of accommodation of 1D is found.

The correct answer is D. The full hypermetropic correction necessary to keep the child straight should be given in the case of an accommodative esotrope.

7 Dynamic retinoscopy:
- A Measures refractive error;
- B Can highlight the presence of astigmatism;
- C Should be performed monocularly;
- D Must be performed from a fixed working distance;
- E Uses an accommodative target at 6m.

The correct answer is B. Dynamic retinoscopy assesses the lag of accommodation, binocularly, using an accommodative target at the child's working distance. If the lag of accommodation is different in the two meridians, it can indicate the presence of accommodation.

8 Which statement is *not* true? When accommodation takes place:
- A The ciliary muscle contracts;
- B The lens becomes more convex;
- C The ciliary muscle has been stimulated by acetylcholine;
- D The tonus of the ciliary muscle alters;
- E The focus point of the eye may 'lag' behind the position of the object of interest.

The correct answer is D. The tonus level remains the same whether or not accommodation takes place.

9 Instilling a cycloplegic agent:
- A Can help a practitioner to perform the Mohindra technique;
- B Can be facilitated by the use of a local anaesthetic;
- C Can produce miosis, which lasts longer than the cycloplegia;

D Always leaves a small amount of residual accommodation;
E Results in an increase in the power of the crystalline lens.

The correct answer is B. Use of proxymetacaine 0.5 per cent can help reduce the stinging when a cycloplegic drug is instilled subsequently.

10 Which of the following is *not* true? The Mohindra technique:
A Works better in scotopic conditions;
B Works better monocularly;
C Requires a known level of accommodation to be present;
D Can induce myopia;
E Can be performed while the infant is feeding.

The correct answer is C. It is thought that by performing the Mohindra technique monocularly, in the dark, the accommodation is relaxed, but it is not known by exactly how much.

11 Tonic accommodation:
A Is not thought to be dependent on refractive error;
B Is abolished by the use of 1 per cent cyclopentalate;
C Must be assumed to be the level of accommodation present for the results of the Mohindra technique to be reliable;
D Is about 2.50D;
E Cannot be abolished fully.

The correct answer is C. Tonic accommodation (about 1.00DS) can be abolished fully by the use of atropine. It is assumed that the relaxed level of accommodation reached with the Mohindra technique allows reliable retinoscopic results to be calculated.

12 Which of the following is *not* true? Anisometropia:
A May not be permanent if demonstrated at birth;
B May be found to be of different amounts when a cycloplegic is used, compared with when a cycloplegic is not used;
C Should always be corrected fully in cases where a correction is deemed clinically necessary;
D Is only significant at levels of over 1.50DS;
E Is of less concern in myopic children.

The correct answer is D. 1.00DS of anisometropia can be clinically significant, particularly in hypermetropic children.

Chapter 5

1 Which statement is true?
A Myopia has a high prevalence in all Asian populations;
B The prevalence of myopia is greater in Caucasian than in Chinese populations;
C The prevalence of myopia in Eskimos increased by over 50 per cent in one generation;
D Both A and C;
E Both A and B.

The correct answer is C. The prevalence of myopia is greater in Chinese than in Caucasian populations. Tibet and Melanesia have much lower prevalences of myopia than Hong Kong, Japan and Taiwan. After the introduction of a 'westernised' lifestyle, the prevalence of myopia in Eskimos increased by over 50 per cent in one generation.

2 The prevalence of myopia in Caucasian children at 6 years of age is approximately:
A 30 per cent;
B 6 per cent;
C 15 per cent;
D 25 per cent;
E 2 per cent.

The correct answer is B. In Caucasian children the prevalence of myopia at 6 years of age is approximately 6 per cent. In Chinese 6-year-old children the prevalence is around 30 per cent.

3 The odds ratio for developing myopia if both parents are myopic is:
A 3;
B 2;
C 4;
D 6;
E 8.

The correct answer is D. The odds ratio for developing myopia if both parents are myopic has been reported as between 5 and 7.3.

4 The heritability of refractive error has been reported to be:
A 0.25;
B 0.33;
C 0.82;
D 0.73;
E 0.50.

The correct answer is C. The heritability of refractive error has been reported to be 0.82 or greater.

5 Which of the following is false? Myopia has been found to have an association with:
A Parental history of myopia;
B Higher intelligence levels;
C Increased use of visual display units;
D Chinese race;
E Occupation.

The correct answer is C. Increased use of visual display units has been associated with asthenopia symptoms, but not with myopia.

6 Which of the following is *not* true? Juvenile onset myopia is:
A Correlated with an increase in axial length;
B Correlated with a steeper cornea;
C The most common aetiology of myopia;
D Likely to progress;
E Likely to have a parental history of myopia.

The correct answer is B. Juvenile-onset myopia is correlated with an increase in axial length. The cornea does not change significantly with the development of myopia.

7 Which of the following is *not* associated with high myopia?
A Down's syndrome;
B Congenital stationary night blindness;
C Microspherophakia;
D Stickler's syndrome;
E Diabetes.

The correct answer is E. Diabetes is not known to be associated with high myopia. All the other conditions are associated with high myopia.

8 Which statement regarding use of bifocal or multifocal spectacle lenses in reduction of myopia progression is true:
A The rationale for using bifocal or multifocal lenses stems from myopes who have an increased lag of accommodation during near work;
B The use of bifocal or multifocal lenses results in reduction of retinal blur at near;
C The use of bifocal or multifocal lenses results in reduction of accommodative demand;
D Combination of A and C;
E Combination of A, B and C.

The correct answer is E. Bifocal or multifocal spectacle lenses reduce retinal blur at near and reduce accommodative demand. Myopes have been found to have an increased lag of accommodation during near work.

9 The COMET study is investigating the reduction of myopia progression with:
A Contact lenses;
B Bifocal spectacle lenses;
C Multifocal spectacle lenses;
D Pirenzepine;
E Atropine.

The correct answer is C. The COMET study is the Correction of Myopia Evaluation Trial and is investigating the reduction of myopia progression with multifocal spectacle lenses.

10 Antimuscarinics are believed to reduce myopia progression by:
A Reducing the accommodative demand;
B Their action on the ciliary muscle and iris;
C Their action on M1 receptors in the retina;
D Their action on M4 receptors in the retina;
E All of the above.

The correct answer is C. The finding that myopia progression is reduced with pirenzepine, a relatively selective M1 antimuscarinic, suggests that myopia progression is mediated via the M1 receptor in the retina.

11 The CLAMP study is investigating the reduction of myopia progression with:
A Contact lenses;
B Bifocal lenses;
C Multifocal spectacle lenses;
D Pirenzepine;
E Atropine.

The correct answer is A. The CLAMP study is the Contact Lens and Myopia Progression study and is investigating the reduction of myopia progression with rigid gas-permeable contact lenses.

12 Interventions to reduce myopia progression in humans have included:
A Timolol;
B Atropine;
C Contact lenses;
D Multifocal spectacle lenses;
E All of the above.

The correct answer is E. Timolol, atropine, contact lenses and multifocal lenses have all been investigated as a possible intervention for myopia progression.

Chapter 6

1 What is the percentage volume of the eye at birth with respect to its adult value?
A 25 per cent;
B 40 per cent;
C 50 per cent;
D 75 per cent;
E 100 per cent.

The correct answer is C. The eye at birth is 70 per cent the axial length of the adult eye, but only 50 per cent its volume.

2 In humans, ocular dominance columns are thought to develop over what period in early life?
A 6 years;
B 6 months;
C 6 days;
D 6 weeks;
E Fully developed at birth.

The correct answer is B. The ocular dominance columns are thought to develop over 6 weeks in cats, which is considered to be the equivalent of 6 months in humans.

3 Smooth pursuit and head tracking are known to reach full maturity by:
A 6 months;
B 6 weeks;
C 2 months;
D 5 months;
E None of the above.

The correct answer is E. Smooth pursuit and head-tracking movements are thought not to have reached maturity by 6 months.

4 Stereoacuity has been shown to improve up to what age?
A 6 months;
B 6 years;
C 5 years;
D 18 years;
E No improvement seen from levels at birth.

The correct answer is C. Subtle improvements in stereoacuity have been reported up to 5 years of age.

5 Heterotropia caused by unilateral blindness in an adult is most likely to be:
A Exotropia;
B Esotropia;
C Cyclotropia;
D Both A and B;
E Hypertropia.

The correct answer is A. Monocular blindness in late childhood or adulthood is likely to result in an exotropia.

6 A wide interpupillary distance tends towards which phoria?
A Exophoria;
B Esophoria;
C Cyclophoria;
D Hypophoria;
E Hyperphoria.

The correct answer is A. Wide interpupillary distances may predispose towards exophoria.

7 The most likely explanation for Duane's retraction syndrome is:
A Thickening of the lateral rectus muscle;
B Fibrosis of the lateral rectus muscle tendon;
C Abnormal connection between the facial nerve and the lateral rectus;
D Sixth nerve palsy;
E Abnormal misdirection of a branch of the third nerve that supplies the medial rectus to the lateral rectus.

The correct answer is E. Neurological misdirection is now the favoured theory for the development of Duane's syndrome, and the thickening and fibrosis occur as a result of this.

8 Which of the following is *not* a typical feature of oculocutaneous albinism?
A Loss of melanin;
B Nystagmus;
C Fewer fibres decussate at the optic chiasm;
D Photophobia;
E Incomplete foveal differentiation.

The correct answer is C. It seems an increased number of fibres decussate at the chiasm.

9 Spasmus nutans:
A Does not resolve with time;
B Is a horizontal nystagmus accompanied by head nodding;
C Is a double levator palsy;
D May result from dorsal midbrain defects;
E Typically presents between 3 and 18 years.

The correct answer is D. Spasmus nutans is a vertical nystagmus accompanied by head nodding, seen in infants between the ages of 3 and 18 months, and may resolve spontaneously.

10 Which of the following cranial nerves is *not* affected by Moebius syndrome:
A Facial;
B Abducent;
C Accessory;
D Glossopharyngeal;
E Hypoglossal.

The correct answer is C. Moebius syndrome affects the VIth, VIIth, IXth and XIIth cranial nerves, not the XIth or accessory nerve.

11 Which of the following is *not* a feature of third nerve aberrant regeneration?
A Elevation of the upper lid on down gaze;
B Abduction of the affected eye on attempted up gaze;
C Pupil constriction on adduction;
D Retraction of the globe on attempted up or down gaze;
E The mechanism for the regeneration is uncertain.

The correct answer is B. On attempted up gaze the affected eye adducts.

12 The most common acquired ocular motor nerve palsy is that of:
A IVth;
B IInd;
C IIIrd;
D VIth;
E VIIth.

The correct answer is D. A lateral rectus palsy (VIth nerve) is the most commonly acquired ocular motor nerve palsy.

Chapter 7

1 Persistent epicanthal folds may give the impression of:
A Exotropia;
B Superior oblique overaction;
C Inferior oblique overaction.
D Exophoria;
E Superior oblique underaction.

The correct answer is C. The impression of an inferior oblique overaction may be cancelled by gentle pinching of the bridge of the nose, so lifting the epicanthal folds.

2 The term associated phoria refers to:
A The movement seen under the cover in the cover test;
B The phoria measured by a Maddox rod;
C The phoria measured in a fully compensated heterophoria;
D The size of prism needed to align the nonius strips on a fixation disparity unit;
E The phoria found in increased levels in dyslexia.

The correct answer is D. Associated phoria is indicative of the uncompensated element of a heterophoria and is represented by the prism needed to realign the nonius strips.

3 Binocular vision recovery to a base-out prism may be demonstrated:

A From birth;
B At 6 months of age;
C Only in amblyopes;
D Not before 6 years of age;
E After the plasticity period.

The correct answer is B. Base-out prism recovery may be demonstrated from 6 months of age.

4 Which of the following is *not* a stereopsis test?

A TNO;
B Titmus;
C Lang;
D Frisby;
E Base-out prism.

The correct answer is E. Response to the base-out prism indicates the presence of motor fusion.

5 Which *one* of the statements about abnormal retinal correspondence (ARC) is true?

A Bagolini lens streaks cross through the light target, even though strabismus is present if ARC is harmonious;
B Lightly ingrained ARC is stable and unchanging;
C The angle of esodeviation increases as a fixation point is moved towards the nose in ARC;
D Lang's two-pen test is a quantitative assessment of ARC;
E Patients with deeply ingrained ARC need occlusion therapy.

The correct answer is A. Assuming the angle of deviation matches the angle between the corresponding points, the lines appear to pass through the spotlight, though a break in the centre of the line seen by the aberrant eye indicates the degree of suppression in that eye (which is related to the angle of deviation).

6 Which of the following represents a suitable period of occlusion for a 15-month-old infant?

A 10 minutes daily;
B 30 minutes daily;
C 4 hours daily;
D Full time;
E 6 hours daily.

The correct answer is B. 30 minutes occlusion daily may be appropriate for infants between 9 and 24 months of age.

7 Which of the following is *not* necessarily a contraindication to occlusion therapy?

A Reversal amblyopia;
B Intractable diplopia;
C Psychological distress;
D Decompensating heterophoria;
E Age of the patient.

The correct answer is E. Recent research suggests there is some benefit to occlusion even beyond the plastic stage. Dissociation may break down an unstable phoria, which leads to intractable diplopia.

8 Partial occlusion refers to:

A The use of intermittent occlusion;
B The use of occlusion for a short period;
C The use of an opaque occluder;
D The use of a translucent occluder of variable density;
E Use of a hand-held occluder.

The correct answer is D. Partial occlusion is not completely opaque, but removes some form of light sense, as is the case with a translucent occluder.

9 Penalisation refers to:

A Total occlusion by optical means;
B Cycloplegia;
C Reduction of acuity by occlusion;
D Partial occlusion by optical means;
E The preferred method of management when loss of binocular control is feared.

The correct answer is D. Partial occlusion as a result of optical change rather than occlusion is referred to as penalisation.

10 Penalisation may be carried with all the following except:

A Modified contact lens prescription in front of the fixating eye;
B Fogging lens in front of the fixating eye;
C Modified prescription lenses in front of the fixating eye;
D Frosted lens in front of the fixating eye;
E Atropine in the fixating eye.

The correct answer is D. A frosted lens has the effect of occlusion other than by optical means so is not strictly a penalisation method.

11 Which might be appropriate for the management of convergence excess?

A Negative addition segment;
B Convergence exercises;
C Exercising negative relative accommodation;
D Exercising positive relative convergence;
E Positive addition segment.

The correct answer is E. A positive segment reduces the accommodative demand and hence the related convergence, and so reduces the esotropic movement for near targets.

12 Which of the following is and/or are unlikely to help a near exophoria?

A Flipper lenses;
B Stereograms;
C Exercising negative relative accommodation;
D Exercising positive relative accommodation;
E Flipper prisms.

The correct answer is D. Accommodation in excess of the angle of convergence (thereby exercising positive relative accommodation) helps in esophoria.

Chapter 8

There are no questions for Chapter 8.

Chapter 9

1 The critical period for visual development:

A Lasts throughout childhood;
B Is the same as the sensitive period;
C Is identical for all visual modalities;
D Spans the first 10–16 weeks of infancy;
E Has no bearing on congenital cataract management.

The correct answer is D. The critical period is the period of early infancy (up to 10–16 weeks), during which abnormal visual circumstances cause irreversible change in the developing visual system.

2 Amblyopia:

A Affects 20 per cent of the population;
B Can be classified into two different subgroups;
C Can be treated by atropine penalisation of the fellow eye;
D Does not occur in myopic anisometropia;
E Is never bilateral.

The correct answer is C. Atropine can be used to bring about cycloplegia in the fixing eye and so encourage the use of the amblyopic eye, particularly where compliance with occlusion is a problem.

3 With regard to cataract morphology:

A Anterior polar cataracts are associated with a poor visual prognosis;
B Bilateral lamellar cataracts require early surgical intervention;
C Nuclear cataracts are usually managed by providing appropriate refractive correction;
D Sutural cataracts are often visually insignificant;
E Posterior lenticonus can be steroid induced.

The correct answer is D. Sutural cataracts are often not dense or visually significant. Similarly, anterior polar cataracts are not visually significant, but can cause refractive error and may progress. Lamellar cataracts, if bilateral, often do not require intervention until late in the first decade or early second decade of life. Nuclear cataracts require early surgical intervention in a large majority of cases. Posterior subcapsular cataracts can be steroid induced, but posterior lenticonus is a congenital lens anomaly.

4 In the post-operative management of infants with congenital cataracts:

A Minimal occlusion therapy is usually needed after unilateral cataract surgery;
B Early optical correction is critical;
C Aphakic glaucoma always occurs within weeks of surgery;
D Vitreous wicks can be managed conservatively;
E Strabismic amblyopia is unusual in bilateral cases.

The correct answer is B. Early optical correction, whether by the use of contact lenses, aphakic glasses or primary intraocular lens implantation, is essential for a good visual outcome.

5 In non-organic visual loss:

A There is a gender bias towards boys;
B Severe visual loss is usually associated;
C Referral is usually instigated by an optometrist;
D There is no association with social conflict;
E The visual prognosis is usually poor.

The correct answer is C. Optometrists instigate most referrals of this common condition. It is usually associated with moderate visual loss, often reflects social conflict and carries a good prognosis.

6 In retinopathy of prematurity (ROP):

A Premature babies born at or less than 31 weeks gestational age are at risk of ROP;
B Uncontrolled oxygen administration is currently the main cause of ROP;
C Infants at risk of ROP undergo screening by neonatologists;
D Infants with stage 1 and stage 2 ROP can be discharged safely;
E ROP is treated by laser photocoagulation of neovascular tissue.

The correct answer is A. The current RCOphth guidelines state that infants at or below 31 weeks gestational age and/or 1500g or less in weight should be screened for ROP. Uncontrolled oxygen administration used to be the main cause for ROP until this association was recognised in the 1950s. Oxygen administration is now regulated and the main risk factors for ROP are low birth weight and low gestational age. Oxygen fluctuation, nevertheless, remains an important risk factor. The role of the neonatologist in ROP is to identify babies at risk and submit them for screening by a trained ophthalmologist. Ophthalmologists follow up these babies at fortnightly intervals until vascularisation is complete or, if they develop any ROP, at weekly intervals until the ROP regresses and vascularisation is complete. When ROP reaches threshold (stage three for five contiguous clock hours, or eight discontiguous clock hours with plus disease), laser photocoagulation is applied to all the avascular retina as continuous light burns from the ora serrata to the anterior margin of the neovascular ridge, but generally treatment of the ridge is avoided because of the risk of haemorrhage from the neovascular vessels.

7 In treated ROP:

A Laser treatment is always successful in restoring normal visual function;
B Children can be discharged safely from further follow-up;
C Normal emmetropisation is usually observed;
D The retina recovers to give a normal appearance;
E Intracerebral haemorrhage may result in reduced vision despite a fundus of normal appearance.

The correct answer is E. Many extremely premature babies at risk of developing ROP have co-existing intracerebral, subependymal or intraventricular haemorrhages that often result in cortical visual impairment. Laser treatment has a high success rate in terms of preventing progression to stage four or five ROP, but in approximately 20 per cent of treated patients the disease may continue to progress despite treatment. Despite successful treatment there is a high incidence of refractive error, strabismus and amblyopia in these children.

This requires follow-up throughout early childhood. Laser treatment in itself may result in retinal scarring, which may be restricted to the periphery or may result in dragging of retinal vessels and traction on the retina.

8 With regard to the incidence of retinoblastoma:
A It is more common in girls than in boys;
B Strabismus is the most common presenting feature;
C It has a worldwide incidence of approximately one in 20,000;
D Hereditary forms usually present at 6 years of age;
E Most tumours are inherited.

The correct answer is C. This is the most common intraocular malignant neoplasm in children. Hereditary forms of the tumour represent around 40 per cent of cases and usually present in the first year of life and often in the first 6 months. Leucocoria is the most common mode of presentation (60 per cent), followed by strabismus (20 per cent).

9 Regarding the management of retinoblastoma:
A Children with retinoblastoma are best managed by external beam irradiation;
B Patients show greatest survival when treated by a team of ophthalmologists and oncologists at their nearest hospital;
C External beam radiation is applied if the tumour is shown to have invaded the optic nerve head after the eye is enucleated;
D Examination of the parents is not required in unilateral retinoblastoma;
E Younger siblings of an affected patient should be entered into a screening programme that involves examinations under anaesthesia.

The correct answer is E. External beam radiation used to be the most common modality used to treat medium-to-large or bilateral macular retinoblastoma. It has become less common now that chemotherapy combined with local modalities, such as laser, cryocoagulation or focal irradiation with a plaque, has become the favoured treatment. Enucleation is still a common modality for treatment, particularly when an eye has become blind from an extensive tumour or where there is extensive anterior segment involvement that gives rubeosis and secondary glaucoma. External beam radiation to the orbit is used if the cut end of the optic nerve shows tumour, but invasion of the optic nerve head alone is an indication for chemotherapy. Since retinoblastoma is a rare malignancy, children with tumours are best managed in a few specialised centres at which clinicians have greater experience, rather than at their local eye units. Genetic counselling is a complex issue, and 15 per cent of unilateral retinoblastomas may be hereditary. Thus, in these patients, examination of parents can occasionally reveal old spontaneously regressed retinoblastomas or retinomas (a benign form of the tumour), which indicates the child has the hereditary form of the disease.

10 Which of the following is *not* associated with direct blunt trauma to the eye?
A Posterior embryotoxon;
B Lens dislocation;
C Cataract;
D Retinal commotio;
E Hyphaema.

The correct answer is A. Posterior embryotoxon is a common congenital anomaly of the anterior segment and is not associated with trauma.

11 With regard to retinal haemorrhages after shaken-baby syndrome:
A Pre-retinal haemorrhages disappear most quickly;
B Intracranial bleeding always coexists;
C They may provide a clue as to the timing of injury;
D Superficial retinal haemorrhages disappear completely within 24 hours;
E Their pathogenesis is very well understood.

The correct answer is C. Retinal haemorrhages may provide a clue as to the timing of an inflicted injury. Superficial retinal haemorrhages absorb very rapidly – usually within a few days, but not usually in 24 hours. If they are noted, this is an indicator that the causative injury was relatively recent. Other types of haemorrhages, such as intraretinal or preretinal haemorrhages, may take much longer to disappear (up to 3 months) and are thus less helpful. The correlation with intracranial damage is not invariable. Of children who with non-accidental injury-related subdural bleeding, 20–30 per cent do not exhibit retinal haemorrhages. Similarly, there are rare cases of retinal haemorrhages that occur without concurrent intracranial bleeding. The pathogenesis of the retinal haemorrhages observed in shaken-baby syndrome is not understood fully.

12 Which of the following is *not* associated with shaken-baby syndrome?
A Intraretinal haemorrhages;
B Perimacular folds;
C Subdural haemorrhage;
D Vitreous haemorrhage;
E Angioid streaks.

The correct answer is E. Angioid streaks are irregular breaks in Bruch's membrane beneath the retina, but are unrelated to the shaken-baby syndrome. They are associated with a number of systemic conditions, including pseudoxanthoma elasticum and sickle cell anaemia.

Chapter 10

1 Duane's retraction syndrome (DURS) is normally caused by:
A VIth cranial nerve palsy;
B Anomalous blood supply to the lateral rectus muscle;
C Aplasia of the VIth cranial nerve nucleus;
D Absent lateral rectus muscle;
E An acquired brainstem tumour.

The correct answer is C. DURS has been shown to be associated with abnormalities of the VIth cranial nerve nucleus.

2 Which of the following is *not* a feature of Moebius syndrome?
A Absence of pectoralis major muscle;
B Loss of corneal sensation;
C Corneal ulceration;
D Entropion;
E Hypermetropic astigmatism.

The correct answer is D. Entropion is not a feature of Moebius syndrome.

3 In the congenital fibrosis of extraocular muscle (CFEOM) syndromes:

A The replacement of striated muscle with fibrous collagenous tissue is characteristic;
B Surgery does not usually improve head posture;
C The forced duction test reveals normal passive movement of the eye;
D Squint surgery restores normal ocular movements;
E The condition shows relentless progression.

The correct answer is A. Striated muscle is replaced by fibrous collagenous tissue in CFEOM syndromes.

4 Which of the following statements concerning double elevator palsy (DEP) is correct?

A DEP is so-called because of the apparent paralysis of the upper eyelid levator palpebrae superioris muscle and the superior rectus muscle;
B The involved eye is always hypotropic;
C DEP is not compatible with normal binocular function;
D An absent Bell's phenomenon is a regular feature;
E Acquired DEP may be caused by a brain tumour.

The correct answer is E. Acquired DEP has been observed as a result of the brain tumour pineocytoma.

5 Which of the following statements concerning neuromuscular disorders is correct?

A Transient congenital myasthenia gravis is caused by maternal transfer of antibodies to acetylcholine;
B Myotonic dystrophy is a mitochondrial disorder;
C All cases of congenital myasthenia resolve by 12 weeks;
D In CFEO muscle biopsy reveals fibrosis of the extraocular muscles;
E Progressive external ophthalmoplegia can be associated with heart defects.

The correct answer is E. Cardiac conduction defects are common in PEO.

6 Which of the following is true in anterior segment dysgenesis?

A The presence of posterior embryotoxon results in a 50 per cent risk of glaucoma;
B Rieger syndrome is associated with dental anomalies;
C Iridogoniodysgenesis anomaly results from mutations in the CYP1B1 gene;
D Axenfeld anomaly results in an abnormal pupil;
E Glaucoma does not develop until the end of the first decade.

The correct answer is B. Peg-like teeth are a feature of Rieger syndrome.

7 Which of the following is true in Peter's anomaly?

A It is always unilateral;
B Cataract is not a feature;
C Surgical management is straightforwards;
D There is a defect in the posterior cornea;
E Glaucoma is not an associated feature.

The correct answer is D. A defect in the posterior cornea that involves Descemet's membrane occurs in this condition.

8 In sclerocornea, which of the following is correct?

A The cornea is always totally opaque;
B Both eyes are usually affected symmetrically;
C Malformation syndromes may be associated;
D The cornea has a steep curvature;
E Visual behaviour of affected children is good.

The correct answer is C. Sclerocornea is associated with a variety of malformation syndromes, including Mietens–Weber syndrome and Rothmund–Thompson syndrome.

9 Which of the following is true in primary trabecular dysgenesis (primary congenital glaucoma)?

A It is usually autosomal dominant in inheritance;
B Affected eyes typically exhibit high hypermetropia;
C Surgical success rates are poor;
D Corneal clouding is a feature;
E Anisometropia is uncommon.

The correct answer is D. The formation of Haab's striae (splits in Descemet's membrane) and associated corneal clouding are characteristic of this condition.

10 Which of the following is true of aniridia?

A Only the anterior segment of the eye is affected;
B Glaucoma is rarely associated;
C If cataract occurs it is always an insignificant anterior polar opacity;
D The underlying gene defect is in PAX6;
E All affected children are at risk of Wilms' tumour.

The correct answer is D. Aniridia is a whole eye disorder caused by a defect in the gene PAX6 on chromosome 11.

11 Which of the following is true in microphthalmia and anophthalmia?

A The axial length of the eye is one standard deviation below (the mean of) age-matched normal eyes;
B In simple microphthalmia, only the anterior segment is abnormal;
C In anophthalmia there is always complete absence of ocular tissue;
D Microphthalmia may arise from a variety of genetic mechanisms;
E Coloboma is not associated with microphthalmia.

The correct answer is D. Microphthalmia arises from over 100 monogenic entities and a number of chromosomal abnormalities.

12 Which of the following statements concerning albinism is correct?

A Nystagmus worsens with age;
B The fovea is normal;
C Iris transillumination is unique to albinism;
D There are three main autosomal recessive forms of oculocutaneous albinism (OCA);
E Visual evoked potentials are unhelpful in making the diagnosis.

The correct answer is D. There are three main autosomal recessive forms of OCA – types 1, 2 and 3.

Chapter 11

1 Which of the following statements is *not* correct? Spectacle frames selected for children should:

A Ensure an anatomically correct fit;
B Place the lenses correctly in front of the eyes;
C Be comfortable, stable and not damage the forming nasal features;
D Not inhibit the natural development of the nasal structure;
E Be made using components designed for adult frames.

The correct answer is E. Spectacle frames that are marketed as being suitable for children should not be miniature or 'scaled-down' adult frames, or be made from components for adult frames.

2 Which of the following statements is *not* correct? When comparing the main features of a spectacle frame designed for a child with one designed for an adult, the:

A Crest height is larger;
B Frontal angle is larger;
C Splay angle is larger;
D Frontal width is smaller;
E Angle of side is smaller.

The correct answer is A. The crest height of a child's frame is usually smaller (lower) than that designed for an adult.

3 With reference to the development of children's facial measurements, which of the following is *not* correct?

A Crest height becomes more negative with age;
B Bridge projection becomes more positive with age;
C Frontal angle reduces with age;
D Splay angle reduces with age;
E Head width increases with age.

The correct answer is A. It is usual to expect the crest height to become more positive with age.

4 With reference to children's facial measurements, which of the following statements is *not* correct?

A Children's faces do not grow at a steady rate;
B Children's facial structures differ in proportion from those of adults;
C A child's nose alters considerably during development;
D Only two dimensions remain practically unchanged – the angle of crest and the apical radius;
E The facial measurements of Afro-Caribbean children do not significantly differ from those of Caucasian children.

The correct answer is E. There are significant differences between the facial measurements of Afro-Caribbean and Caucasian children.

5 With reference to the facial measurements of children with Down's syndrome, which of the following statements is *not* correct?

A Down's syndrome children show a slight, but insignificant, increase in crest height with age;
B The bridge projection in Down's syndrome appears to increase with age;
C Children with Down's syndrome have frontal angles that are smaller than normal and splay angles that are larger than normal;
D Older Down's syndrome children have interpupillary distances that are smaller than normal;
E The head width of a Down's syndrome child is larger than normal in younger children, but smaller than normal in older children.

The correct answer is B. The bridge projection in Down's syndrome appears to decrease with age.

6 Which type of bridge is most suitable for an infant or toddler?

A A keyhole bridge;
B An adjustable pad bridge with large nose pads;
C A 'w' bridge;
D A regular bridge with a low crest height and a negative bridge projection;
E A regular bridge with a high crest height and a positive bridge projection.

The correct answer is D. When dispensing to children, the bridge of the frame must be compared with the child's bridge. They should have the same shape and be of equal width. A regular bridge with a low crest height and a negative bridge projection is often the most suitable design for an underdeveloped nasal structure.

7 With reference to spectacle frame measurements, which of the following statements is *not* correct?

A Crest height is defined as the distance, measured in the assumed spectacle plane, between the lower limbus and the nasal crest;
B The careful selection of crest height can be used to control the vertical position of a frame;
C Bridge projection is defined as the horizontal distance between the assumed spectacle plane and the eyelashes in their most projecting position;
D The careful selection of bridge projection can be used to control the horizontal position of a frame;
E Bridge height is synonymous with crest height.

The correct answer is D. Option E is an incorrect statement, as bridge height is measured with reference to the bridge width line and crest height is measured with reference to the horizontal centre line – they are not the same.

8 With reference to the Comoframe, which of the following statements is *not* correct?

A It can be used by older children to reduce the risk of facial and ocular trauma during sporting activities;
B It can be used during the treatment of amblyopia by occlusion;
C It can be used to correct infantile aphakia;
D It is available as a trial frame for the refraction of young babies;

E It is most suited for general paediatric dispensing.

The correct answer is E. It is not designed for use in general paediatric dispensing.

9 With reference to polycarbonate, which of the following statements is *not* correct?
A Polycarbonate has a high impact resistance;
B Polycarbonate does not warp, chip or discolour with age;
C Polycarbonate has a relatively high refractive index ($n_d = 1.586$) with a relatively high V-value ($V_d = 47$);
D Polycarbonate is one of the lightest lens materials available;
E Polycarbonate absorbs UV radiation below 380nm.

The correct answer is C. The refractive index of polycarbonate is in the region of 1.586, but its V-value is low at around 30.

10 With reference to polycarbonate, which of the following statements is correct?
A Compared with CR39 or glass, the surface quality of polycarbonate is excellent;
B The V-value of polycarbonate is high and does not cause visual problems when viewing off-axis;
C Polycarbonate has a scratch resistance equivalent to that of spectacle crown glass;
D Surface coatings reduce the impact resistance of polycarbonate;
E Polycarbonate has limited use in practice because it is available only in a white, single-vision form.

The correct answer is D. Surface coatings reduce the impact resistance.

11 To achieve an appropriate fit a particular patient requires a frame with a 2° pantoscopic tilt. In primary gaze, the pupil centres correspond with a point 2mm above the horizontal centre line. The optical centres of the correcting lens should be placed:
A 2mm above the horizontal centre line;
B 1mm above the horizontal centre line;
C On the horizontal centre line;
D 1mm below the horizontal centre line;
E 2mm below horizontal centre line.

The correct answer is B. A 2° pantoscopic tilt means the optical centre of the lens should be decentred downwards from the pupil centre by 1mm. The optical centre should therefore be placed 1mm above the horizontal centre line.

12 Which of the following is correct. Specialist lenses are available for use in cases of:
A Convergence weakness exophoria;
B Accommodative esotropia;
C Non-accommodative esotropia;
D Hyperphoria;
E Incyclophoria.

The correct answer is B. The Rodenstock Excelit AS is available for the treatment of accommodative esotropia.

Chapter 12

1 Contact lenses should be fitted only if:
A The child wants lenses;
B The parents want the child to have lenses;
C Slit-lamp examination can be carried out;
D Combination of A and C;
E Combination of B and C.

The correct answer is D. If only the parents want the child to have lenses, there is little chance of lens wear being successful. If a slit-lamp examination is not possible, the chance of inserting lenses is low and aftercare may not be carried out safely.

2 A child who wants contact lenses, but who is too nervous, can be helped towards wearing them by:
A Telling them they look better in lenses;
B Everting the eyelids;
C Having the parent instil artificial tears for a few weeks;
D Instilling drops in the practice;
E Making a follow-up appointment many months ahead.

The correct answer is C. If the parent is able to instil a drop that the child finds comfortable it will give him or her more confidence to cope when a contact lens is inserted in the practice.

3 Which of the following is true?
A Most children can be fitted with RGP lenses;
B Children should not be fitted with RGP lenses;
C It is inadvisable to use local anaesthetic drops when fitting children with RGP lenses;
D RGP lenses should always be the first choice when fitting children;
E RGP lenses are more uncomfortable for children than for adults.

The correct answer is A. Children are just as likely to be able to wear RGP lenses as adults. Where the practitioner suggests that RGP lenses are the best choice, most children are comfortable and continue to wear them.

4 Which of the following is correct?
A An eye with unilateral ametropia always does well with a contact lens;
B Orthokeratology works better on children under 10 years of age;
C Fitting RGP lenses has been proved to retard myopia progression;
D High myopes do well with lenses because the image becomes magnified.
E Patching always improves the vision in a unilaterally hypermetropic eye.

The correct answer is D. Spectacle magnification M is expressed as

$$M = 1/(1 - aF)$$

where F is the power in dioptres of the correcting lens and a is the distance in metres from the correcting lens to the entrance pupil of the eye [Bennett AG (1985), *Optics of Contact Lenses*, Fifth Edition (London: Association of Dispensing Opticians]; a is less for a contact lens than for a spectacle lens and where F is negative (in myopia), M becomes greater. Larger objects are easier to see, which makes the visual acuity with contact lenses better.

5 Which is correct?

A Aphakes have better acuity in spectacles;
B Aphakes have better acuity in contact lenses;
C Aphakes have a wider field of vision in spectacles;
D Combination of A and C;
E Combination of B and C.

The correct answer is A. In the formula

$$M = 1/(1 - aF)$$

F is positive for aphakia and thereby produces a smaller image in a contact lens than in a spectacle lens. The acuity is therefore better in spectacles than in contact lenses. The field of vision is wider in contact lenses.

6 Contact lenses may need to be fitted together with IOLs in infants because:

A Bifocal IOLs are not yet available;
B The IOL may decentre in infants;
C There is post-operative astigmatism;
D The power of the IOL is initially too high;
E The power of the IOL is initially too low.

The correct answer is E. The power of the IOL inserted is too low for the young infant to allow for eye growth. Until the eye has grown, the extra plus may be given in the form of a contact lens.

7 Which of the following is incorrect about silicone rubber lenses?

A The first trial lens should be 0.2mm steeper than K;
B The first trial lens should be approximately 0.7mm more than horizontal visible iris diameter (HVID);
C They have very high oxygen permeability;
D They are useful in children with dry eyes;
E They cannot be made with an ultraviolet inhibitor.

The correct answer is A. Lenses should be fitted 0.2mm flatter than K, especially as they tighten once they are fitted, so it is safer to fit a flatter lens to begin with.

8 Which of the following is correct about RGP lenses in infants?

A They should be fitted with increased edge clearance;
B They should not be fitted if the lids are squeezed tightly;
C They should be fitted 3mm smaller than HVID;
D They should only be fitted under a general anaesthetic;
E They cannot be made with an ultraviolet inhibitor.

The correct answer is B. If rigid lenses are forced into a tightly shut eye, there is a risk of a corneal abrasion.

9 Which of the following is incorrect?

A Children with nystagmus have difficulty seeing with RGP lenses;
B Patients with Marfan's syndrome have flat corneas;
C Lenses that fit a microphthalmic aphakic infant may fit an adult microphthalmic aphake;
D Nanophthalmic eyes can have prescriptions of more than +20DS;
E Buphthalmic eyes tend to be more sensitive than normal.

The correct answer is A. RGP lenses do not affect the vision of patients with nystagmus, although they may reduce the amplitude of the nystagmus.

10 Which of the following is correct?

A Tinted lenses help congenital aniridics to see better;
B Albinos always see better if their astigmatism is corrected;
C Cosmetic iris lenses improve the cosmesis in cases of unilateral coloboma;
D Reducing the amount of light that enters the eye improves the visual acuity in albinos;
E Patients with achromatopsia always see better with a red tint.

The correct answer is C. A coloboma in one eye, especially if the iris is a light colour, is very noticeable. A cosmetic lens can therefore be beneficial.

11 Aphakic patients cannot be fitted with silicone hydrogel lenses because:

A They are too expensive;
B The material is too rigid;
C They are not manufactured in the necessary parameters;
D They need replacing too often;
E They do not correct enough astigmatism.

The correct answer is C. Silicone hydrogel lenses are only available in low powers, which are not suitable for aphakes.

12 Which of the following is *not* true?

A Microphthalmic corneas show worst neovascularisation;
B Lipid leakage can lead to amblyopia in a young eye;
C Aphakic eyes should have their intraocular pressure checked regularly;
D As the aphakic eye grows, the contact lens radius increases and the power decreases.
E Infants have a high blink rate.

The correct answer is E. Infants' blink rates tend to be lower than adults' and, as a result, soft lenses may dry and fall out.

Chapter 13

1 Blind and partially sighted registration statistics for the UK are compiled from data supplied by which of the following organisations?

A WHO;
B DoH;
C Local authority social services departments;
D Local Education Authorities;
E RNIB.

The correct answer is C. National figures are compiled and published by the DoH, but local social service departments supply the statistics on which these figures are based.

2 The proportion of children on school rolls in England with statements of special educational need (SEN) is approximately:

A 0.31 per cent;
B 3.1 per cent;
C 20 per cent;
D 31 per cent;
E 60 per cent.

The correct answer is B. About 20 per cent of children on school rolls in England have SEN, but only 3.1 per cent have a statement of SEN.

3 Specialist support services for the schooling of children with visual impairment (VI) are usually arranged by:

A A general practitioner;
B An orthoptist;
C An ophthalmologist;
D A qualified teacher of the visually impaired (QTVI);
E A school nurse.

The correct answer is D. While a number of professionals may become involved in the provision of support to children with VI, the QTVI has the major responsibility for making arrangements.

4 Which of the following statements about the low vision assessment of a child with VI is false?

A Assessment of accommodative function is important;
B Assessment of reading function with words or sentences on a log scale is preferable;
C Assessment of refraction is rarely helpful, since most children with VI are emmetropic;
D Assessment of binocular status can be valuable;
E Assessment of contrast sensitivity (CS) can help predict 'real world' functioning.

The correct answer is C. Assessment of refraction is essential. Many children with VI have significant refractive errors.

5 Which of the following statements about the 'Hiding Heidi' test is false?

A The response to the test can be either verbal, pointing or based on preferential looking;
B The test measures chromatic CS;
C Contrast levels on the cards are 1.25 per cent, 2.5 per cent, 5 per cent, 25 per cent, 50 per cent and about 100 per cent;
D The test employs a low-contrast face stimulus;
E The test may be used on younger children or in cases where comprehension for a letter-based CS test is difficult.

The correct answer is B. The low-contrast face stimuli measure luminance CS, not chromatic CS.

6 For the fluent reading of text with a print size of N10, a child is likely to require a minimum near visual acuity threshold of:

A N5;
B N6;
C N8;
D N10;
E N20.

The correct answer is A. An acuity reserve of at least 2:1 is considered necessary for fluent reading, and thus a threshold near acuity of at least N5 is required to read a print size of N10.

7 Which of the following statements about magnification devices to help with reading in childhood VI is false?

A When using a stand magnifier, high emergent vergence is often necessary;
B A wide range of magnification is available with stand magnifiers;
C When prescribing a high reading addition, the estimated add equals the working distance (in dioptres) minus half the amplitude of accommodation;
D When dispensing a reading addition in bifocal format, the segment should usually be placed at the lower pupil margin;
E The limited magnification provided by bar and brightfield magnifiers makes these devices unsuitable in most instances.

The correct answer is E. Bar and brightfield magnifiers do have limited magnification, but this can be offset to some extent when used at a close working distance (i.e., with relative distance magnification) and, unless the VI is severe, these devices can be very useful.

8 Which of the following statements about telescopic devices is false?

A A spectacle-mounted full-field telescope may be useful for copying from the blackboard;
B A handheld telescope may assist an older child with independent travel;
C Binoculars are often easier for a younger child to handle;
D A bioptic telescope offers the potential for both distance spotting with magnification and unmagnified orientation through the spectacle carrier lens;
E Telescopes are sometimes rejected in the classroom because they are considered too conspicuous.

The correct answer is A. A bioptic device could be used for board work, but a full-field telescope is unsuitable.

9 Adaptations in the classroom that may be of value to a child with VI include which of the following?

A A reading stand or angled desk;
B Large print;
C Local task lighting;
D Black felt tip pens for writing;
E All of the above.

The correct answer is E. All of the adaptations may help.

10 A CCTV or other electronic aid for a child with VI is most likely to be funded by which one of the following organisations?

A The Local Social Services Department;
B The Local Education Authority (LEA);
C National or local charities;
D Employment Services;
E Hospital Eye Service.

The correct answer is B. The LEA has responsibility to ensure that children with VI have access to the curriculum, and this responsibility may mean that the LEA funds specialist equipment.

11 Which of the following statements about prescribing a tint for a child with VI is false?
- A A tint of about 15 per cent light transmission factor (LTF) removes the presence of discomfort glare in most cases;
- B A tint with selective short-wavelength attenuation can be useful in selected cases;
- C A red-free green tint is helpful in children with cone dystrophy;
- D The Corning CPF photochromic lenses are yellow, amber or red in colour;
- E Transitions photochromic lenses can be used in selected cases.

The correct answer is C. Short-wavelength attenuation with a low LTF may be helpful in a case of cone dystrophy, but long wavelength absorption (i.e., red free) is unlikely to help.

12 With respect to the provision of reports after a paediatric low vision assessment, which of the following is false?
- A The content of the report should include details on visual function;
- B The report should try to link visual function to relevant examples of functional vision;
- C The QTVI should receive a copy of the report;
- D Consent to release patient information is not required where a child is under 16 years of age;
- E The report should make recommendations on the use of spectacles and low vision devices, adaptive equipment, lighting and glare control.

The correct answer is D. A child 16 years of age or older can give consent to the release of information. Children under 16 years of age also have the right to consent under the 'Gillick' test (an understanding of 'nature, purpose and hazards'), although more commonly parents or guardians provide consent.

Chapter 14

1 Which of the following conditions has been identified by the National Screening Committee (NSC) as having the potential to cause severe vision defect?
- A Strabismus;
- B Glaucoma;
- C Anisometropia;
- D Astigmatism;
- E Myopia.

The correct answer is B. Glaucoma, along with cataract and retinoblastoma, has been identified as a significant potential congenital cause of vision loss.

2 The aim of the neonatal fundus screen in premature and babies with low birth weight is to detect retinopathy of prematurity (ROP) at which stage?
- A Stage one;
- B Stage two;
- C Stage three;
- D Stage four;
- E Stage five.

The correct answer is C. Stage three ROP should be detected by an effective screening programme.

3 Before what pre-term age do babies automatically qualify for ROP screen?
- A 26 weeks;
- B 29 weeks;
- C 30 weeks;
- D 31 weeks;
- E 36 weeks.

The correct answer is D. Low birth weight babies of less than 1500g or pre-term babies of less than 31 weeks' gestational age are automatically screened for ROP.

4 The NSC recommends that examination of red reflex should be undertaken perinatally before what age?
- A 4 weeks;
- B 5 weeks;
- C 7 weeks;
- D 8 weeks;
- E 11 weeks.

The correct answer is C. The NSC have recommended red-reflex assessment before 7 weeks, together with an assessment of visual behaviour and detection of squint.

5 Absence of red reflex may indicate the presence of:
- A Congenital cataract;
- B Strabismus;
- C Amblyopia;
- D Keratoconus;
- E Microphthalmia.

The correct answer is A. Congenital cataract prevents light reflecting from the retina through the pupil and a red reflex is not seen.

6 Congenital cataracts occur in:
- A 1 in 1000–2000 births;
- B 1 in 4000 births;
- C 1 in 8000 births;
- D 1 in 9000 births;
- E 1 in 10,000 births.

The correct answer is E. Congenital cataract occurs in one in 10,000 births (excluding births in which there are multiple abnormalities).

7 Sure Start is the government initiative to:
- A Provide new health centres;
- B Introduce new premises for screening programmes;
- C Integrate health education and family support;
- D Introduce localised screening programmes;
- E Expand vision screening within schools.

The correct answer is C. Sure Start has been set up to increase integration between education, health care and family support services.

8 **The NSC recommends that the only screening to be carried out before the age of 4 years should be that for:**
A Media opacities and ROP;
B Glaucoma and media opacities;
C Media opacities and amblyopia;
D Amblyopia;
E Strabismus.

The correct answer is A. The NSC recommends that the only screening carried out before the age of 4 years should be for ROP and media opacities.

9 **The advantage of school entry screening is:**
A The potential for 100 per cent coverage;
B All children can read by this age;
C School nurses can perform the screen;
D It is the ideal age to detect media opacities;
E Parents comply fully with any advice based on findings.

The correct answer is A. School entry provides a captive audience and low attendance rates elsewhere make what is often assumed to be ineffective and haphazard suddenly more appealing.

10 **LogMAR-based vision tests are preferential to Snellen-based tests because:**
A Pre-literate children can perform the test;
B The test is portable;
C The scoring system has linear progression;
D They are cheaper;
E They measure CS function.

The correct answer is C. The equal magnification between the lines and equal spacing between the letters provide one of several advantages over Snellen acuity. Other advantages include a more reliable prediction of near vision capability based on direct correlation with the distance target size (1.0 at 6m should correlate with 1.0 at 25cm on the near test card).

11 **What percentage of boys have red–green colour vision deficiency?**
A 0.5 per cent;
B 5 per cent;
C 8 per cent;
D 0.002 per cent;
E 20 per cent.

The correct answer is C. 8 per cent of boys have some red–green defect. The bias towards males is because of an X-linked inheritance. As boys have only one X chromosome, they are far more likely to express the trait.

12 **One of the benefits of the identification of colour vision deficit is:**
A Appropriate career choice advice;
B Early detection permits early treatment;
C Use of coloured overlays may assist reading;
D Warning of a future inability to drive;
E Identifies the need for special training.

The correct answer is A. Certain careers in which colour coding is essential require full colour perception.

Chapter 15

1 **According to the Denver Developmental Screening Test, a child might be expected to respond to voices from others by what age?**
A From birth;
B At 3 months of age;
C At 5–6 months of age;
D At 12 months of age;
E At 24 months of age.

The correct answer is C. Voice response develops early on in life and a delay may indicate a sensory or cognitive impairment.

2 **Most researchers believe a child to be capable of using two or more related words by what age?**
A At 3 months of age;
B At 6 months of age;
C At 12 months of age;
D At 20–24 months of age;
E At 36 months of age.

The correct answer is D. Rudimentary sentence structuring should be possible by a child's second birthday.

3 **Which of the following communication development milestones is least reliant on visual input?**
A Interpersonal communication;
B Response to aural cues;
C Group interaction;
D Distance correspondence;
E Orientation relative to another.

The correct answer is B. Auditory signal response is related to visual input, but is the least reliant in the list. Auditory responses develop, albeit in a modified manner, in the absence of visual cues.

4 **Which of the following behaviours may indicate the need for assessment by a speech-language specialist?**
A Lack of response to others talking by 1 month of age;
B Inability to follow simple instructions by 10 months of age;
C Inability to understand simple questions by 12 months of age;
D Inability to use simple sentences by 3 years of age;
E Inability to be understood by a stranger at 12 months of age.

The correct answer is D. Communication difficulties might be shown by an inability to use simple sentences by the age of 3 years and intervention by a speech-language specialist at this stage may be crucial in aiding development or in isolating an underlying cause.

5 **The percentage of early learning estimated to be based upon visual input is what?**
A 10–20 per cent;
B 20–40 per cent;
C 50–60 per cent;
D 60–80 per cent;
E 80–90 per cent.

The correct answer is E. Most early learning has been estimated as dependent upon visual stimuli.

6 Which of the following statements concerning eidetic imagery is correct?
- A It is a result of progressive semantic-processing development;
- B It is most likely found in adults;
- C It is exclusive to autistic children;
- D It becomes less significant as semantic processing develops;
- E It is related to the concentration of photoreceptors in the retina.

The correct answer is D. As word meaning becomes more significant it seems that the ability to associate memory in purely pictorial terms is compromised.

7 Which of the following might be inappropriate to establishing the best environmental orientation for a child patient?
- A Informal surroundings;
- B Greeting before entering the consulting room;
- C A white coat;
- D Use of new equipment, provided it is introduced appropriately;
- E Slow and fluent movement.

The correct answer is C. A less formal setting may improve co-operation in young patients. A white coat, with connotations of doctors and dentists, may detract from this.

8 Which of the following actions might *not* be appropriate when examining an 8-month-old patient?
- A Addressing the child as well as the parent;
- B Lots of music and bright pictures to relax the child;
- C Keeping individual procedures as brief as possible;
- D Making the appointment outside a natural feeding time;
- E Gathering information from a parent or guardian prior to the consultation.

The correct answer is B. Music and lighting may constitute significant distractions and make the examination more difficult.

9 'Stranger fear' is classically associated with which age group?
- A Birth to 9 months of age;
- B 9 months to 3 years of age;
- C 3–5 years of age;
- D 5–11 years of age;
- E 11–18 years of age.

The correct answer is B. As the first social interactions develop, a distinct fear of strangers often coincides with the formation of strong social bonds with a familiar figure, usually a parent or guardian.

10 A parent wishes to know the outcome of an assessment of their 17-year-old daughter. Which of the following is correct?
- A Until 18 years of age a parent has full access to child health records;
- B A child has no rights under the Data Protection Act;
- C After his or her 16th birthday, the patient needs to give consent for details of the examination to be passed on;
- D A parent has no access to their children's medical records;
- E The parent needs to consult the general practitioner for permission.

The correct answer is C. After 16 years of age the patient has the right to patient confidentiality and needs to give permission for any points raised in the consultation to be passed on, even to a parent.

11 Pronoun confusion and excessive questioning may be a result of what?
- A Excessive questions by carers earlier in life;
- B An inability to cope with impairment;
- C A signal of mental instability;
- D A result of previous assessment being not detailed enough;
- E A sign of poor vision.

The correct answer is A. Excessive interrogation by well-meaning clinicians early in the life of a child with sensory impairment has been shown to have an adverse effect on their subsequent language development.

12 Which specialised language might be most appropriate for a deaf–blind child?
- A British Sign Language;
- B Paget;
- C Makaton;
- D Lip-reading;
- E Hands-on signing.

The correct answer is E. Hands-on signing is primarily a tactile code, while all the other languages listed have a significant visual component.

Index